OB/GYN

Mentor

Your Clerkship &
Shelf Exam Companion

FOURTH
EDITION

OB/GYN

Mentor

Your Clerkship &
Shelf Exam Companion

FOURTH
EDITION

Michael D. Benson, MD
Clinical Assistant Professor of Obstetrics
and Gynecology
Feinberg School of Medicine
Northwestern University
Chicago, Illinois

 F.A. Davis Company • Philadelphia

F. A. Davis Company
1915 Arch Street
Philadelphia, PA 19103
www.fadavis.com

Printed in the United States of America

Last digit indicates print number: 10 9 8 7 6 5 4 3 2 1

Senior Acquisitions Editor: Andy McPhee
Developmental Editor: Andy Pellegrini
Manager of Content Development: George W. Lang
Art and Design Manager: Carolyn O'Brien

As new scientific information becomes available through basic and clinical research, recommended treatments and drug therapies undergo changes. The author(s) and publisher have done everything possible to make this book accurate, up to date, and in accord with accepted standards at the time of publication. The author(s), editors, and publisher are not responsible for errors or omissions or for consequences from application of the book, and make no warranty, expressed or implied, in regard to the contents of the book. Any practice described in this book should be applied by the reader in accordance with professional standards of care used in regard to the unique circumstances that may apply in each situation. The reader is advised always to check product information (package inserts) for changes and new information regarding dose and contraindications before administering any drug. Caution is especially urged when using new or infrequently ordered drugs.

Library of Congress Cataloging-in-Publication Data
Benson, Michael D.
    OB/GYN mentor : your clerkship & shelf exam companion / Michael D. Benson. -- 4th ed.
        p. ; cm.
    Rev. ed of: Obstetrical pearls. 3rd ed. c1999.
    Includes bibliographical references and index.
    ISBN 978-0-8036-1693-6 (pbk. : alk. paper) 1. Obstetrics--Handbooks, manuals, etc. 2. Gynecology--Handbooks, manuals, etc. I. Benson, Michael D. Obstetrical pearls. II. Title.
    [DNLM: 1. Genital Diseases, Female--Handbooks. 2. Obstetrics--Handbooks. 3. Pregnancy Complications--Handbooks. WP 39 B4739o 2009]
    RG531. B46 2009
    618.2--dc22
                                                                2008051819

This book is dedicated to my patients, who teach me something new every day, and to my wife, Bonnie, who has shown true fortitude during her childbirth experiences.

I would also like to acknowledge the tireless work of my friend and colleague, William C. Banzhaf, MD, who edited and proofread this book. However, any mistakes are my own.

FOREWORD

Medical education has changed dramatically over the past decade. Medical students and residents first look to the Internet for information. Such resources as PubMed and the Cochran Database have become invaluable references. For those individuals being initiated into the field of Obstetrics and Gynecology, the problem is not inadequate information resources but information overload. In his book *OB/GYN Mentor*, Dr. Michael D. Benson has provided the "nuggets" necessary for medical students and residents to gain an important overview of the specialty. Each chapter is written in outline form. This lends itself to reading small sections at a time during a busy schedule. Each chapter also contains a feature titled "Mentor Tips," which is useful for the leader of the team to engage the learner in group discussions to highlight key clinical issues. The reader is given authoritative selected references for supplementation. Finally, there are self-test questions to allow the readers to assess whether they have assimilated the necessary knowledge. Overall, the book is easy to read and provides guidance to help overcome the conundrum of information overload.

I have had the privilege of knowing Dr. Benson since he was a resident with us in the Department of Obstetrics and Gynecology at Northwestern University. His dedication and talent as an educator have had a positive influence on numerous medical students and residents over the years, many of whom have chosen Obstetrics and Gynecology for their careers. Dr. Benson has exemplified the quality of gratitude for his own education by imparting his wisdom and knowledge to future generations of physicians, and this book is a prime example of this commitment.

Sherman Elias, MD
John J. Sciarra Professor and Chair
Department of Obstetrics and Gynecology
Northwestern University Feinberg School of Medicine
Chicago, Illinois

PREFACE

I am particularly excited about *OB/GYN Mentor*, in which we intend to provide the best preparation possible for the OB/GYN clerkship rotation and shelf exam. Written in a succinct outline format, the text is intended to convey information necessary for thriving in the clerkship *and* the first 2 years of residency in the most efficient manner possible. Reflecting the experience of its authors, the content reflects a mixed heritage of private practice and academic medicine. Always skeptical of the idea that "we do it this way because we have always done so and it seems to work," the book incorporates the latest in evidence-based medicine. However, as medicine is an art as well as a science, there are many common practices that seem to help patients but do not yet have evidence for support. Where possible, this practical advice is given, and the absence of strong scientific support is noted.

In an effort to be sure to provide both depth and breadth of information, I have tried to tie the scope of the book to an external and well respected teaching standard. The Association of Professors of Gynecology and Obstetrics (APGO) has created such objectives for OB/GYN clerkships (http://www.apgo.org/bookstore/). Throughout *OB/GYN Mentor*, we have included cross-references to the relevant objectives. Each APGO citation in the *Mentor* text (for example: 40A) points to a certain objective. This feature shows our readers exactly how each *Mentor* discussion helps to meet the relevant objectives.

On a personal note, after 20 years in a hybrid private practice and academic career, I can still say that I am glad that I picked Obstetrics and Gynecology as a specialty. Having delivered perhaps 4,000 babies thus far, I find that each delivery remains an affirmation of life and, in some small way, immortality. For anyone with a mystical sense, nothing can beat witnessing birth. Yet the specialty offers even more. I can look at my schedule and immediately recognize many of the patients of whom I have taken care for a decade or more. I am privileged to know their hopes, triumphs, and tragedies. Occasionally I can even help. The ties to the community and the genuine opportunity to reduce suffering simply are not offered to the same degree in other specialties. Of course, the opportunity to perform surgery and use science in daily practice only adds to the satisfaction of a career in Obstetrics and Gynecology.

Michael D. Benson, MD

CONTRIBUTORS

William C. Banzhaf, MD
Clinical Assistant Professor of Obstetrics and Gynecology; Associate
Residency Program Director, Feinberg School of Medicine, Northwestern
University, Chicago, Illinois

Chapter 4: Succeeding in Your Clerkship

Michael D. Benson, MD
Clinical Assistant Professor of Obstetrics and Gynecology, Feinberg
School of Medicine, Northwestern University, Chicago, Illinois

Linda H. Holt, MD
Clinical Assistant Professor of Obstetrics and Gynecology, Feinberg
School of Medicine, Northwestern University, Chicago, Illinois

Chapter 6: Menopause

Sigal Klipstein, MD
Board Certified in Reproductive Endocrinology and Infertility; Attending
Physician, Northwest Community Hospital, Arlington Heights, Illinois

Chapter 10: Infertility, Endometriosis, and Chronic Pelvic Pain

Reviewers

Kellie Bryant, MS, RN, NP, CCE
Assistant Professor
School of Nursing
Long Island University – Brooklyn Campus
Brooklyn, New York

Jennifer Kossoris
Medical Student
University of Chicago
Chicago, Illinois

Dawn Morton-Rias, PD, PA-C
Assistant Professor
Dean, College of Health Related Professions
Physician Assistant Program
SUNY Downstate Medical Center
Brooklyn, New York

Robert J. Solomon, MS, PA-C, DFAAPA
Professor of Physician Assistant Sciences
Community College of Baltimore County Essex
Physician Assistant Program
Baltimore, Maryland

ACKNOWLEDGMENTS

I would like to thank the contributors to this book, Drs. Holt, Banzhaf, and Klipstein. A special thanks goes to Dr. Banzhaf as residency director for Northwestern residents rotating through Evanston Hospital. He reviewed every chapter and made numerous improvements and suggestions. I would also like to acknowledge the efforts of Dr. Patricia Garcia, Director of Undergraduate Medical Education in our department. Her commitment to making the program oriented to improving clinical skills and patient interaction beyond just the didactics will make new doctors more empathic and better communicators than in days past. Finally, I would like to thank Dr. Sherman Elias, Chair of Obstetrics and Gynecology at Northwestern, for his support and encouragement over the years (and for a foreword that made me blush).

Michael D. Benson, MD

CONTENTS

PART
three
CORE TOPICS IN OBSTETRICS 319

THE BASICS

CLINICALLY RELEVANT ANATOMY

Michael D. Benson, MD

I. Abdominal Wall

  A. Muscles (Fig. 1.1)

    1. External oblique: attached to eight lower costal cartilages and to anterior half iliac crest and inguinal ligament

    2. Internal oblique: attached to three lower costal cartilages and midline (linea alba) and to iliac crest and inguinal ligament

    3. Transversus: lies beneath internal oblique and attached from lower six costal cartilages and to iliac crest and inguinal ligament

    4. Rectus: strap-lie muscles that traverse vertically from top of pubis to fifth, sixth, and seventh costal cartilages

  B. Key structures (see Fig. 1.1)

    1. Ligaments

      a. Linea alba: fibrous midline structure upon which muscle aponeurosis from either side meet

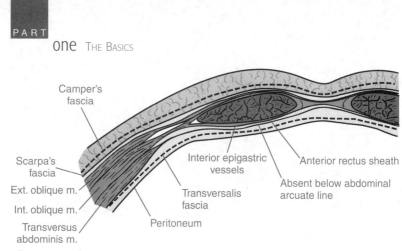

Camper's
fascia

Scarpa's
fascia

Ext. oblique m.

Int. oblique m.

Transversus
abdominis m.

Interior epigastric
vessels

Transversalis
fascia

Peritoneum

Anterior rectus sheath

Absent below abdominal
arcuate line

FIGURE 1.1 Cross-section of abdominal wall.

    b. Inguinal ligament: tendinous lower border of aponeurosis of obliquus externus and extends from anterosuperior iliac spine to pubic tubercle

    c. Cooper ligament: fibrous band that extends along superior aspect of symphysis

2. Rectus sheath: each muscle is enclosed in a fibrous sheath, or aponeurosis, that forms the key structural enclosure of abdominal wall; this sheath needs to be reapproximated during surgery; surgically meaningful fascia consists of fusion of aponeuroses of obliquus, transversus, and rectus muscles and passes in front of rectus muscle; it is a shiny white sheet that separates abdominal fat from underlying abdominal musculature

    a. A second, thinner fascial layer lies behind rectus sheath; this layer exists only above arcuate line

        i. Arcuate line: transverse line (actually visible) at which the posterior, fascial sheath ends—approximately one-third the distance from pubis to umbilicus

        ii. Camper fascia: thin, white fibrous tissue marking a plane in subcutaneous adipose tissue

        iii. Scarpa fascia: even thinner fibrous tissue running through adipose layer

3. Vessels
   a. Inferior epigastric vessels: lie beneath rectus muscle; arise from external iliac immediately above inguinal ligament
   b. Superficial epigastric vessels: lie in subcutaneous tissue lateral to underlying rectus muscles; branch of inferior epigastric
4. Inguinal canal: weakness in abdominal fascia—common site for hernias; contains round ligament and ilioinguinal nerve
   a. Exit: subcutaneous (external abdominal) ring
   b. Entrance: abdominal (internal abdominal ring)
5. Femoral canal: lies exterior to bony pelvis and beneath inguinal ligament
   a. As external iliac artery exits canal, it becomes femoral artery
   b. From lateral medial is NAVEL: femoral *n*erve, *a*rtery, *v*ein (vein most medial).
C. Surgical incisions: Figure 1.2

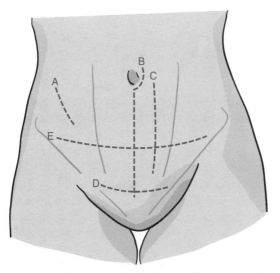

FIGURE 1.2 Abdominal incisions. *A*, McBurney. *B*, Lower midline. *C*, Left lower paramedian. *D*, Pfannenstiel. *E*, Transverse (aka Maylard).

II. External Genitalia (Fig. 1.3)

A. Mons pubis: fat pad that lies above symphysis pubis (pubic bone) and is covered with hair

B. Labia majora (homologous to male scrotum): skin folds parallel to the urethral-rectal access that lies outside vaginal opening; outer surface covered by sweat and glands and hairs; inner surface contains sebaceous glands

C. Labia minora: flaps of skin immediately adjacent to vaginal opening (inside labia majora)

D. Clitoris (homologous to penis): firm protuberance anterior to urethra, with abundant nerves and vessels; key organ in sexual sensitivity

E. Vestibule: area bound by labia minora and encompasses urethral meatus and vaginal opening

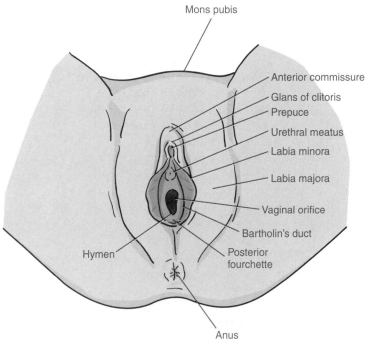

FIGURE 1.3 **External genitalia.**

F. Skene ducts: lie alongside last centimeter of urethra and open into vestibule; minor role in lubrication

G. Hymen: fold of skin that forms ring around vaginal opening; presexual configuration varies significantly; after sex, hymeneal ring typically consists of very irregular fleshy irregularities around vaginal opening

H. Bartholin glands: located between labia minora and vaginal orifice; have some role in sexual lubrication

III. Anatomy of the Perineum

A. Overview: inferior boundary of pelvis; superficial and deep transverse muscles divide perineum into urogenital triangle anteriorly and anal triangle posteriorly (Fig. 1.4)

B. External layer of muscles (muscles of vulva)

    1. Muscles of perineal body (central tendinous point of perineum)—lies beneath skin and between vagina and anus; three muscles below meet at this point

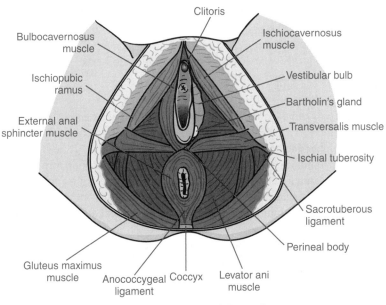

FIGURE 1.4 **Musculature of the perineum.**

a. Bulbocavernosus muscle: attached to symphysis anteriorly and perineal body posteriorly

b. External anal sphincter: attached to tip of coccyx posteriorly and perineal body anteriorly

c. Superficial and deep transverse muscle: passes transversely from ischial tuberosity to meet in midline at perineal body

2. Ischiocavernosus: arises from ischial tuberosity and terminates at symphysis pubis and base of clitoris; provides most of voluntary urethral sphincter control and erectile function of clitoris

C. Internal layer of muscles (pelvic floor)

1. Levator ani

a. Comprises three components: iliococcygeus, puborectalis, and pubococcygeus

b. Muscle inserts anteriorly into pubis, laterally into ischial tuberosity, and posteriorly into coccyx; meets in midline; provides support for pelvic viscera; raises rectum; constricts vagina

c. Tendineus arch or white line of pelvic fascia: fascial thickening extending from lower part of symphysis pubis to spine of ischium—forms part of lateral attachment of levator ani

2. Coccygeus: extends from ischial spine to lower vertebrae of sacrum and coccyx

IV. Bony Anatomy (Fig. 1.5)

A. Bony pelvis: comprises right and left innominate bone joined anteriorly to each other at symphysis pubis and posteriorly to either side of sacrum

1. Innominate bone (two—right and left); large bone forming semicircle; meets contralateral bone anteriorly and pubic rami ("branches") and sacrum posteriorly; consists of three bones that fuse during adolescence; all three meet and fuse to form acetabulum, socket-like receptacle for head of femur.

a. Ilium (hip bone)

i. Ala (wing): iliac crest—classic hip bone palpable on examination

(1) Arcuate line: dividing line between ala and body— smooth rounded, internal lower border of ala

      (2) Iliac fossa: smooth concave surface of ala

    ii. Body: forms upper portion of acetabulum—merges with ischium inferiorly and pubis medially

b. Ischium (you sit on this)

    i. Body: forms two-fifths of acetabulum

      (1) Ischial spine: protrudes from posterior surface; palpable as pointed "bump" beneath posterior wall on vaginal examination

      (2) Greater sciatic notch: large "notch" above spine

      (3) Lesser sciatic notch: smaller "notch" below spine

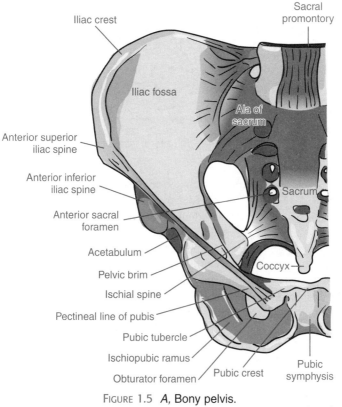

FIGURE 1.5 *A,* Bony pelvis.

(continued)

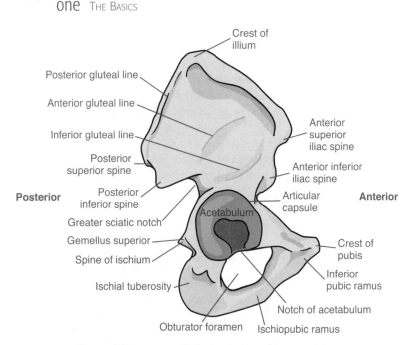

FIGURE 1.5 (continued) *B,* Lateral view of bony pelvis.

      ii. Superiori ramus: posterior lower portion of ischium
         (1) Connected above to body of ischium and to inferior rami medially and superiorly
         (2) Ischial tuberosity: lower edge of superior rami of ischium; most dependent part of pelvis when seated
      iii. Inferior ramus: extends medially and upward from superior ramus to join with pubic rami
   c. Pubis (pubic bone—joined in midline)
      i. Body: forms one-fifth of acetabulum
      ii. Superior rami: extend from body to midline where they form midline joint with contralateral pubis
      iii. Inferior rami: extend downward from superior rami to meet inferior rami of ischium
 2. Sacrum: wedge-shaped bone situated between the two innominate bones, the last lumbar vertebrae (L5) above and coccyx below
   a. Five or six segments with four foramina—permitting egress of S1–S4 spinal roots

    b. Promontory: anterior protuberance at top of sacrum

3. Coccyx: formed by three to five coccygeal vertebrae; often fused to form a joint with sacrum (sacrococcygeal joint)

4. Pelvic joints

    a. Pubic symphysis: synarthrodial (immovable)—does move slightly with shock or childbirth; joined by fibrocartilage

    b. Sacroiliac: diarthrodial (movable) with irregular surfaces; as with all movable joints, articular surfaces covered with cartilage; joint held together by anterior and posterior sacroiliac ligaments and interosseous ligaments

    c. Hip: diarthrodial (movable), ball and socket type; acetabulum forms socket (comprises all three components of innominate bone)

5. Foramen (natural opening, typically in bone)

    a. Greater sciatic foramen

       i. Boundaries

          (1) Front and above: greater sciatic notch (posterior aspect of ilium)

          (2) Behind: sacrotuberous ligament

          (3) Below: sacrospinous ligament

       ii. Contents: superior and inferior gluteal vessels and nerve, internal pudendal vessels and nerves, sciatic nerve

    b. Lesser sciatic foramen

       i. Boundaries

          (1) Front: lesser sciatic notch

          (2) Above: sacrospinous ligament

          (3) Behind: sacrotuberous ligament

       ii. Contents: obturator internus, obturator internus nerve, and internal pudendal vessels and nerve; piriformis muscle

    c. Obturator foramen

       i. Boundaries: circled entirely by bones of ischium and pubis

       ii. Contents: obturator nerves and vessels within obturator canal—usually located in lateral aspect of foramen

V. Miscellaneous Anatomic Terms of Pelvis (Fig. 1.6)

    A. Pelvic brim: circumference of plane dividing pelvis into true and false; comprises arcuate line (line that divides ala of ilium from body), pectineal line, and upper margin of pubis

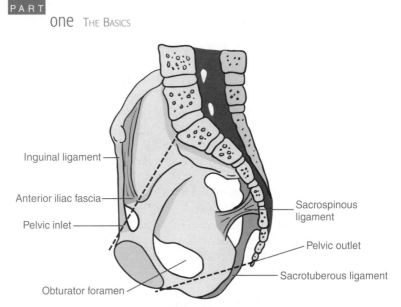

FIGURE 1.6 **Pelvic inlet and outlet.**

Inguinal ligament

Anterior iliac fascia

Pelvic inlet

Obturator foramen

Sacrospinous ligament

Pelvic outlet

Sacrotuberous ligament

B. False (greater) pelvis: expanded portion of pelvis above pelvic brim

C. True (lesser) pelvis: portion below pelvic brim

D. Axis of pelvis: corresponds to curve of sacrum and coccyx
   1. Pelvic inlet: plane from top of pubis to sacral promontory
   2. Pelvic outlet: plane from bottom of pubis to tip of coccyx

VI. Internal Organs (Fig. 1.7)

A. Vagina: muscular tube lined by squamous epithelium very responsive to estrogen; rugae are ridges that are redundant tissue that permit vagina to expand when distended and collapse when not

B. Cervix: typically 3–4 cm long with a longitudinal canal—openings are internal os and external os; inserts into vagina along anterior vaginal wall; vaginal portion known as portio and covered with squamous epithelium; cervical canal lined by glandular epithelium; transformation zone is area where the two cell types meet and tends to move outward following childbirth

C. Uterus: lining is glandular epithelium called endometrium; wall composed of smooth muscle known as myometrium; typically

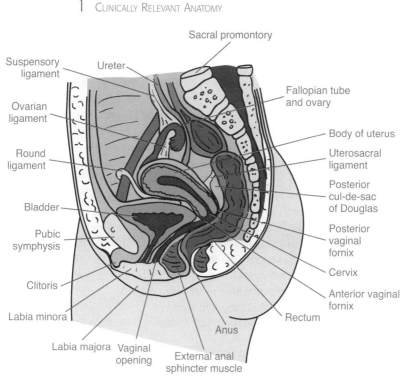

FIGURE 1.7 **Pelvic viscera.**

receives 1% of cardiac output—during pregnancy, may receive as much as 20% of increased cardiac output; can expand internal volume by 1000%

D. Fallopian tubes: lined by ciliated columnar epithelium—not merely passive structure; from uterus outward: interstitial (within wall of uterus); isthmus (uniform width); ampulla (expanding ovarian end), and infundibulum (terminal portion of tube with finger-like projections)

E. Ovaries: surface covered by cuboidal germinal epithelium; capsule beneath consists of fibrous tissue known as tunica albuginea; cortex lines beneath—composed of stromal tissue and epithelial cells; medulla is central portion of ovary with blood supply and nerves; ovary connected to uterus by ovarian suspensory ligament; infundibular pelvic ligament provides blood supply

F. Bladder: lined by squamous epithelium with walls composed of smooth muscle; anterior to uterus

G. Space of Retzius: potential space lying outside peritoneal cavity bounded anteriorly by symphysis and posteriorly by bladder

H. Ureters: vulnerable during gynecologic surgery; insert into trigone of bladder—pass as close as 8–12 mm to uterus; lie entirely behind peritoneum; ureter runs beneath ovarian vessels housed in ovarian suspensory ligament, above the internal iliac (hypogastric) artery and beneath the uterine artery

I. Urethra: 2.5–5 cm long, running beneath symphysis and anterior to vagina

J. Peritoneum: thin, transparent lining containing abdominal viscera including ovaries, small intestine, and kidney; retroperitoneal (behind and outside peritoneal cavity) organs include kidneys, large vessels, and ureter; peritoneal cavity will sometimes define disease course such as abscess spread or bleeding by confining source within or outside cavity

   1. Parietal: lines abdominal wall

   2. Visceral: covers organs of abdomen—bladder, uterus, fallopian tubes

VII. Key Supports, Vessels, Nerves, and Lymphatics of Pelvis

A. Supports: all pelvic supports contain nerves branches and blood vessels that supply the relevant viscera

   1. Uterosacral ligament: extends from posterior aspect of cervix to anterior surface of sacrum; contains inferior hypogastric plexus nerve bundles as well as sympathetic and parasympathetic innervations from lumbar and sacral spinal segments

   2. Broad ligament: fold of peritoneum arising from pelvis floor between rectum and bladder and attaches along lateral wall of uterus; bounded superiorly by fallopian tube

   3. Round ligaments: consisting of fibrous tissue and muscle, they are attached to uterus immediately below ovarian ligament; they sweep laterally and traverse the inguinal canal to end in the labia majora

   4. Cardinal ligaments: lateral support of cervix and top of vagina that extend to obturator fossa on pelvic sidewall

   5. Ovarian ligament: fibrous band of tissue from medial (inferior) pole of ovary to lateral aspect of uterus

  6. Ovarian suspensory (infundibulopelvic) ligament: peritoneal fold attaching to top of ovary and containing the ovarian vessels
  7. Urachus: embryonic remnant of umbilical cord that remains as visible, fibrous cord in parietal perineum traveling from umbilicus to bladder, roughly in midline
B. Vessels: veins are generally paired with arteries (Fig. 1.8)
  1. Iliac arteries
    a. External iliac: continues on to travel through obturator fossa and becomes the femoral artery upon leaving pelvis
    b. Internal iliac: provides much of the blood supply to pelvic viscera; arises at level of lumbosacral articulation; divides at greater sciatic notch

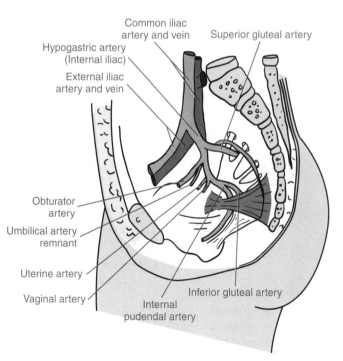

FIGURE 1.8 **Pelvic arteries.**

    2. Internal iliac (hypogastric)

      a. Anterior division: provides structure for umbilical circulation in fetal life

        i. Gives rise to superior vesical, middle vesical, inferior vesical, middle hemorrhoidal, obturator, internal pudendal, inferior gluteal, uterine, vaginal

      b. Posterior division: not major blood supply of pelvis

        i. Gives rise to iliolumbar, lateral sacral, superior gluteal

    3. Ovarian vessels

      a. Left: typically arises from left renal artery

      b. Right: usually arises directly from aorta

C. Nerves of the pelvis

    1. Somatic innervation: controls skeletal muscles and external sensory receptors; relates primarily to sensory perceptions of external genitalia and voluntary skeletal muscle of the pelvic floor; provided largely by the pudendal nerve, which arises from the S2–S4 segments of the spinal cord

    2. Autonomic innervation: controls function of internal viscera; both sympathetic and parasympathetic systems innervate all organs and act in balanced opposition

      a. Sympathetic outflow: mediates flight or fight; utilizes adrenaline (epinephrine) and noradrenaline as neurotransmitters; receptors classified as alpha or beta receptors; presynaptic neurons arise in spinal cord and end a short distance in paravertebral sympathetic ganglion

      b. Parasympathetic outflow: mediates relaxation; utilizes acetylcholine as neurotransmitter; nerve endings that release ACh are known as cholinergic fibers; receptors divided into muscarinic and nicotinic; presynaptic neurons arise in motor centers of cranial nerves III, VII, IX, and X and the spinal cord nerve roots of S2–S4; typically these neurons are long and end in ganglions close to the target organs

    3. Pain

      a. Uterine pain: mediated through sympathetic afferent nerves passing through spinal roots T11–L2

      b. Cervical pain: mediated through parasympathetic afferent fibers passing through S1–S3

      c. Perineal pain: mediated through pudendal nerve

D. Lymphatics: largely follow venous distribution and drainage; by organ
  1. Perineum, vulva, lower vagina
    a. Superficial femoral nodes
    b. Superficial inguinal nodes (two groups); some drain into deep femoral nodes, one of which is gland of Cloquet lying within femoral canal
      i. Upper group parallel to inguinal ligament
      ii. Lower group along upper part of great saphenous vein
  2. Upper vagina, cervix: drain into internal iliac (hypogastric), obturator, and external iliac groups and then to common iliac and para-aortic chains
  3. Uterus and ovaries: follow drainage of ovarian vessels into para-aortic chains

MENTOR TIPS

Surgical Considerations
- Scarpa fascia is often confused with rectus fascia—scarpa is much thinner.
- Ureter at risk for injury during clamping of infundibulopelvic ligament and of uterine arteries—particularly close to the uterus; remember ureter is retroperitoneal. It lies along the posterior leaf of the broad ligament.
- During tubal ligation, the fallopian tube should be distinguished from the round ligaments by finding the tubes' fimbriated ends. Surgical note: round ligaments can be confused with the fallopian tube during tubal ligation.
- If asked to palpate a firm mass in the bladder during laparotomy, that mass is the Foley bulb.
- Camper and Scarpa fascia may not be visible, particularly on repeat incisions. Alternately, the Camper fascia might be so evident that it might fool the novice into thinking it is actually the tougher anterior rectus sheath.
- Pfannenstiel and Mallard incisions are typically made in the same transverse location. The Pfannenstiel incision involves dissecting the anterior rectus sheath off the underlying muscles superiorly and inferiorly and then dividing the muscles in the midline. In contrast, the Mallard incision carries the transverse incision down through the muscles. There is not a clear-cut difference in healing, although some surgeons prefer the Mallard incision when there has been a previous incision,

as scarring can make the dissection of the fascia off the underlying muscle more difficult.
- Gynecologists almost uniformly refer to the anterior rectus sheath as "fascia." When they discuss closing the fascia, they are not referring to Camper or Scarpa fascia, which provide no structural integrity.
- When placing a self-retaining retractor into the abdominal cavity, be sure blades do not rest on the psoas major muscle (arising from the lumbar spine) because the obturator nerve runs on its surface and compression will prevent adduction.
- Tension-free vaginal tape procedures indicated for urinary stress incontinence utilize either the space of Retzius or the obturator foramen to place the support mesh.

Clinical Considerations
- A single anatomic name can apply to more than one structure—arcuate line of innominate bone is less important than arcuate line of abdominal wall (marking lower border of posterior rectus sheath).
- Anterior superior iliac is the most prominent point of the bone palpable.

Differences Between Female and Male Pelvis
- Less massive.
- Ilia less sloped.
- Anterior iliac spines more widely separated (more lateral prominence of hips).
- Pelvic inlet larger and more nearly circular.
- Sacrum shorter and wider.
- Sciatic notches wider and shallower.
- Pelvic outlet wider.
- Coccyx more movable.

Resources

DeCherney AH, Nathan L. (eds). Current obstetric and gynecologic treatment, 9th ed. New York, Lange, 2003.

Gray H: Gray's anatomy, 15th ed, 1901. Reprinted by Barnes and Noble Books, New York, 1995.

Netter F, Colacino S: Atlas of human anatomy. New York, Elsevier Health Sciences, 1989.

Rock KA, Jones HW. (eds). Te Linde's operative gynecology, 9th ed. Philadelphia, Lippincott Williams and Wilkins, 2003.

Chapter Self-Test Questions

Circle the correct answer. After you have responded to the questions, check your answers in Appendix A.

1. Pick the sacral nerve roots that mediate the pain of labor.

   a. T10–L2, S2–S4

   b. L1–5; S1, 2

   c. T11–L2, S1–S3

   d. T11–L4, S1–S4

2. Which of these is a muscle of the pelvic floor?

   a. Bulbocavernosus

   b. Levator ani

   c. Anal sphincter

   d. Deep transversalis

3. Define the pelvic brim:

_____

_____

4. Define the pelvic outlet:

_____

_____

5. Enumerate the differences between the female and male pelvises (8):

_____

_____

_____

_____

_____

_____

_____

_____

See the testbank CD for more self-test questions.

History and Physical Examination

Michael D. Benson, MD

I. Rationale for History and Physical Examination

A. First assessment of patient

B. Should point to next steps in diagnosis and treatment

C. Serves as starting point for establishing rapport with patient

D. The history is a "work product" that serves as basis for billing for physician services; much of the format comes from a standard (Current Procedural Terminology) created by the American Medical Association at the request of the U.S. Health Care Financing Administration in the 1970s; this standard is used by physicians, hospitals, insurance companies, and government to codify physician services

E. Structure of a history is standardized and formal; history is derived from traditional medical practice over the prior century

F. Formal structure has practical benefit—easier to remember

II. Components of History 🔲

A. Chief complaint (CC)

    1. Concise statement describing symptom, problem, diagnosis, or condition that is reason for patient's encounter

    2. Often stated in patient's own words

B. History of present illness (HPI)

    1. Chronologic description of course of patient's condition from first onset to present

    2. Seven descriptors

        a. Location

        b. Quality

        c. Severity

        d. Timing

   e. Context
   f. Modifying factors
   g. Associated signs and symptoms
   3. Almost all HPIs in obstetrics and gynecology begin with age, gravidity and parity, and last menstrual period (LMP) in first sentence
C. Past history
   1. Illnesses and medical problems (include current problems not directly addressed in HPI)
   2. Operations and injuries
   3. Hospitalizations
   4. Current medications
   5. Allergies
   6. Immunizations
D. Social history
   1. Substance abuse
      a. Tobacco
      b. Alcohol
      c. Illicit drug use
   2. Marital status and household members
   3. Employment
   4. Educational attainment
   5. Sexual history
E. Family history
   1. Health status (or cause and age of death) of parents, siblings, children
   2. Specific history of relevant diseases
   3. Other family history that may be hereditary or place patient at risk
F. Review of systems (ROS)
   1. Helps define problem, clarify differential diagnosis, and identify need for testing
   2. Covers 14 systems: (1) constitutional; (2) eyes; (3) ears, nose, mouth, throat; (4) cardiovascular; (5) respiratory; (6) gastrointestinal; (7) genitourinary; (8) musculoskeletal; (9) integumentary (skin and/or breast); (10) neurologic; (11) psychiatric; (12) endocrine; (13) hematologic/lymphatic; and (14) allergic/immunologic

III. Physical

Body areas and organ systems are grouped differently for the purpose of organizing the record.

  A. Body areas
  1. Head (and face)
  2. Neck
  3. Chest (breasts and axilla)
  4. Abdomen
  5. Genitalia, groin, buttocks
  6. Back
  7. Four extremities

  B. Organ systems
  1. Eyes
  2. Ears, nose, mouth, throat
  3. Cardiovascular
  4. Respiratory
  5. Gastrointestinal
  6. Genitourinary
  7. Musculoskeletal
  8. Skin
  9. Neurologic
  10. Pschiatric
  11. Hematologic/lymphatic/immunologic

IV. Impression/Assessment 1C, 2C, 4B

  A. Problem list 4A
  1. Active
  2. Inactive
  3. Resolved

  B. Differential diagnosis presented as needed for each problem

V. Plan 4D

  A. Testing planned
  B. Medications prescribed
  C. Procedure/surgery recommended
  D. Patient education
  E. Follow-up plans including time of return visit or reassessment

VI. Special Aspects of History for Obstetrics and Gynecology

  A. Menarche
  B. Last menstrual period

C. Period frequency, duration, amount, associated symptoms (pain, etc.)

D. Contraception method

E. Sexual preference

F. Number of sexual partners (in previous year)

G. Domestic violence

H. Sexually transmitted diseases/abnormal Pap test results

I. Pregnancy history

    1. Miscarriages (spontaneous abortions)

    2. Elective abortions

    3. Pregnancies longer than 20 weeks

        a. Gestational length

        b. Route of delivery

        c. Gender

        d. Live-born (or not); complications in early life

        e. Country, city, and name of hospital (add physician if local and patient remembers easily)

VII. Special Aspects of Examination for Gynecology 🔲

Obstetrical examination is discussed in Chapter 19.

A. Mechanics of the physical examination

    1. Inspection of vulva: note lesions, hymen anomalies (uncommon)

    2. Speculum examination

        a. Separate labia with nondominant hand

        b. Gently place closed speculum into vagina

        c. Keep any pressure on the speculum directed downward, against posterior wall of vagina, to avoid more sensitive urethra

        d. When back of vagina is reached, slowly separate bills of speculum

        e. If cervix not visible, close speculum, withdraw slightly, and reopen—process might have to be repeated to identify cervix

        f. Prior to removal, rotate speculum 90° to check for lesions on anterior and posterior vaginal walls (rare)

    3. Obtaining Pap smear

        a. With cervix in view, Pap smear is obtained, using either broom or spatula and endocervical brush

    b. Collection device rapidly placed in collection medium (Thin Prep, Sure Pap) or spread across slide and fixed (traditional)

    c. Any additional tests, such as bacterial swabs, taken after Pap smear sample obtained

  4. Bimanual examination

    a. With nondominant hand, place forefinger (or occasionally second and third finger) inside vagina

    b. Palpate cervix

    c. Place dominant hand on lower abdomen

    d. Between two hands, assess uterus for size and irregularities; palpate either side of uterus in adnexal region (containing tubes and ovaries)

    e. For those who have not yet had coitus or those with small vaginal openings, a rectal-abdominal examination might be more comfortable

  5. Rectal-vaginal examination

    a. Change gloves

    b. Place forefinger of nondominant hand in vagina while placing third finger in rectum simultaneously

    c. Palpate area behind uterus and posterior vaginal wall while also maintaining dominant hand on abdominal wall

    d. May also test for occult blood as appropriate

       i. Traditional occult blood testing using the guaiac smear (a popular trade name is Hemocult) probably has little sensitivity or specificity as a one-time test administered in the office

       ii. Newer, immunochemical tests using markers for specific human blood are much more sensitive and specific

B. Common (and uncommon findings) on examination

  1. Vulva: note lesions, hymen anomalies (uncommon)

  2. Vagina: lesions rare; herniations common

    a. Cystocele: protrusion of anterior vaginal wall downward

    b. Uterine prolapse: descent of uterus toward introitus

    c. Rectocele: protrusion of posterior vaginal wall toward introitus

    d. Enterocele: difficult to discern; herniation of small bowel into upper, posterior portion of vaigna

    e. Herniation assessment: typically, patient asked to cough or perform Valsalva maneuver while only half the speculum is inside vagina

        i. Posterior bill placed to assess for uterine prolapse and cystocele

        ii. Anterior bill placed to check for rectocele, enterocele

3. Cervix: true pathologic condition rarely seen

    a. Parous cervical os appears larger and oval-shaped in contrast to nulliparous cervix, which is typically round and small

    b. Lumpy surface irregularities on cervix that reflect light are typically nabothian cysts—plugged cervical glands; entirely benign and do not require follow-up

    c. Polyps may be seen protruding through cervix; invariably benign, they might be removed if causing bleeding or heavy discharge

    d. Cervical cancer is very uncommon—appearance can be varied from polypoid, friable lesion to more subtle irregular color or texture of cervix (even less common endocervical cancers often very hard to observe on physical examination)

4. Uterus

    a. Enlargements typically described in terms of gestational age—a difficult judgment for students; comparison with fruits (orange, grapefruit) also common

        1. Typically smaller in nulliparous and menopausal women

        2. Enlargements, particularly irregular masses, most often the results of fibroids (leiomyoma)

    b. Note whether uterus tipped anteriorly (most common), mid-position, or posteriorly (not indicative of disease but useful to know for any procedures—do not discuss this finding because it does not have any implications for patient's health)

    c. Note any tenderness with or without movement ("cervical motion tenderness" is actually tenderness of uterus upon any movement of the cervix)

5. Adnexa (tubes and ovaries) and rectal-vaginal examination

    a. Tubes almost never palpable on examination

    b. Ovaries rarely palpable if normal size and consistency

    c. Enlargements and tenderness should be noted

    d. Masses and tenderness on rectal-vaginal examination should be noted separately

VIII. Advice From a Mentor's Perspective `1B, 2A, 5A-C`

A. Shake hands, make eye contact, and introduce yourself

B. Do not claim to be what you are not: if you are a medical student, say so

C. Feel free to make small talk, if you wish, during the examination; statements/questions about the weather, travel, and the like can help distract the patient during unpleasant parts of the examination

D. Humor works well when it works, but with novices who do not have long-term relationships with their patients it can sound arrogant or condescending; patients can think the humor is at their expense; avoid it

E. Avoid politics entirely

F. Wash your hands *before* and *after* examining the patient

G. If you are using a metal speculum, warm it with warm water and touch it to the inside of the patient's knee to check temperature if you are not sure—ask patient if too hot or cold

H. As a general rule, take a very abbreviated history if friends or relatives are in the room—avoid sexual, pregnancy, and substance use history or anything else that might embarrass the patient; medical students have to use judgment in this regard and do not have the same freedom as senior physicians to ask relatives to leave

I. Never wear gloves except when actually examining the patient; do not wear gloves (clean or not) in the hallway or to touch common objects such as doorknobs or to take items out of your pocket

J. Do not chew gum or candy or eat in front of the patient; do not sit on the patient's hospital bed

K. Be very circumspect about documentation

    1. Abnormal findings: be sure to check with a resident or attending physician before committing abnormal findings to the record; a perceived abnormality might not be abnormal; and any abnormal finding should be communicated directly to a physician in a position to follow-up

    2. Potentially embarrassing or illicit behavior: also check with a senior physician before committing it to the record; for example, a remote history of drug use might interfere with the patient's ability to obtain insurance in the future

    3. When in doubt about the wisdom or appropriateness of documentation—ask

L. Examiners with gem-bearing rings should probably remove them before the examination because they can dig into patients' thighs

M. Keep focused on what you need to know, skip irrelevant items, and do not overtax the patient; if need be, save documentation to record later, although this is less efficient

N. The 45-second review of systems (assuming only two positive and brief responses)

    1. Have you had any change in your weight in the past year?

    2. Do you have any trouble with your head, eyes, ears, nose, or throat?

    3. Any chest pain, palpitations, coughing, or shortness of breath?

    4. Any nausea, vomiting, or diarrhea?

    5. Any abnormal vaginal bleeding or pain on urination (do not use medical terms such as "dysuria")?

    6. Muscle aches or joint pain?

    7. Breast pain or lumps?

    8. Weakness or numbness in your arms or legs?

    9. Depression or anxiety?

    10. Hot flashes or easy bruising?

O. Tips on review of systems

    1. Judgment has to be used here; some patients will have an entirely positive review of systems that has nothing to do with their reason for seeking medical help

    2. Two areas of concern

      a. GI symptoms—this area is very often positive and classically leads to a long discussion irrelevant to the patient's reason for seeking medical care; obviously, women with abdominal pain need to be asked about constipation

      b. Depression and anxiety—these are usually important questions but can result in a long digression; often, though, the digression might be relevant so, again, judgment is needed;

treatment of depression and anxiety is definitely part of obstetrics and gynecology

P. Self-consciousness
   1. Your interaction with the patient is chiefly to benefit you—not the patient
   2. Many medical students feel very awkward because they are imposing (which they are, to an extent); to mitigate the imposition, be polite, interested, and attentive to patient comfort (helping them up, getting water, etc.)
   3. Most patients who deal with medical students actually want to help; some are also lonely and/or afraid and derive real benefit from interaction with someone who is interested
   4. Ultimately, toughen up; to be of any use as a physician, medical students simply have to learn these skills even if they cannot be of immediate benefit to the patient

Q. "Relax"
   1. Never, ever tell a patient this
   2. The instruction to relax is usually given to a naked patient, upon whom a bright light is shining, who is about to have a foreign body placed in a potential bodily opening
   3. Rather than use this term, specify what the patient should do
      a. "Let your knees flop out to either side."
      b. "Remember to breathe."
      c. "Try not to move too much."

R. Tell the patient the results of your assessment `2D`
   1. Remember to address each of the patient's presenting concerns
   2. Give results of the examination (including "normal')
   3. Specify each and every test that is being done and why
   4. Avoid adding extraneous or irrelevant remarks or findings as patients will not know how to interpret these statements

S. Compliance issues; `4C` issues include expense, transportation, and establishing empathy (obtaining patient understanding; obtaining cooperation)

MENTOR TIPS

• Review the sections above under "Advice From a Mentor's Perspective." They contain wisdom based on clinical experience.

Chapter Self-Test Questions

Circle the correct answer. After you have responded to the questions, check your answers in Appendix A.

1. Which does not form a separate organ system in the review of systems?

a. Eyes

b. Neurologic

c. Genitourinary

d. Lymphatic

2. The history and physical examination serve which of the following purposes?

a. Provide a basis for billing for physician services

b. Establish patient rapport

c. Develop a differential diagnosis

d. Lay foundation for follow-up testing

e. All of the above

3. Structure of history and physical examination is formulated by which of the following?

a. Insurance industry

b. Medicare

c. Health Care Financing Administration

d. American Medical Association

4. Which is *not* a symptom descriptor?

a. Timing

b. Location

c. Prior medical treatment

d. Associated signs and symptoms

See the testbank CD for more self-test questions.

3 CHAPTER

LEGAL AND ETHICAL ISSUES

Michael D. Benson, MD

I. **Ethical Issues in Patient Care.** There are five ethical principles; occasionally they may conflict in the course of clinical care 6G

A. *Nonmaleficence:* "First, do no harm"; requires some perspective; generally, the likely benefit of proposed intervention should outweigh risk; as risks and benefits are invariably different, patient often has to make this judgment

B. *Beneficence:* duty to promote well-being of others

C. *Autonomy:* right of self-determination; patient must not be coerced or have choices limited by external constraints; a key issue that comes up occasionally is soundness of mind—patients in pain or with specific disease processes may have their reasoning ability impaired

D. *Justice:* equals should be treated equally; GE this can be a cultural and a social problem; whereas in Western societies, men and women should be treated equally (at least in principle), in many Western societies, racial and ethnic preferences are often assigned; in particular, federally funded research studies in the United States require a breakdown of study participants by race and ethnicity

E. *Veracity:* obligation to deal honestly

F. Conflicts among these five key principles occur daily in clinical practice and often have no clear-cut answers; for instance, the risk of death to a fetus from a vaginal trial of labor after a prior cesarean is estimated to be 1 in 500, yet many expectant mothers prefer this attempt to a scheduled repeat cesarean (which might involve more postdelivery pain for the mother than a successful vaginal birth after cesarean [VBAC])

G. Ethical dilemmas under debate involve stem cell research; status of embryos not used during fertility treatments; multifetal reduction for the benefit of one or two fetuses in multiple pregnancies; and right to die

II. Informed Consent

A. Involves an ethical and legal obligation underlying any decision by the patient to accept treatment; always a consideration but generally more formally documented in decisions to proceed with surgery **6A**

B. Basis for physician-patient relationship

   1. Informed consent forms the basis of the professional relationship; it is key to establishing trust

   2. Must be individualized; some patients wish to abdicate their autonomy and instruct "Doc, just do what you think is best"; although most physicians appreciate the sentiment, and it represents direct instructions from the patient, the relationship is often better served in the long term if an attempt is made to honor the patient's autonomy

   3. Disease and circumstances may intervene; unconscious patients and those with illnesses that can affect reasoning always pose special problems; when possible, family members or those with legal power of attorney should be consulted

C. Who can consent

   1. Varies from state to state and is a formal legal definition

   2. Examples of special categories of individuals who might (or might not) be able to consent **6D**

      a. Minors (persons younger than age 18 years)

         i. Parental permission might be required

         ii. Patient (minor) assent (empowers child or adolescent commensurate with capacity)

      b. Married minors

      c. Emancipated minors (living independently and self-supported)

      d. Incapacitated individuals

         i. Power of attorney can dictate delegation of consent

         ii. In absence of power of attorney, law may give preference—typically spouse, adult child, parents

   3. Need for consent may be waived (varies by state); presumes no evidence exists for patient's opposition to treatment

a. Unconscious patients

b. Patients in need of immediate treatment

D. Conflicting interests—mother and fetus occasionally have competing priorities 6F

1. Cesarean occasionally recommended for fetal benefit although it may pose increased risks of injury to mother

2. Most mothers gladly accept additional risk for any fetal benefit

3. Rarely, the risks might be extreme and the mother may decline treatment that would be of great benefit to fetus—court might have to decide

E. General principles for obtaining consent (always use terminology and language that patient is most likely to understand while retaining professional decorum)

1. Diagnosis (the condition or symptoms to be treated)

2. Rationale for treatment

3. Alternatives (including no intervention)—not all alternatives necessarily need be presented but certainly some should

4. Benefits—likelihood, extent, and duration

5. Risks—likelihood, extent, and duration

a. Not all risks can be enumerated or anticipated

b. Some statement should be made to this effect (such as "risks include but are not limited to...."); although a relevant legal consideration, the concept that all risks cannot be anticipated or even enumerated for practical reasons is important for patients

6. Treatment of complications

7. Likely outcomes of no intervention

8. Time for questions

F. Common barriers to obtaining effective informed consent

1. Patient anxiety: as a rule, the more serious or disruptive the condition, the greater the anxiety

2. Time: some conditions require urgent treatment and leave the patient with little time to reflect

3. Language: even when patient and physician speak the same language, differences in educational attainment and professional vocabulary can impede communication

G. Techniques for improving communication 5A

1. Say important things first

2. Say important things repeatedly

3. Ideally, important things should be said in more than one visit; this allows patient to reflect without pressure of time

4. In addition to asking for questions, physician should question patient about key points; caution must be used as this can appear condescending, so an explanation should be given such as, "I want to be sure I have explained the key points...."

5. Generally, the most experienced clinician or the one who will likely have the longest contact with the patient should be the one obtaining informed consent; this responsibility is often delegated to junior house staff or nursing staff and is not ideal

6. Usually best to explain everything and answer questions with the patient alone; presence of friends and family members can change the interaction in unpredictable ways and change patient's willingness to confide or ask questions; however, as patients often want an important other to help process information, offer to repeat the discussion with significant others present 5B

7. Avoid interrupting patients—the most long-winded patient will usually not go on for more than 90 seconds or so without pausing

8. "Physician, know thyself!" 5C all physicians have strengths and weaknesses in personal interactions; simply being aware of them is helpful in improving communication with patients

III. Professional Ethical Issues (adapted and modified, in part, from the American College of Obstetricians and Gynecologists [ACOG] Code of Professional Ethics)[1]

A. Physician conduct and practice

1. Recognize limits of knowledge and experience (the most dangerous people are those who do not know what they do not know)

2. Maintain educational currency

3. Represent credentials truthfully

4. Those with infectious diseases should limit their activities appropriately, with emphasis on protection of patients

5. Should not provide services while impaired (this covers full range of impairments)

B. Conflict of interest: serious issue that is receiving increasing attention

    1. Use caution in promoting commercial products—should avoid bias and appearance of bias

    2. Offer prescribed treatments solely on basis of patient's best interests

    3. Receipt of compensation from third parties should be disclosed when material

  C. Professional relations

    1. Treat other health professionals with dignity, respect, and honesty

    2. Refer or cooperate with other health professionals when interests of patients demand it

IV. Legal Issues

  A. Error in medical practice is summed up by *To Err Is Human*, an Institute of Medicine study published in 1999 that attributed 100,000 deaths annually in the United States to medication errors alone[2]

    1. Common sources of error are carelessness, fatigue, miscommunication, ignorance (health-care provider does not possess relevant factual knowledge), and failure to follow up

    2. Many types of errors are predictable

    3. Objective should be to reduce error rate—elimination of error is unreasonable expectation

  B. Medical malpractice

    1. Legal elements of liability

      a. Duty: physician-patient relationship; must prove that physician had duty to treat patient

      b. Duty breached: standard of care not followed

      c. Injury (damages): medical errors occasionally result in no injury; no legal liability results

      d. Causation (injury caused by breach of duty): there are cases in which medical errors occurred and there was a bad outcome, but if the specific errors did not cause the injury, then no legal liability occurred (this is definitely not to say that a lawsuit, settlement, or trial will not result)

    2. Standard of care

      a. In most cases defined as treatment and care that would be provided by the majority of reasonably prudent physicians in the same specialty under the same or similar circumstances

b. Often difficult to define precisely

c. Not necessarily "best practice" or "most up-to-date"

d. Because medicine is specialized field, common practice is to utilize medical experts to define standard of care for juries

3. Legal process

  a. Discovery (varies some in different states):

    i. Plaintiffs, defendants, and fact witnesses deposed

      (1) Witnesses served with subpoena (court order to appear for questioning)

      (2) Questioning typically done by opposing counsel—plaintiff by defense attorney, defendants by plaintiff attorneys

    ii. Expert witnesses: in most states, defense and plaintiff expert witnesses deposed to discover their opinions

      (1) Depositions often define and limit opinions that experts can offer at trial

      (2) Expert opinion testimony often governed by state law and precedent rather than the usually more stringent federal laws

  b. Settlement: given the nearly universal unpredictable nature of juries, both sides have a compelling reason to settle prior to trial

    i. Although nationwide, physicians found innocent in roughly 80% of jury trials, many cases are settled in advance and these statistics are harder to obtain

    ii. Although settlements have to be reported to National Practitioner Data Bank, they are often kept confidential (and out of the media)

  c. Trial

    i. Jury selection (can be hugely important as no one has a jury composed strictly of one's peers)

    ii. Opening arguments (plaintiff first)

    iii. Presentation of witnesses with cross-examination

    iv. Closing arguments

    v. Jury deliberation

    vi. Verdict

  d. Components of awards

    i. Economic: cost of medical care and lost wages

ii. Noneconomic: emotional distress, pain, and suffering

iii. Discussion of "caps" (limits) on damages typically centers on limits of "noneconomic damages"

4. Consequences for the practitioner

a. Physicians become more careful

b. Malpractice litigation often causes huge emotional distress for the practitioner—cases usually take years to make their way through the legal system

c. All payments in malpractice litigation are reported to National Practitioner Data Bank; data available to hospitals and state licensing boards

d. Most important: payments have effect on professional insurability

i. Can cause premiums to rise substantially

ii. Can cause insurer to drop coverage

iii. Problems with insurability can force individuals to go to a different state, retire early, or stop practice altogether

C. Emergency Medical Treatment and Active Labor Act (EMTALA)

1. Patients must be stabilized at institutions providing emergency care before transfer or transport to another institution

2. "Stabilization" of pregnant women in labor means delivered of both fetus and placenta

3. Patients should be seen by physician before being transferred to another facility

4. Fines for violation can be substantial and expose institution and health-care providers to legal liability

D. Health Insurance Portability and Accountability Act (HIPAA) 6B

1. Federal law governing disclosures of health information

2. Communicable diseases such as HIV and psychiatric conditions are held separate and require special consent for disclosure

3. Regardless of federal law, health-care providers have a high duty to keep medical information confidential—federal law passed because health-care professionals did not live up to their confidentiality obligations; even the fact that a patient is in the office should not be disclosed to anyone outside the office; in obstetrics and gynecology, privacy assumes even greater importance than in some other specialties

E. Reportable medical findings—specific circumstances may trump privacy concerns (varies from state to state—HIPAA waived) 6C

1. State law may require reporting some events to state agencies or referring patient for specific assistance (referring patient to shelter for domestic violence)
   a. Domestic violence
   b. Neglect or abuse of minors or elders
   c. Sexually transmitted disease
2. Good medical care might require intervention (even in the absence of specific state law)—suicidal and homicidal ideation when risk of injury to self or others substantial
3. When in doubt, ask a more experienced health professional

F. Mitigation of medical errors
   1. Be sure to stay well educated and current; ignorance can injure or kill
   2. Do not order laboratory tests without a very specific plan for checking the results; it is often helpful to involve patients directly and have them call after a specific amount of time has elapsed to check; no news should never be "good news"—it should mean that the patient should call to check
   3. The only time a laboratory test will not be done or a drug not administered in the hospital is if its omission would make a really big difference in outcome; if a patient is to be cross-matched before surgery, make sure the crossmatch is done; if an antibiotic for a septic patient is ordered, make sure it is given
   4. Close the communication loop: it is not uncommon for physicians to speak softly or give an order to a room filled with nurses, and it is not uncommon for the order not to be carried out in such circumstances; if a communication is important (i.e., the patient's life or well-being depends on it), ask the person with whom you are communicating to repeat the instructions to ensure they are correct
   5. Consult: if you are unsure about what to do in a specific situation, do not hesitate to ask a colleague for advice
   6. Do not let a theory about the cause of a patient's condition stand in the way of the facts: if a differential diagnosis list cannot explain all of a patient's problems, expand the list of possibilities
   7. Temperature, pulse, blood pressure, respiratory rate, and oxygen saturation are good starting points: if any one is abnormal, determine the cause

MENTOR TIPS

- Informed consent is the culmination of patient education and communication. A clear understanding of the risks, alternatives, and benefits of the available medical interventions is key for establishing a good physician-patient relationship.
- Ethical dilemmas often have more than one acceptable answer (and often a variety of equally difficult or bad choices).
- Patient privacy should be paramount in everything.

References

1. American College of Obstetricians and Gynecologists (ACOG): Code of professional ethics. ACOG, Washington, DC, 2008. http://www.acog.org/from_home/acogcode.pdf
2. Institute of Medicine: To err is human: Building a safer health system. Institute of Medicine, Washington, DC, 1999. http://www.iom.edu/CMS/8089/5575.aspx

Chapter Self-Test Questions

Circle the correct answer. After you have responded to the questions, check your answers in Appendix A.

1. Patient's mother calls the office and asks for a doctor's note for her daughter, who missed a day of school because of a family vacation. You should:

   a. Write the note

   b. Write the note only after the daughter comes in for an examination

   c. Decline to write the note, explaining that you can do so only for patients who are both examined and actually have a medical illness

2. You are doing an endometrial biopsy, and the patient cries out in pain. You pause and ask if you should continue. The patient says yes. You should:

   a. Follow the patient's wishes and finish the procedure

   b. Abandon the attempt and repeat it only after accommodations for the patient's comfort have been made

3. A laboring patient with an epidural is experiencing substantial pain. You discover that the epidural pump was not hooked up and that the prophylactic antibiotic intended for her IV is infusing into her epidural space. After notifying the anesthesia service you should:

   a. Disclose the error to the patient and explain what remedial steps are being taken

   b. Not disclose the error, file an incident report, and reassure the patient that the anesthesia service will appear and remedy the situation

   c. Not disclose the error, seek the compliance of the anesthesiologist, tell no one, and remedy the situation

4. A patient whom you are treating for depression seeks an increase over the phone in her antidepressant medication because she is increasingly upset over her recent breakup with her boyfriend. She confides that she has obsessive thoughts about him and is driving by his house daily. On further questioning she admits that she "is thinking about killing him" and when asked admits without hesitation that she would stab him. You should:

   a. Contact the police department of the municipality in which she resides and have the police secure immediate psychiatric evaluation in the closest emergency room—voluntarily or involuntarily

   b. Increase the dose of medication as the patient asks

   c. Insist that the patient come to the office at the first available appointment for re-evaluation before increasing the medication dosage

   d. Refer the patient to a specific psychiatrist and call that psychiatrist to let him or her know that that referral was made

5. A laboring patient experiences spontaneous rupture of membranes at 3 cm. At time of examination, the umbilical cord is felt prolapsing through the cervix. At the moment, the fetal heart rate tracing drops to 60, where it remains for the next few minutes. The patient is promptly moved to the operating room where she declines a cesarean. She is informed that the baby will die or suffer serious injury in the next several minutes if she does not have the procedure. She refuses. Her significant other supports her decision. The next thing you do is:

   a. Proceed with surgery

   b. Respect her wishes while continuing to try to have her change her mind

c. Proceed with surgery over the patient's objections while attempting to get an emergency court order to support this action

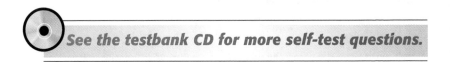

See the testbank CD for more self-test questions.

SUCCEEDING IN YOUR CLERKSHIP

William C. Banzhaf, MD

I. Before Your Clerkship

A. Review basic science relevant to ob/gyn: breast and pelvic anatomy (organs, vessels, nerves); embryology; physiology and endocrinology of menstruation; and surgical technique (if you have had your general surgery rotation)

B. Review clerkship protocols and materials

    1. Obtain clerkship written materials in advance, if possible

        a. Rotation schedule (Ob, Gyn, night float, etc.)

        b. Didactic: lecture schedule usually takes priority over clinical activities (some programs cluster these on a given day, others spread them out)

    2. Speak with students who have completed the rotation

    3. Contact residents in advance (demonstrates initiative): this lets you review expectations, and lets them know when to expect you

C. Develop positive attitude, and keep an open mind: even if you think you have no interest in ob/gyn

    1. Knowledge of physiology of pregnancy relevant to all specialties: all areas of medicine interface with pregnant women

    2. Ob/gyn has many important elements

        a. Primary care: annual pelvic examination and Pap smear, contraception, breast health (many women consider ob/gyn physician to be their primary care physician)

        b. Surgery

        c. Obstetrics

        d. Long-term relationships with patients and community

        e. Dynamic, procedure-oriented specialty

3. Common "myths"

  a. Long hours

   i. Most surveys show ob/gyn physicians work similar number of hours as other specialties

   ii. Residency duty hours (80-hour workweek) is comparable with other specialties during training

  b. Females only: perception that female patients prefer same-sex provider and thus males less competitive for residency positions and jobs; most female patients want competence, character, and compassion, with gender a secondary issue

  c. Malpractice: liability reform has improved the climate in many areas; no specialty is immune

II. During Your Clerkship

A. General rules

  1. Be on time, and be available: the majority of your clinical experience, both in the operating room (OR) and Labor and Delivery, will require your ready availability; do not make residents or attending physicians have to find you to participate in surgery or deliveries

  2. Aggressively pursue clinical experience: follow as many patients as possible; for obstetric patients, stay in the room as much as possible during the second stage of labor (pushing)

  3. Evaluate and emulate the work habits of the postgraduate year 1 and 2 (PGY-1, PGY-2) students, and embrace the concept that you are part of the team

  4. Legible, complete documentation eases resident workload and allows for more student teaching and supervision; do not be too proud to do scut work: these chores are necessary parts of quality patient care, and doing them will endear you to all members of the team

  5. Remember that all members of the team can advance your learning: nurses, lactation consultants, social workers; treat them with dignity and respect (as an equal), and you will benefit

  6. Arrive early enough so that postpartum/postoperative rounds and notes are completed before morning sign-out

7. If you must leave for required off-service activities, such as lecture, inform the relevant resident and/or attending physician, particularly if it involves leaving during a surgery or delivery (other assistance may need to be arranged)

8. Many issues in ob/gyn are personal, intimate, and confidential; be mindful of this when deciding where, when, and with whom you have conversations regarding patient care; a prime example of this principle is discussed later (history-taking in the presence of the patient's family or friends)

9. Ask questions but not during stressful situations such as emergency surgeries or postpartum hemorrhages

10. Never invent information: do not be afraid to say "I did not do it" or "I don't know"

11. Read constantly

B. History

1. With new patients, take standard comprehensive history with ob/gyn focus

   a. Age
   b. Gravidity and parity
      i. Parity given as T (term), P (preterm), A (abortions: elective or spontaneous), L (living children)
   c. Obstetric history
   d. Last menstrual period (LMP)
   e. Contraception history
   f. Genetic and ethnic background (important for prenatal diagnosis and cancer screening)
   g. Sexually transmitted infections (STIs), abnormal Pap smear results, incontinence

2. For patients in labor, review prenatal record first, and perform abbreviated history and physical examination (H&P), focusing on prenatal course and labor history

3. Use this time to develop rapport with the patient

4. Do not let a language barrier stop you: if necessary, find a translator

5. Obtaining a history from a patient when a friend or family member is present may be completely unreliable

   a. This pertains particularly to the following subject areas but should be generalized to the entire history

    i. Social history: tobacco, alcohol, and substance use have varying amounts of stigma; patients are often not candid in front of friends and relatives (including and particularly husbands, mothers, and sisters)

    ii. Reproductive history: many women do not disclose to their mates past abortions (or even abortions in which the current mate is the father)

    iii. Past medical history: in the presence of friends or relatives, patients may not disclose such data as cosmetic surgery, medications, psychiatric history, and sexually transmitted diseases

b. Patients often give consent to have others present during interview: "he/she knows everything—he/she can stay"

    i. While the patient may believe this to be the case, it is often not, and there is no way to know unless the patient is interviewed privately

    ii. No information obtained in front of a friend or relative can be relied upon completely

    iii. In many cases, a third party is required for practical reasons (translation, serious illness or pain, impaired mental status)

c. The issue of patient privacy on questioning about history is not fully appreciated across hospitals, the medical profession, and allied health professionals

    i. Nurses routinely do a rather complete history with relatives present on admission to the hospital—this is probably a bad practice but still commonplace

    ii. Because privacy is not fully recognized by health professionals, it is certainly not always expected or accepted by patients—asking friends and relatives to leave the room may not be looked upon favorably by the patient

    iii. The Health Insurance Portability and Accountability Act (HIPAA) does not cover patients disclosing potentially embarrassing information in the presence of family and friends

    iv. It is an open moral and ethical question whether health professionals should ask questions in the presence of others about which the patient may be embarrassed or inclined to lie

d. Medical students should:
   i. Ask friends and relatives to leave—(caution: medical students have little to no authority)
      (1) Patient has often been asked same questions
      (2) Medical students have the least confidence, knowledge, and authority on the team
   ii. If getting all friends and family to leave is not an option, ask the questions with them present
      (1) Ask patient if it is "okay to go over history now"
      (2) Regard information as potentially unreliable
   iii. Omit the most classically sensitive questions, such as those pertaining to substance use, pregnancy, and sexually transmitted infections
   iv. With or without the preceding, get most or all of past medical history from medical records

e. Approaches for medical students
   i. Priority for a medical student has to be on not alienating patient and family
   ii. For a medical student, history reliability is a secondary issue
   iii. An element of common sense should prevail
      (1) One approach not appropriate in all circumstances—individualize
      (2) Timing is everything—often patients will be alone shortly after arrival as friends and relatives help with admission, park the car, and so on

C. Physical examination
   1. Use standard physical examination skills, focusing on three components
      a. Breasts
         i. Inspection, palpation, expression of nipple, axillary lymph nodes
      b. Abdomen
         i. Inspection, auscultation, palpation, uterine fundal height measurement if pregnant
      c. Pelvis
         i. Inspection of vulva (external genitalia)
         ii. Speculum examination: inspection of vagina and cervix
         iii. Bimanual examination: palpation of uterus, tubes, and ovaries (vaginal fingers elevate cervix toward

abdominal wall to allow structure to be palpated between both hands)

2. These examinations should always be chaperoned

D. Assessment and plan

1. As with other areas of medicine, integrate history, physical examination, and relevant laboratory tests/imaging/fetal monitoring results to arrive at a differential diagnosis and a management plan

2. Form an assessment and plan with every patient encounter, even for brief outpatient visits, labor room visits, or postoperative evaluations; the process will soon become second nature, maximize your analysis skills, and optimize patient care

3. Document your findings and assessment clearly and concisely; avoid lengthy "templates" (particularly in emergencies); volume of information less important than quality

4. Mentally rehearse your presentations prior to reporting to the resident/attending physician; your best patient workup will go unrecognized if not well presented; always begin with age, race, gravidity/parity, and LMP: e.g., patient is a 27-year-old Caucasian female, G2 P0010, LMP June 1, who presents with....

E. Conferences and grand rounds

1. Sit in the front; you will learn more and demonstrate enthusiasm and initiative

2. For case presentations: although it may traditionally be a resident responsibility, volunteer to present at least the history and physical examination

3. Volunteer to do literature searches

4. Do not be afraid to ask questions

MENTOR TIPS

- Read a book on obstetrics and gynecology before the clerkship begins—this will provide some basic knowledge and perspective that will help you better understand what you see.
- A key paradox of clinical clerkships is that patients are helping you more than you are helping them. Be polite and helpful to the extent possible. Keep history and physicals brief by knowing what information you want in advance.
- Read in advance about the next day's activities.

Chapter Self-Test Questions

Circle the correct answer. After you have responded to the questions, check your answers in Appendix A.

1. Your patient's husband calls about his wife's pregnancy test result, which is positive. You should do which of the following?

   a. Give him the results.

   b. Call him back and say you cannot release any information.

   c. Have staff call him back and advise him that you would be happy to talk with him as long as his wife calls and gives her consent for you to talk with him.

   d. Not reply at all.

2. Prior to beginning your ob/gyn clerkship, which basic science subjects should be reviewed?

   a. Embryology

   b. Breast and pelvic anatomy

   c. Neuroanatomy

   d. All of the above

   e. a and b

3. In the ob/gyn physical examination, particular focus should be given to which of the following components?

   a. Breast examination

   b. Pelvic examination

   c. Abdominal examination

   d. All of the above

4. In gynecology clinic, your patient asks you about the possible drug interactions between her seizure medicine, Tegretol, and birth control pill. You remember that there may be an interaction, but you are not sure what it is. Which of the following should you do?

   a. Tell her there is an interaction, but you do not remember what it is.

   b. Tell her you do not know.

   c. Tell her you do not know but that you will look it up and let her know in a few minutes.

   d. Ask the resident or attending physician what the interaction is.

See the testbank CD for more self-test questions.

CORE TOPICS IN GYNECOLOGY

5

CHAPTER

MENSTRUAL CYCLE

Michael D. Benson, MD

I. The Normal Menstrual Cycle 45A

A. The menstrual cycle serves two functions: to make an oocyte available for fertilization and to prepare the uterus for a possible pregnancy; if pregnancy does not occur, the thickened lining of the uterus is shed in the form of menstrual bleeding and is then regenerated during the next cycle

   1. Menarche

   a. First menstrual cycle

   b. Average age in United States is 12 years

   c. Rarely, females can ovulate before first period

   d. Menarche does not denote full fertility

   2. Menopause: begins 1 year after all periods cease; fertility substantially reduced years before (see Chapter 6)

   3. Blood loss (average is 30 mL; heavy is more than 80 mL)

   4. Cycle characteristics

a. Length of cycle: the number of days between the first day of one cycle and the first day of the next cycle; typical interval is 28 days, although anywhere from 21 to 35 days can be considered normal

b. Duration of menses: 3–5 days, with extremes between 1 and 8 days

c. Regularity: many fertile, nonpregnant women who are not on hormones have at least one irregular cycle per year

B. Physiology of menses

1. Follicular phase

a. During menses, estrogen and progesterone, secreted by the ovary, at lowest level

b. Slowly, the amount of estrogen secreted begins to increase

c. At the same time, approximately 12 oocytes begin to mature

d. As the oocytes are prepared for release, the cells around them produce fluid that collects in a cyst or follicle

e. Estradiol peaks day 12–13

f. Progesterone peaks 4–8 days post ovulation

g. Ovulation

    i. Oocytes mature until the follicle containing one of them reaches an average of 18–25 mm in diameter

    ii. The dominant follicle (fluid-filled sphere) breaks open, releasing the oocyte into the abdomen

    iii. Remaining follicles then collapse and disappear

    iv. Rarely, two oocytes might be released if two follicles become large enough simultaneously

    v. After ovulation, oocyte floats into end of the fallopian tube, where mild contractions, along with the motions of the tiny hairs lining the tube, move the egg toward the uterus

    vi. Fertilization usually occurs in the outer portion of the tube, close to the ovary

    vii. Fertilized or not, oocyte takes a day or two to traverse the tube

    viii. If a pregnancy has not occurred, egg is resorbed in the uterus

h. Symptoms of ovulation

    i. Mittelschmerz (ovulation pain)

(1) Some women know when they ovulate because they feel a pain on one side of the pelvis
(2) Usually only a mild discomfort for several hours
(3) Rarely, the pain can be so severe that it may at first appear to be a serious problem such as appendicitis
ii. Vaginal bleeding
(1) Women occasionally have some vaginal spotting at the time of ovulation—typically for a few hours
(2) Can be mistaken for menses
iii. Internal (intraperitoneal) bleeding—rarely, if significant blood vessel traverses cite of ovulation, substantial bleeding requiring surgical intervention can occur (pain, orthostatic vital changes, occasional gastrointestinal [GI] distress, no fever)
i. Follicular phase is the variable portion of menstrual cycle
2. Luteal phase
a. Corpus luteum—after ovulation, cells surrounding oocyte rapidly coalesce to form this structure within the ovary
i. Produces progesterone for 12–14 days
ii. Progesterone secreted by ovary helps to stabilize uterine lining and prepare it for a possible pregnancy
iii. In the absence of conception, corpus luteum stops producing progesterone after 14 days and lining of uterus is shed
iv. If fertilization occurs, corpus luteum produces progesterone steadily for several weeks until placenta takes over
b. Luteal phase almost always lasts 12–14 days; not variable in duration
C. Hypothalamic control
1. Menstrual cycle regulated by hypothalamus
a. Secretes pulses of gonadotropin-releasing hormone (GnRH) in varying amounts at changing frequencies
i. Carried to anterior pituitary by hypophyseal portal circulation
ii. GnRH, in turn, modulates the pattern with which pituitary secretes the two gonadotropins: follicle-stimulating hormone (FSH) and luteinizing hormone (LH)

(1) FSH
  (A) During follicular phase FSH secreted in steadily increasing amounts
  (B) This causes ovarian follicles to develop and produce larger amounts of estrogen
(2) LH
  (A) When the amount of circulating estrogen reaches a specific level over a certain period, pituitary secretes a large burst of LH called the LH surge
  (B) This surge causes ovulation to occur and corpus luteum to form

D. Disrupted cycle regularity
  1. Hypothalamus regulates satiety and cortisol release
    a. May partly explain association of eating disorders with menstrual irregularity
    b. Substantial stress can result in cessation of menses
  2. Relationships among hypothalamus, pituitary, ovary, and uterus may explain why two women may begin menstruating at the same time after several months of living together, although an alternative possibility is unidentified aerosol secretion
  3. Female athletes frequently stop menstruating because hormonal and neurologic alterations disrupt the hypothalamic release of GnRH (exertion equivalent of running 20 miles or more per week)
E. Home ovulation detection kits turn positive on LH surge, indicating that ovulation is about to occur

II. Menarche and Puberty `42A, 44`
A. Timing:
  1. Information for key events in female puberty varies slightly among researchers
  2. In Western nations, average age of first menses has decreased by 3–4 months per decade for the past 100 years
  3. It is thought that better nutrition and less disease have led to this earlier onset of puberty
B. Sequence of events in process
  1. Breast development (begins on average at age $10^1/_2$ years; normally occurs between ages 8 and 13 years)
  2. Appearance of pubic hair and axillary hair

3. Growth spurt
  a. Growth of various body parts proceeds at different rates: first, feet and hands; next, lower legs and forearms; often last, thighs and upper arms
  b. Young teenagers may feel they have "big feet" out of proportion to the rest of their body
  c. Short-lived problem
  d. Axillary hair often appears during growth spurt
4. Menarche: average is age 12 years; normal between ages 9 and 16 years
5. Time span: from first sign to menarche can take 1.5–8 years
C. Marshall and Tanner stages
  1. In the 1960s Marshall and Tanner gave a detailed description of the stages of breast and pubic hair growth (Table 5.1)
  2. Despite such apparently precise classifications, much variation in final appearance of breast tissue and pubic hair
  3. Asian women tend to have less body hair, whereas Mediterranean women tend to have more body hair
  4. About one-fourth of all women have some hair on the abdomen, particularly in the midline
D. Body mass index (BMI) and puberty
  1. Average height at menarche: 5 feet, 2 inches
  2. Average weight at menarche: 105 pounds (this is increasing)
  3. As girls mature, ratio of fat to body water increases; by the time of first period, weight is characteristically 27% fat and 52% water

TABLE 5.1 Marshall and Tanner's Classification of Breast and Pubic Hair Growth

Stage	Breast	Pubic Hair
1	Prepubertal	No hair
2	Breast buds	Wisps of hair on labia
3	Further breast enlargement	Hair on mons pubis in midline
4	Areola forms distinct mound on breast	Hair spreads outward
5	Breast fills out—areola forms single contour with breast	Hair forms inverse triangle, reaching inner thighs

4. Effect of weight

    a. Girls 20%–30% over their ideal weight tend to have an earlier menarche than otherwise; girls heavier than this tend to have a later menarche

    b. Girls lighter than they should be or who exercise regularly and strenuously during early adolescence also tend to have menarche at later age

5. Heavy exercise can delay periods (even indefinitely): swimmers and runners have an average age of menarche of 15 years

E. Family history: mother's menstrual history has some influence, barring extremes of weight and exercise

F. Abnormalities in puberty: an evaluation should be made if the first signs of puberty begin before age 7 or do not appear by age 13 years

III. Delayed Puberty/Primary Amenorrhea 42B

A. Definitions

    1. Primary: complete absence of bleeding

        a. No period by age 14 years in absence of development of secondary sexual characteristics

        b. No period by age 16 years in any circumstance

    2. Secondary: cessation of established menses for three cycle lengths or 6 months

B. Etiology

    1. Anatomic

        a. Müllerian dysgenesis

            i. Secondary sexual characteristics normal

            ii. Absent menarche

            iii. Müllerian ducts fail to develop or fuse during embryonic development resulting in partial or complete absence of fallopian tubes, uterus, cervix, and vagina (upper two-thirds)

        b. Distal genital tract obstruction

            i. Transverse vaginal septum

            ii. Imperforate hymen

        c. Treatment

            i. Surgical correction of obstructions

            ii. Creation of functional vagina, involving plastic surgery, dilators to enlarge perineal skin dimple, and hormonal contraceptives

2. Elevated FSH—Turner syndrome
  a. *45,X*
  b. Also known as gonadal dysgenesis
  c. 98%–99% demise in utero
  d. Mosaic cell lines more variable stigmata
  e. Signs and symptoms include shortness, edema of hands and feet, widely spaced nipples, low hairline, low-set ears, and webbed neck
  f. Health problems can include sterility, coarctation of aorta, and failure to develop secondary sexual characteristics
  g. Treatment includes growth hormone for height, hormone replacement therapy, and egg donation for pregnancy
3. Diminished FSH: treatment typically hormonal contraception (more specific therapy as required by diagnosis)
  a. Kallman syndrome
    i. Hypothalamus does not produce GnRH
    ii. Also known as hypothalamic hypogonadism
    iii. Impaired or absent sense of smell
  b. Pituitary adenomas
  c. Idiopathic panhypopituitarism
  d. Anorexia nervosa
  e. Constitutional delay
4. Androgen insensitivity syndrome
  a. *46 X,Y* karyotype (genotypic male)
  b. Abnormal androgen receptors—testosterone not recognized
  c. Clinical presentation
    i. Female gender identity (phenotypic female)
    ii. Female sexual development
    iii. Sparse axillary/pubic hair
    iv. Blind vaginal pouch (lower third present)
  d. Treatment
    i. Removal of testes as soon as diagnosis is made after age 18 years (to permit normal secondary sexual characteristics to develop)
    ii. 5%–10% chance of malignancy occurring
    iii. Testes may be in inguinal canal
    iv. Hormonal contraception therapy following testes removal

IV. Precocious Puberty

A. Same sex (isosexual—feminized early)
   1. Incomplete
      a. Premature thelarche (breast development, age 8 years) and adrenarche (axillary hair earlier than age 8 years) require no therapy
      b. Premature pubarche (isolated appearance of pubic hair earlier than age 8 years)
         i. Elevated adrenal androgen
         ii. Half may have organic brain disease (structural abnormalities or injuries to hypothalamus)
   2. Complete
      a. Also known as:
         i. True
         ii. GnRH-dependent precocious puberty
      b. Results from early maturation of hypothalamus with release of pulsatile GnRH
      c. Most idiopathic—treatment is with GnRH agonists
      d. Some due to organic brain disease—anatomic abnormalities, injury
   3. Peripheral
      a. Also known as pseudo-precocious puberty or GnRH-independent precocious puberty
      b. Etiology
         i. Ovarian tumor (granulosa cell estrogen secreting tumor most common)
         ii. Adrenal tumor that produces estrogen
         iii. Hypothyroidism
         iv. McCune-Albright syndrome
            (1) Also known as polyostotic fibrous dysplasia
            (2) Involves bone fractures and deformity of legs, arms, and skull; café-au-lait spots on skin; precocious puberty; and low LH and FSH
      c. Diagnosis involves history and physical (including height and weight over time); LH and FSH; androgens; brain computed tomography (CT) or magnetic resonance imaging (MRI); thyroid-stimulating hormone (TSH); estrogen; and pelvic/abdominal ultrasound or CT
      d. Treatment is etiology-specific

B. Virilization

   1. Heterosexual precocious puberty

      a. Elevated androgens

      b. May come from androgen-producing tumor of ovaries or adrenals

      c. May be manifestation of congenital adrenal hyperplasia (adrenal enzyme defect in hormone synthesis pathway)

   2. Virilization and hirsutism evaluation (in absence of heterosexual precocious puberty)

      a. Definitions 44B

         i. Hirsutism

            (1) Excessive male-pattern hair growth

            (2) Generally stable course; slow progression

            (3) Can be associated with acne

         ii. Virilization

            (1) Generalized masculinization

            (2) Generally sudden onset; rapid progression

            (3) Includes severe hirsutism, balding, voice deepening, and enlargement of clitoris

      b. Etiology 44C

         i. Ovarian

            (1) Polycystic ovaries

            (2) Androgen-producing tumors (Sertoli-Leydig, hilus cell)

         ii. Adrenal

            (1) Congenital adrenal hyperplasia

            (2) Rare androgen-producing tumors

            (3) Cushing syndrome

         iii. Exogenous medication (particularly oral or topical testosterone or androgens used for body building)

         iv. Idiopathic

      c. Evaluation 44D

         i. History and physical examination

            (1) Onset, progression

            (2) Hair distribution

            (3) Other stigmata of virilization

         ii. Laboratory

            (1) Polyostotic fibrous dysplasia (DHEAS): if >8 mcg/mL consider adrenal neoplasm

(2) Serum testosterone (total and free)—if total >200 ng/dL consider ovarian neoplasm

(3) 17 α-hydroxyprogesterone (to evaluate for congenital adrenal hyperplasia)

d. Treatment

   i. Contingent on diagnosis; most cases of hirsutism are idiopathic; cosmetic treatments are appropriate (laser, depilatory agents, etc.)

V. Hygiene

A. Feminine hygiene products

  1. Sanitary napkins ("pads"): before commercial absorbent pads to place within underwear, women used articles of clothing, typically rags, to absorb menstrual blood

  2. Tampons

    a. Primarily composed of cotton and polyacrylic rayon

    b. Difference in absorbency among various products depends on their composition; absorbancy published on outside of box

    c. In general, a tampon should not be left in place for more than 12 hours, and it is prudent to change them more frequently

    d. Invisible from outside the body

    e. Eliminate odor—by preventing menstrual blood from reaching air, tampons eliminate odor sometimes associated with sanitary napkins

    f. Insertion of tampons does not cause a woman to lose her virginity, although tampons can tear a hymen that has a particularly small opening

    g. Not uncommon for tampons to be inserted and forgotten

     i. Definitely not recommended to forget; very improbable that toxic shock syndrome will develop; most likely outcome of forgetting to remove a tampon is development of a malodorous discharge that ceases when the tampon is removed (see Chapter 3)

     ii. Many women presenting with a chief complaint of retained tampon will not actually have a tampon present

    h. Addition of deodorants to napkins and tampons can cause allergic reactions in some women, manifested by redness and itching of the vulva; symptoms generally become worse with repeated exposure to the same product

B. Douching

  1. Controversial

    a. Not necessary for good health

    b. Many women feel cleaner and fresher afterward

    c. Probably no harm in doing it once a week or so (not daily)

    d. Has been linked to higher risk of pelvic inflammatory disease (PID) (evidence and association are weak)

    e. Products

      i. Medicated and scented products are expensive and can cause contact dermatitis

      ii. Preferable solution for douching consists of 1 tbsp of white vinegar or 2 tsp of salt per quart of water

C. Perineal hygiene

  1. Avoid scents and sprays: almost never necessary for good hygiene and frequently lead to hypersensitivity and skin irritations

  2. Good hygiene begins with drying off thoroughly after a bath or shower and wearing undergarments made of fabric that "breathes" (such as cotton) and clothes that are not too tight

  3. Young girls should be taught to wipe perineum from front to back after urinating or defecating

    a. A good hygiene practice in itself, this was previously thought to be important in preventing urinary tract infections

    b. It now appears that the issue is more complex, but this technique remains a good recommendation

D. Menses and sex

  1. Although some sexually transmitted diseases do seem to thrive during menses, the responsible organisms would probably have been spread by sex even at a different time in the cycle

  2. No compelling health reason to avoid sex during menses

  3. More of a problem for some is the extreme messiness of sexual contact during the days of heavy flow: diaphragm can make sex more hygienic during the period—should be inserted an hour or so before sex and removed immediately afterward if the period is entirely normal and contraception not a concern

VI. Dysmenorrhea 46A

A. Primary dysmenorrhea is painful periods with an onset within a few years of menarche

1. Presumably physiologic in origin—attributed to increased prostaglandin production during ovulatory cycles

2. For this reason, young teens, who tend to be anovulatory for the first few years after menarche, may eventually develop dysmenorrhea when they start to ovulate

3. Prostaglandin-induced uterine contractions and/or retrograde menses with peritoneal irritation/inflammation

B. Secondary dysmenorrhea is painful menstruation that starts well after ovulatory cycles have begun, typically after age 20 years; suggests underlying pathology, but this is often speculative

C. Etiologies 46B

1. Endometriosis (see Chapter 10)

2. Adenomyosis

   a. Endometrium grows into (invades) myometrium, with isolated islands of bleeding within the smooth muscle

   b. Difficult to diagnose without hysterectomy; suggested by:

      i. Slightly but diffusely enlarged uterus on examination

      ii. Findings of thickened myometrium on hysterosonogram or other imaging study

      iii. Possibly identifiable by MRI

3. Associated with other pain conditions such as irritable bowel syndrome

4. Significant pelvic adhesions such as those arising from pelvic inflammatory disease

5. Pelvic congestion syndrome—pain from pelvic varicosities

6. Fibroids

D. Diagnosis

1. Because treatment is usually empiric medical management, diagnostic work-up has limited utility

2. U.S. Food and Drug Administration (FDA)-approved use of GnRH agonist has omitted previous need for laparoscopy to prove endometriosis

3. Diagnostic evaluation

   a. Physical examination: most helpful, particularly if site of pain or localized tenderness can be established

   b. Hysterosonogram: can occasionally identify intrauterine lesions

    c. Laparoscopy: can confirm endometriosis or pelvic varicosities

E. Treatment of dysmenorrhea 46C

    1. Medical treatment

        a. Hormonal contraception

            i. Inhibits ovulation—very effective

            ii. All routes of dosing equally effective

        b. Nonsteroidal anti-inflammatory agents

            i. Inhibit prostaglandin production

            ii. Include two over-the-counter agents:

                (1) Ibuprofen (e.g., Advil)—two 200-mg tablets every 4 hours

                (2) Naproxen sodium (e.g., Aleve)—two tablets orally to start and then one 220-mg tablet every 8 hours

            iii. These drugs can cause gastric ulcers with overuse—very uncommon with occasional use for dysmenorrhea (for this reason COX-2 inhibitors offer no real advantage)

    2. Surgical treatment

        a. Endometrial ablation: has not been specifically studied for relief of pain but likely to be beneficial

        b. Destruction of the medial aspects of the uterosacral ligaments, which carry much of the uterine innervation

        c. Presacral neurectomy

            i. Removal (or interruption) of superior hypogastric plexus

            ii. Constipation and urinary retention are side effects

        d. Hysterectomy

VII. Infrequent Menstruation/Acquired Amenorrhea 43A-D, 45B-E

A. An abnormally long interval between menstrual periods may be defined as a cycle longer than 35 days; most ovulatory cycles result in withdrawal bleeding within this time span.

B. Oligomenorrhea: bleeding at intervals >40 days

C. Pregnancy: the single most common (and important) cause of infrequent and delayed menses is pregnancy, and urine pregnancy tests should be performed if there is any suspicion of pregnancy (usually there is)

D. Anovulation: also known as abnormal or dysfunctional uterine bleeding (AUB, DUB)—the next most common reason for delayed menses after pregnancy

E. Causes of oligomenorrhea/acquired amenorrhea (other than pregnancy)
  1. Hypothalamic amenorrhea: pituitary not stimulated to release gonadotropins
    a. LH and FSH low
    b. Treated with estrogen and progestin (combined hormonal contraceptives or estrogen and progesterone similar to menopause treatment) unless patient wishes to conceive
    c. Associated with anorexia nervosa and heavy exercise
  2. Thyroid dysfunction
    a. Either hyper- or hypothyroidism can interfere with regular menses
    b. Abnoromal levels of thyroid releasing hormone secreted by hypothalamus can interfere with pulsatile secretion of GnRH
    c. TSH is typically all that is needed to screen
  3. Hyperprolactinemia
    a. Produced by benign pituitary tumor; can be microadenoma or macroadenoma
    b. Prolactin disrupts menses because of feedback inhibition of secretion of GnRH
    c. MRI of pituitary for levels of >100
      i. Macroadenomas that can compress nearby vital structures more common with substantial elevations
      ii. As there is not a strict relationship between amount of prolactin elevation and pituitary size, some recommend MRI for any elevation
      iii. Almost a third of women have incidental pituitary microadenomas at time of autopsy
    d. Treatment
      i. Medical
        (1) Bromocriptine (Parlodel)
          (A) Dopamine agonist; typically twice daily dosing by mouth (2.5-mg tablets); vaginal dosing may reduce side effects (dizziness, GI distress)
        (2) Cabergoline
          (A) Dopamine agonist
          (B) 0.25 mg twice weekly up to 1 mg twice a week
          (C) Titrate dose by prolactin level

      (D) Dose increase only every 4 weeks

      (E) Can stop after 6 months of normal prolactin levels with continued follow-up of normal levels

    ii. Surgical: reserved for removal of significant macroadenomas that threaten compromise of adjacent structures

4. Polycystic ovarian syndrome (see Chapter 10): treated with combined hormonal contraception for those who do not desire pregnancy

5. Elevated androgens (uncommon)

  a. Cushing syndrome

  b. Polycystic ovarian syndrome

6. Premature ovarian failure (see Chapter 10)

  a. Consistently elevated LH and FSH before age 40 years

  b. Signifies sterility, although on rare occasions pregnancy has occurred without treatment

  c. Treat with estrogen and progestin (by contraceptives or hormone replacement therapy) to prevent osteoporosis and heart disease

  d. May be an autoimmune disorder

    i. Calcium and phosphorus

    ii. Fasting glucose

    iii. TSH (get thyroid antibodies if abnormal)

    iv. Adrenal antibodies to 21-hydroxylase

7. Sheehan syndrome: necrosis of pituitary due to hemorrhagic shock during childbirth—practically never seen in United States

8. Asherman syndrome: scarring of uterus following dilation and curettage

  a. May present as amenorrhea or hypomenorrhea

  b. Hysterosonogram makes diagnosis

  c. Treated by hysteroscopic lysis of adhesions

9. Infection: tuberculosis (seen more commonly in developing nations); schistosomiasis; severe PID (rare)

10. Idiopathic: most patients with irregular menses do not have a specific diagnosis; associated with obesity

11. Medications: dopaminergic psychiatric drugs; hormonal contraception; chemotherapy

12. Evaluation of oligomenorrhea/acquired amenorrhea

  a. Urine pregnancy test

    b. History—exercise, eating disorders, stress, symptoms referable to thyroid disease, pituitary mass, medication

    c. Physical examination—BMI, thyroid, hirsutism

    d. Laboratory tests

       i. TSH and prolactin initially

       ii. LH and FSH if no result from progestin challenge test

    e. If TSH and prolactin normal (usually they are), administer progestin for 10 days; withdrawal bleeding should occur within 7 days of drug cessation; suggests production of endogenous estrogen (and that LH and FSH will be normal)

    f. If progestin challenge test fails to produce bleeding, LH and FSH should be checked

F. For acquired amenorrhea, treatment is empiric depending on patient wishes

    1. For those with a specific cause, treat medical condition

    2. For those desiring conception, ovulation induction

    3. For those not desiring pregnancy

       a. Hormonal contraception

       b. Hormonal replacement therapy

       c. Progestin treatment alone:

          i. Two approaches:

             (1) Every month days 16–25 or

             (2) If no period for 35 days after first day of LMP, take daily for 10 days

          ii. Two medications

             (1) Medroprogesterone acetate (Provera)—10 mg

             (2) Micronized progesterone (Prometrium)—400 mg (supplied as 100-mg or 200-mg capsules)

VIII. Menorrhagia `45C-E`

A. Definitions

    1. Menorrhagia: excessive uterine bleeding occurring regularly

       a. > 80 mL of blood loss (very hard to quantify)

       b. Period longer than 7 days

    2. Metrorrhagia: bleeding <21 days but irregular

    3. Polymenorrhea: bleeding <21 days but regular

B. Etiology

    1. Uterine neoplasms

a. Endometrium
   i. Benign: uterine polyps
   ii. Premalignant or malignant: adenocarcinoma of the uterus (see Chapter 16)
b. Myometrium
   i. Benign: uterine leiomyomata (fibroids) 53A-D
      (1) Present in up to 30% of women by age 35 years
      (2) Location
         (A) Submucous: impinging on uterine cavity
         (B) Intramural: occupying middle portion of uterine wall
         (C) Subserosal: lying just beneath serosal covering of uterus
      (3) Usually asymptomatic
         (A) Most common symptom is bleeding
         (B) Pain much less common—can cause pain if outgrows blood supply and necrosis ensues— so called "degenerating fibroid"
         (C) Other symptoms: pelvic pressure, abdominal enlargement, fertility and pregnancy problems (miscarriage, prematurity)
      (4) Cause unclear—some appear estrogen-dependent
         (A) Not premalignant
         (B) May shrink in menopause
         (C) May grow during pregnancy
      (5) More common in African Americans
      (6) Treatment commonly recommended for menorrhagia, other significant symptoms, or rapid growth (to help exclude sarcoma)
   ii. Malignant: uterine sarcomas (very rare)
2. Disorders of endometrium (endometriosis, adenomyosis)
3. Anovulation (can cause heavy regular periods as well as infrequent heavy periods)
4. Bleeding disorders (uncommon)
   a. Platelet dysfunction (idiopathic thrombocytopenia purpura)
   b. Von Willebrand disease
      i. Defect in protein (von Willebrand factor) that aids platelet adhesion
      ii. Four types

        iii. Most common screens
- (1) Von Willebrand factor antigen assay
- (2) Ristocetin-induced platelet agglutination assay
- (3) Factor VIII levels (von Willebrand factor slows factor VIII degradation)

        iv. Treatment
- (1) Desmopressin (release of von Willebrand factor from endothelium)
- (2) Factor VIII concentrate

  5. Idiopathic—as with irregular menses, most patients with menorrhagia do not have a specific diagnosis

  6. Rare causes (estrogen-producing tumors, cervical cancer, thyroid disorders, copper intrauterine device [IUD])

C. Diagnosis

  1. Ultrasound
- **a.** Hysterosonogram more sensitive for detecting intrauteruine lesions such as fibroids (particularly submucous) and endometrial polyps
- **b.** Thin catheter placed through cervix and sterile saline infused into uterus during transvaginal ultrasound

  2. Endometrial biopsy
- **a.** Small (3-mm outer diameter) aspiration curette placed through cervix into uterus
- **b.** Suction applied (typically with pulling back on small syringe)
- **c.** Typically recommended for women 40 years or over with increase in frequency or flow of menses
- **d.** Primary goal to obtain endometrial histology to rule out endometrial hyperplasia or cancer

  3. Complete blood count
- **a.** Hemoglobin: most women complaining of heavy or long menses are not anemic; some have significant anemia, and a few are dangerously anemic
- **b.** Platelet count: can help exclude thrombocytopenias

  4. Differential diagnosis
- **a.** Genital tract malignancies
- **b.** Genital tract lacerations or lesions
- **c.** Genital tract infections (cervix and uterus in particular)
- **d.** Bleeding from urethra or rectum

D. Treatment
  1. Nonsteroidal anti-inflammatory drugs (NSAIDs) (reduce bleeding by 20%–40%)
  2. Hormonal contraception (birth control pills)
  3. GnRH agonist (Lupron)
    a. Results transient
    b. Treatment beyond 6 months generally not recommended (osteoporosis is significant concern)
    c. Tolerability improved with concomitant treatment using norethindrone acetate 5 mg/day
    d. Commonly used for endometriosis and uterine fibroids
  4. Uterine artery embolization
    a. Chiefly used for treatment of fibroids
    b. Causes substantial short-term pain—many patients hospitalized overnight for pain management
  5. Dilation and curettage, hysteroscopy
    a. Chiefly a diagnostic method when endometrial biopsy cannot be performed
    b. May be used to remove benign endometrial polyps in women who wish to remain childbearing
  6. Endometrial ablation
    a. Very effective treatment
    b. Not generally recommended for women with large fibroids, adenomyosis
    c. While not a reliable method of sterilization, can only be offered to those who are absolutely sure they do not want to become pregnant in future
    d. A minority of patients (20%–40%) experience amenorrhea
    e. Four commonly used intrauterine methods
      i. Thermachoice: pressurized balloon with hot water
      ii. Novasure: electrocautery
      iii. Hydrothermablation: free-flowing hot water
      iv. Cryocautery: freeze of either cornua under ultrasound guidance
  7. Myomectomy 53D
    a. For those who may wish to become pregnant in future (otherwise hysterectomy more effective)
    b. More likely to be beneficial if fibroid submucous (impinging on uterine cavaity)

    c. If myoma submucous in location, can be done transvaginally via operative hysteroscopy; otherwise most myomectomies performed abdominally (laparotomy versus laparoscopy)

8. Hysterectomy

9. Life-threatening menorrhagia

    a. Exclude pregnancy

    b. Exclude uterine malignancy via endometrial biopsy or dilation and curettage

    c. Transfuse as necessary

    d. Medical treatment to stop bleeding

        i. Conjugated equine estrogens (Premarin) IV 25 mg every 4 hours until bleeding stops for up to 24 hours

        ii. Alternative oral estrogen therapy

            (1) 5 mg conjugated equine estrogen every 6 hours for four doses

            (2) 2 mg estradiol every 6 hours for 24 hours

        iii. Follow 1 day of high-dose estrogen with combined estrogen/progestin therapy (birth control pills) or progestin treatment

10. MRI-guided ultrasound ablation: high-energy focused ultrasound used to destroy fibroid under MRI guidance—role is still evolving

---

MENTOR TIPS

- NSAIDs and hormonal contraception are effective treatments for pain and menorrhagia.
- Endometrial ablation techniques are growing in popularity and are often done as office procedures—patient must be done with childbearing and not have large fibroids.
- Progestin IUD effective for pain and menorrhagia.
- Most cases of menorrhagia, oligomenorrhea, and dysmenorrhea will not have a specific diagnosis after investigation.
- Menstrual complaints (too long, infrequent, irregular, heavy) are very common concerns among women.

Resources

Speroff L, Fritz MA: Clinical gynecologic endocrinology and infertility, 7th ed. Philadelphia, Lippincott Williams and Wilkins, 2005.

Chapter Self-Test Questions

Circle the correct answer. After you have responded to the questions, check your answers in Appendix A.

1. Which is *not* true about menarche?

   a. Pregnancy cannot occur before first period.

   b. Menarche does not denote full fertility.

   c. Average age in United States is 12 years.

   d. Absence of menses by age 16 years merits investigation.

2. Which is true about primary amenorrhea?

   a. Defined as the absence of secondary sexual characteristics by age 14 years.

   b. Secondary sexual characteristics do not appear with müllerian dysgenesis.

   c. Turner syndrome not usually lethal in utero.

   d. Hirsutism associated with androgen insensitivity syndrome.

3. Which is *not* true about precocious puberty for girls?

   a. Isosexual refers to early feminization.

   b. No treatment (or evaluation) required for young girls (<8 years) who develop isolated thelarche or andrenarche.

   c. CT or MRI of brain is often helpful for premature pubarche

   d. Complete precocious puberty usually has a cause.

4. The most common cause of amenorrhea is:

   a. Pregnancy.

   b. Polycystic ovarian syndrome.

   c. Thyroid dysfunction.

   d. Hyperprolactinemia.

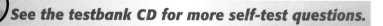

See the testbank CD for more self-test questions.

MENOPAUSE

Linda H. Holt, MD

I. Perspective

A. The menopausal transition is stressful for many women; rapid changes in physiology and psychosocial transitions that accompany this change can be stressful; the symbolic backdrop of aging and declining fertility symbolized by menopause can make menopause a difficult transition

B. For women experiencing difficulty, there are many tools to make the transition smooth and prevent some of the diseases historically assumed to be inevitable with aging

C. Many women make this transition easily without medical intervention

D. Either with or without interventions, most women can anticipate decades of productive life after menopause

II. Definitions 47A

A. *Menopause:* cessation of spontaneous menses resulting from permanent loss of ovarian function due to failure of ovaries to respond to elevated gonadotropins; derived from Greek *men* (month), *pausis* (cessation).

  1. *Perimenopause:* years up to and following menopause, starting with onset of variable menstrual cycle lengths and ending a year after final menstrual period

  2. *Climacteric:* continuum beginning with steep decline in fertility at age 35 years and concluding with end of menses and perimenopausal symptoms

III. Types of Menopause

  A. Naturally occurring menopause

  B. Surgical menopause

C. Premature ovarian failure
  1. Nonidiopathic cases may be triggered by high radiation doses or chemotherapeutic agents
  2. Idiopathic ovarian failure is presumably due to genetic and/or autoimmune processes

IV. Epidemiology

  A. Life expectancy for a woman in the developed world is approximately 80 years; hence, a large proportion of women live more than a third of their lives in postmenopausal status
  B. Average age of menopause 51 years, normal range early 40s to middle to late 50s; earlier in smokers, underweight women; some geographic and ethnic differences but fairly consistent over historic time and in various populations

V. Differential Diagnosis

  A. Look for other causes of amenorrhea and hypogonadism; e.g., pregnancy, hyperprolactinemia, absence or blockage of lower genital tract, pan hypopituitarism, thyroid disorders, hypothalamic amenorrhea
  B. Follicle-stimulating hormone (FSH), estradiol, thyroid-stimulating hormone (TSH), prolactin, human chorionic gonadotropin (hCG) levels may be helpful
  C. Workup indicated at early ages; may not be necessary by late 40s if other signs and symptoms of menopause

VI. Clinical Concerns 47B–C

  A. Symptoms: early
  1. Hot flashes: sensation of flushing or heat, typically with onset of reddening of skin over head, neck, and chest, often with profuse perspiration; often followed by chills; when occurring at night, called night sweats
    a. Duration: a few seconds to several minutes
    b. Incidence: 68%–82% in United States; 90% following oophorectomy; 60% in Sweden; 10%–20% in Indonesia; 10%–25% in Chinese women
  2. Insomnia: common complaint; brain wave and skin temperature patterns show wakeful episode pattern similar to night sweat sleep disruption
  3. Irritability: common complaint; probably related to sleep disruption and fatigue

    4. Mood disturbances: commonly described as emotional lability, worsening premenstrual dysphoria, and difficulty with concentration and short-term memory

B. Physical changes: occur at an intermediate period in menopause process and may continue beyond menopause

    1. Vaginal atrophy is thinning and reduced moisture production of vaginal, vulval, and periurethral and perivesical mucosa; worse in thin women as obese women have more circulating estrogen from peripheral conversion of androgens; causes vulvovaginal burning, painful intercourse, and urinary frequency and urgency

    2. Urinary incontinence symptoms include urge and stress incontinency, may occur or increase due to combination of aging and hormonal decline

    3. Skin thins out, creating increased wrinkling

    4. Hair may thin, especially in individuals with genetic predisposition to hair loss; female pattern is gradual thinning of scalp hair

C. Diseases with incidence escalating due to menopause transition

    1. Osteoporosis

        a. Defined by World Health Organization as bone density score of -2.5 standard deviations (SDs) below average peak bone mass or presence of osteoporotic-type pathologic fractures; osteopenia defined as -1 to -2.5 SDs below average peak bone mass

        b. Bone loss of roughly 1%/year in women age over 35 years escalates to 2%–3%/year perimenopausally due to loss of estrogen

        c. Bone loss occurs with any hypoestrogenic state; various causes are possible, such as menopause, medications (gonadotropin agonists and aromatase inhibitors), low body mass (anorexia nervosa, runner's amenorrhea), or surgical menopause

    2. Cardiovascular disease: the leading cause of death in American women; incidence rises rapidly after menopause

        a. Loss of endogenous estrogen results in lower total cholesterol and higher low-density lipoprotein (LDL) and resulting plaque accumulation

        b. Weight gain and high rates of metabolic syndrome occur with menopause

    c. Women with polycystic ovaries and insulin insensitivity at very high risk

    d. Effects of exogenous estrogen on cardiovascular system are complex

        i. Oral estrogen increases triglycerides, C-reactive protein, factor VII, prothrombin fragments, and fibrinopeptide A

        ii. Oral estrogen lowers total cholesterol and raises HDL levels, improves glucose metabolism, boosts endothelial vascular function, reduces plasma homocystine levels

        iii. Transdermal estrogen is a mild vasodilator but has little impact on coagulation factors

        iv. Two- to threefold risk in thromboembolic events in oral estrogen users; risk dose-dependent and multiplies with additional risk factors (e.g., smoking, thrombophilias); risk lower with use of transdermal/transvaginal products at equivalent oral doses

3. Alzheimer's disease

    a. Risk increased in early menopause and hypoestrogenic states

    b. Observational, cohort, and case-control studies indicate a reduced risk (RR) of 0.66 (0.53–0.32) of dementia in hormone therapy users[1]

    c. Conjugated equine estrogen (CEE) 0.625/medroxyprogesterone acetate 2.5 doubled the risk of dementia (RR 2.05 (1.21–3.48))[2] and CEE 0.625 increased risk (RR 1.38 (1.01–1.89))[3] in a cohort of women starting therapy several years after menopause, mean age 62 years at initiation

    d. Reason for discrepancies unclear but may relate to age of onset of therapy, form of estrogen used, estrogen antagonism, and downregulation of estrogen receptors in brain by progestins

4. Sexuality

    a. Declining libido common with menopause

        i. Most mammalian species only sexually responsive during fertile periods; hence, anovulation may lower biologic drive

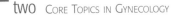
  ii. From early to late menopause, low sexual function increased from 42% to 88% in one large Caucasian population

 b. Longer time to achieve orgasm

 c. Dyspareunia can result from vulvovaginal atrophy

VII. Office Evaluation of the Menopausal Woman

A. General history

 1. Family history

 2. Lifestyle evaluation including social support, substance use, domestic violence screening, exercise, and diet

B. Physical examination

 1. All the basics, plus height, weight, blood pressure (BP), body mass index (BMI); thyroid; breast; cardiovascular; pulmonary; abdominal; pelvic and rectal; extremities; lymphatics; integument

C. Laboratory work

 1. Lipids, TSH, glucose, complete blood count (CBC)

 2. Bone densitometry: 65 years old or with risk factors, female, perimenopausal, Caucasian or oriental, smoker, small frame, low BMI, poor dietary intake, sedentary, family history

 3. Mammography usually annually beyond age 50 years

 4. Magnetic resonance imaging (MRI) if known *BrCa* carrier or first-degree relative

 5. Colon cancer screening: initiate at age 40–50 years per American Cancer Society (ACS) guidelines

D. Counseling

 1. Diet, lifestyle

 2. Weight optimization

 3. Smoking cessation

 4. Exercise: aerobic, cardiovascular, weightbearing

 5. Calcium, vitamin D

 6. Hormone therapy: basic counseling—indications and contraindications

VIII. Hormone Replacement Therapy (HRT) and Principal Hormone Analogues Used in Menopause Transition

A. Estrogen (E) encompasses many compounds that have stimulating effects on target tissues; different estrogens acting through the same receptor can induce different biologic activity; usual assay is rat uterine weight

1. Target tissues—breast, bone, connective tissue, central nervous system, uterus, vulvovaginal, bladder, integument
2. Two well-described receptor systems
   a. Alpha receptors predominate in reproductive organs
   b. Beta receptors predominate in bone and brain
3. Varying compounds of estrogen, other steroid hormones, and selective estrogen receptor modulators can induce differing biologic activity (Table 6.1)

B. Progesterone (P) is a specific chemical compound; progestins are chemical compounds with progestogenic activity; i.e., block effects of estrogen in endometrium (Tables 6.2 and 6.3)
   1. Reduce estrogen receptors in some target tissues by definition endometrium; endometrial protection requires 10 days of progestin exposure[4]
   2. Uterus: can reduce bleeding, downregulate fibroids; progestins can cause atrophy of endometrium including ectopic endometrium in endometriosis and adenomyosis
   3. Induces target cell enzymes that convert estradiol to estrone and can reduce intracellular availability of potent estrogens such as estradiol
   4. Central nervous system can reduce migraines triggered by fluctuating estrogen but can also trigger dysphoric responses
   5. MPA, more so than micronized progesterone, blunts some of estrogen impact on lipids[5]

C. Testosterone
   1. Enhances libido and female-initiated sexual encounter frequency and intensity
   2. Most testosterone preparations do not have specific FDA approval for use in women; known to increase libido but safety concerns remain over long-term effects on cholesterol metabolism
   3. Discussed later in section on additional hormones

D. Selective estrogen receptor modulators (SERMs) are synthetic, nonsteroidal compounds that bind to estrogen receptors and trigger varying estrogen agonist or antagonist effects in differing target tissues

IX. Counseling About Menopause Process and Use of Menopausal Hormone Therapy 47E

A. Definitions
   1. Hormone therapy encompasses estrogen-progestin therapy in women with intact uteri

TABLE 6.1	Estrogen Products Available in United States			
Brand Name	Generic Name	Route of Administration	Daily Doses	Comments
Premarin	Conjugated equine estrogens	PO	0.3, 0.45, 0.625, 0.9, 1.25 mg	Used in Women's Health Initiative (WHI) and many major clinical trials; E2 levels 30–50 pcg/mL at 0.625 mg/day, 40–60 at 1.25/day
Cenestin	Synthetic conjugated estrogens	PO	0.3, 0.45, 0.625, 0.9, 1.25 mg	
Enjuvia	Synthetic conjugated estrogens, B	PO	0.3, 0.45, 0.625, 1.25 mg	10 synthetic estrogens mimicking premarin
Ogen	Estropipate (piperazone estrone sulfate)	PO	0.75, 1.5, 3 mg	E2 35 pg/mL at 0.0625 (0.75) dose, 126 at 2.5 (3) dose
Estrace	Micronized estradiol	PO	0.5, 1, 2 mg	Inexpensive; available in generic, E2 30–50 pg/mL at 1 mg/day, 40–60 pg/mL at 2 mg/day
Femtrace	Estradiol acetate	PO	0.45, 0.9, 1.8 mg	
Estratest, Estratest HS	Esterified estrogens and methyl-testosterone	PO	1.25/2.5, 0.625/1.25 mg	One of few testosterone-containing products not "off label" in women

Alora (twice weekly) Climara (weekly) Menostar (weekly) Vivelle-Dot (twice weekly)	Estradiol patch	Transdermal patch	0.014 (Menostar), 0.025, 0.0375, 0.05, 0.06, 0.075, 1 mg	E2 30–65 pg/mL levels at 0.05 dose, 50–90 at 0.1 mg dose
Estrogel 0.06%	Estradiol gel		1.25 g gel 0.075 estradiol	0.075/day approximately E2 40–100 pg/mL; 3 60–140 pg/mL
Elestrin 0.06%	Estradiol gel		0.87 g gel per pump	0.012 mg/day 1 pump, 0.041 mg/day 2 pumps; E2 10–18 pg/mL at 0.87 g/day, 24–55 at 1.7 g/day gel*
Divigel 0.1%	Estradiol gel	Transdermal gel	0.25 g packet	0.025 mg/day packet or single pump
Premarin vaginal cream	Conjugated equine estrogen cream	Vaginal cream	0.625 mg/g	Typical dose 1 g twice weekly with applicator or can apply externally
Estrace vaginal cream	Micronized estradiol cream	Vaginal cream	1.0 mg/g	Typical dose 1 g twice weekly with applicator or apply externally
Estring	Estradiol	Vaginal ring	0.0075 mg	Used for 3 months; serum levels not detectable; preferred for women with hormone-dependent cancer who need vaginal estrogen
Femring	Estradiol	Vaginal ring	0.05, 0.10 mg	For vasomotor symptoms as well
Vagifem (twice weekly)	Estradiol	Vaginal tablet	0.025 mg	Twice weekly is recommended dose

*Kenwood Therapeutics, Fairfield, NJ; package information for Elestrin, 12/14/06.

TABLE 6.2

Combination Estrogen-Progestin Products Available in United States

Brand Name	Generic Name	Route of Administration	Doses	Comments
Activella	Estradiol and norethin-drone acetate	PO	1/0.5, 0.5 mg	
Prempro	Conjugated equine estrogen/medroxyprogesterone acetate	PO	0.3/1.5, 0.45/1.5 0.625/2.5 0.625/5 mg	Used in Heart and Estrogen/Progestin Re-placement Study (HERS), WHI, and many major trials
Femhrt	Ethinyl estradiol/norethindrone	PO	5/1; 2.5/0.5 mg	Uses form of estrogen used in oral contraceptives at approx. 1/10 dose
Prefest	Estradiol and norgestimate	PO	1 mg of estradiol for 3 days alter-nating with 3 days of 0.9 norgestimate—repeated continuously	
Angeliq	Estradiol and drosperinone	PO	1/0.5 mg	
Climara Pro	Estradiol and levonorgestrel	Transdermal patch	0.045/0.015 mg	Weekly
Combipatch	Estradiol and norethin-drone acetate	Transdermal patch	0.05/0.14	Twice weekly
Compounded transdermals	Typically estriol estradiol, progesterone can in-clude testosterone or dehydroepiandrosterone	Transdermal gels or creams	0.05/0/25 mg Varies	

TABLE 6.3	Progesterone and Progestin Products Available in United States			
Brand Name	Generic Name	Route of Administration	Doses	Comments
Prometrium	Micronized progesterone	PO	100, 200 mg	Lipid impact in Postmenopausal Estrogen/Progestin Interventions trial more favorable than in medroxyprogesterone acetate
Compounded progesterone	Micronized progesterone	PO	Formulated per request	Bioavailability may vary
Provera	Medroxyprogesterone acetate (MPA)	PO	2.5, 5, 10 mg	Inexpensive generics; used in WHI and HERS trials
Aygestin, Micronor	Norethindrone, norethindrone acetate	PO	0.35, 2.5, 5, 10 mg	"Minipill" dosing 0.35 mg daily or 2.5–5 mg for 10–12 days
Prochieve 4%, 8%; Crinone 4%, 8%	Progesterone gel	Per vagina	45–90 mg/day	Secondary amenorrhea (4%) and adjunct to assisted reproduction (8%); absorption half-life 25–50 hours; six doses every other day for secondary amenorrhea in women using estrogen
Compounded progesterone creams and gels	Varies	Transdermal or transvaginal	Varies	Bioavailability varies

2. Estrogen therapy refers to systemic estrogen therapy (unopposed estrogen) usually used only in women who have had hysterectomies

3. Topical estrogen therapy refers to topical, usually vaginal, use for atrophy

B. Treatment of vasomotor symptoms, urogenital atrophy, osteoporosis prevention

C. Benefits of estrogen therapy

1. Estrogen effectively treats vasomotor symptoms

2. Vaginal atrophy reversed with adequate estrogenization; estrogen topically or systemically may alleviate many of these problems

3. Genitourinary symptoms

   a. Incontinence increases with age and is multifactorial; menopause and thinning vaginal and bladder tissues play a contributing factor, and adequate estrogenization may be helpful

   b. Declining estrogen levels in the vaginal, bladder, and vulvovaginal tissues have negative impact

   c. Reduced cellular mitosis, tissue vascularity, thinning of mucosal layer, shift in vaginal flora toward bacterial flora that cause bacterial vaginosis

   d. Clinical sequelae include dyspareunia, urethritis, urethral syndrome, increasing susceptibility to urinary tract infections

   e. Vulval dermatoses, i.e., lichen sclerosis, may become symptomatic with menopause; incidence increases with age

4. Prevention of osteoporosis

   a. Estrogen prevents perimenopausal and hypoestrogenemic bone loss

   b. Estrogen reduces osteoclastic activity

   c. WHI one of few trials powered for fracture reduction and was not in women at high risk for fracture

   d. All site fracture relative risk is reduced to a mean of 0.76 (0.69–0.83) for conjugated equine estrogen combined with medroxyprogesterone acetate versus placebo[6]

   e. Fracture relative risk is reduced to mean of 0.70 (0.59–0.83) for just conjugated equine estrogen versus placebo[7]

    f. Benefits seen mainly with long-term use and if initiated perimenopausally

  5. Mood and sleep disturbances

    a. Subjective improvement in mood, sleep, and general well-being

    b. Estrogen does not treat major depression or major mood disorders but may potentiate antidepressant treatment

  6. Sexuality—complex interaction of aging and menopause

    a. Lack of libido is primary sexual complaint among women with an overall sexual dysfunction rate of as high as 43% (most due to lack of libido) among adult women

    b. Dyspareunia resulting from lack of estrogen adversely affects sexuality; improved lubrication and correction of dyspareunia with either vaginal or systemic estrogen may improve sexual experience

    c. Many women report improvements in sexual interest and function with estrogen and/or testosterone therapy

  7. Decreased risk of colon cancer 30% noted in randomized trials (WHI),[6] observational studies (Nurses' Health Study),[8] and other epidemiologic studies

  8. Reduction in age-related incidence of macular degeneration

D. Risks of hormone therapy

  1. Thromboembolic disease

    a. Increased risk two- to threefold of venous thromboembolism with oral formulations[9]; the Women's Health Initiative study showed an increased mean relative risk of 2.06 (1.57–2.70) with conjugated equine estrogen and medroxyprogesterone acetate and a relative risk of 1.32 (0.99–1.75) with conjugated equine estrogen alone

    b. Risks increase with advancing age

    c. Risks increase in smokers

    d. Transdermal compounds less to negligible risk at low doses[10]

    e. Risks multiplicative with other risk factors (venous stasis, thrombophilias, surgical insult or trauma)

    f. If at risk for thromboembolic disease, either avoid or minimize risk by ruling out other factors via thrombophilia workup and/or venous flow evaluation

  2. Hormone-dependent tumors

    a. Breast carcinoma
- **i.** Epidemiologic studies suggest increased RR 1.1 with estrogen only, 1.4 with estrogen:synthetic progestin therapy
- **ii.** WHI showed attributable risk of 8/1000 woman-years of use with CEE 0.625/MPA 2.5, a decreased risk of breast cancer with CEE 0.625 (RR 0.8) that escaped statistical significance

    b. Endometrial carcinoma two- to tenfold risk
- **i.** Postmenopausal Estrogen/Progestin Interventions Trial—simple hyperplasia 27%, complex hyperplasia 22% after 3 years CEE 0.625

3. Two- to fourfold increased risk of cholecystitis in estrogen users

4. Endometriosis can recur with estrogen and rare endometrioid tumors found in long-term estrogen users; progestins may mitigate risk

5. Blood pressure elevation can occur with oral estrogen therapy rarely; overall, estrogen therapy has little impact on blood pressure

6. Hepatic adenomas very rare

E. Side effects

1. Bleeding: common; occurring in 20%–30% of continuous combined hormone users; can be minimized by reducing dose or cycling hormones to establish predictable bleeding pattern; may require workup with endometrial sampling

2. Breast tenderness: can be due to estrogen or progestin component; can be reduced by discontinuing or reducing dose

3. Headaches: commonly due to hormone fluctuations; may be alleviated by evening out fluctuations (changing from short half-life compound to long half-life compound) or raising or reducing dose; neurologic workup as needed for new-onset, severe, unusual headaches

4. Fluid retention: both estrogen and progestins can cause fluid retention; may respond to decreased dose or changing compound or mild diuretic

F. Contraindications

1. Undiagnosed abnormal genital bleeding

2. Known, suspected, or history of breast cancer

3. Known or suspected estrogen-dependent neoplasia
4. Active deep-vein thrombosis, pulmonary embolism
5. Active or recent arterial thromboembolic disease
6. Liver dysfunction or disease
7. Known or suspected pregnancy

X. Initiating Hormone Therapy

A. Confirm indications, lack of contraindications

B. Counsel and document counseling on risks and benefits

C. Pretreatment laboratory tests

1. Consider endometrial assessment if risk factors for endometrial hyperplasia/cancer (significantly obese, history of anovulatory cycles, polycystic ovary syndrome, unusual bleeding)
2. Mammogram
3. If family history of known thrombophilias (e.g., Leiden factor), test for specific inherited factor

D. Choice of therapy

1. Combination estrogen/progestin if intact uterus
   a. Continuous combined: balanced estrogen/progestin on a daily basis; many combined products available (see Table 6.2); no timed withdrawal bleeds but high rate of breakthrough bleeding
   b. Cyclic (estrogen continuously or with "off" times combined with intermittent progestin) offers predictable, timed bleeding
   c. Duration of progestin must be 12 days to convert proliferative endometrium to secretory
2. Estrogen only if no uterus
3. Oral—convenient; preferred by many patients; wide range of doses and compounds; generics available for some compounds; many oral estrogens and progestins available
4. Transdermal (patches, gels)—less thromboembolic risk at equivalent doses; limited availability of progestin combinations
5. Vaginal (estrogen creams, rings, or tablets of varying doses; progesterone gel)
6. Intrauterine progestin available in Mirena intrauterine system
7. Compounding pharmacies provide varying combinations of estrogens, progesterone, dehydroepiandrosterone (DHEA),

testosterone; available in oral, transdermal, vaginal, and subcutaneous pellet depot preparations

   a. Bioavailability may vary

   b. Controversy at U.S. Food and Drug Administration about extent of regulation

8. Evaluation of breakthrough bleeding necessary only if persistent >6 months or risk factors for hyperplasia

   a. Endometrial biopsy (EMB)—3-mm plastic suction device

   b. Office biopsy correlates well with hysterectomy or dilation and curettage (D&C) specimens

   c. Transvaginal ultrasound

      i. Endometrial thickness positively correlates with presence or absence of pathology in women not receiving HRT

      ii. Thickness <5 mm in postmenopausal women rarely associated with endometrial pathology

      iii. Reassuring varies in women on hormone replacement therapy but an endometrial thickness of 5 mm or greater may warrant investigation (some disagreement on minimum abnormal threshold)

   d. D&C—if unable to perform office EMB

   e. Sonohysterogram or hysteroscopy to evaluate for submucous fibroids or polyps

      i. Sonohysterogram consists of saline infusion into uterine cavity, outlining intrauterine contents such as fibroids or polyps

      ii. Hysteroscopy allows direct visualization and directed biopsy or resection of fibroids or polyps

9. Management of irregular bleeding after endometrium assessed; decrease dose, discontinue, change to cyclic formulation to ensure scheduled bleeding

XI. Additional Hormones and Hormone Analogues Used in Menopause Management

A. Testosterone

1. Symptomatic testosterone deficiency following natural menopause, surgical menopause, chemotherapy, irradiation, premature ovarian failure

2. Improves sexual interest and frequency of female-initiated sexual contact in women with hypogonadism

3. Improves bone density[11]
4. Many are labeled only for use in men and difficult to titrate for women
   a. PO methyltestosterone 10-mg tablets; female dose would be roughly 1/10 of male dose
   b. Combination oral product, esterified estrogen/methyl-testosterone, available for vasomotor symptoms; with 1.25–2.5 mg of methyltestosterone
   c. Transdermal gels: typical female dose 1.25–2.5 mg/day
   d. Transdermal patches available for men; similar dosing
   e. Vaginal preparations
   f. 2% testosterone ointment widely used for vulval dermatoses, specifically lichen sclerosis
5. Side effects are acne, facial hair, deepening voice, alopecia
6. Risks are worsening lipid parameters and possible atherosclerotic changes

B. DHEA and DHEA sulfate are C-19 steroids produced in adrenal glands and ovaries converted into androgens in vivo; some studies suggest benefits in mood, well-being, and libido, and others do not

C. Tamoxifen—SERM indicated for breast cancer treatment and prevention
1. Estrogen-like impact on bone demonstrated in clinical trials but not indicated for osteoporosis treatment or prevention
2. Indicated for treatment of estrogen replacement and breast cancer and prophylaxis of breast cancer in high-risk women
3. Increased risk of thromboembolic events approximately threefold over baseline due to impact on clotting cascade
4. Endometrial carcinogen 1% risk after 5 years of use

D. Raloxifene—SERM indicated for osteoporosis treatment and breast cancer prevention
1. Estrogen-like impact on bone indicated for osteoporosis prevention and treatment
2. Ralifene is indicated in high-risk women for reduction of breast cancer risk
3. Increased thromboembolic events two to three times over baseline; similar to tamoxifen and oral estrogen at 0.625 CEE equivalent dose
4. No increase in endometrial hyperplasia or cancer

5. Approved also for breast cancer prevention

E. Tibolone—SERM not used in United States; available in Europe—androgenic, progestogenic, estrogenic activity via conversion in vivo

XII. Additional, Nonhormonal Therapeutic Alternatives 47D

A. Vasomotor symptoms

1. Selective serotonin reuptake inhibitors (SSRIs)

a. Paroxetine (Paxil) results in a 62% reduction of hot flashes with a dose of 12.5 mg and a 65% reduction for a 25-mg dose

b. Fluoxetine (Prozac) 20% improvement over placebo

c. Serotonin/norepinephrine reuptake inhibitor (SNRI) venlafaxine (Effexor) 60% reduction versus 27% for placebo at 75–150 mg/day, 37% versus 27% at 37.5 mg/day

2. Clonidine reduces 46%–80% depending on dose

3. Progestins modestly effective in some women

4. Gabapentin (Neurontin) reduced 45% versus 29% placebo

5. Herbal regimens—black cohosh, ginseng, chaste-tree berry, dong quai, licorice, sage, red clover, evening primrose, wild yams used in various over-the-counter menopause preparations; individual clinical trials on hot-flash risks have mixed results but do not support consistent improvement over placebo for vasomotor symptoms

6. Phytoestrogens—plant estrogens, primarily phenolic compounds that include isoflavones and lignans; modest impact on flashes demonstrated in some studies

a. Isoflavones—soybeans; brown, black, navy, pinto beans contain isoflavones converted in gut to genistein, daidzein, equol

b. Lignan precursors found in whole grains, seeds, fruits, vegetables, flaxseed, rye, millet, legumes; lignans converted in gut to enterolactone and enterodiol

B. Vaginal atrophy

1. Variety of over-the-counter lubricants available to counteract lack of secretions

a. Oils or ointments serve as barrier protectants of vulval and vaginal tissues; cannot be used with latex condoms; may be less irritating than some of commercial lubricants

      b. Vaginal moisturizer (Replens)

      c. Vulval dermatosis (commonly mistaken for atrophy)—consider vulval biopsy to rule out vulval intraepithelial neoplasia and diagnose dermatoses, such as lichen sclerosis, which can often be treated with topical steroids

C. Sexual dysfunction

    1. Phosphodiesterase inhibitors, such as sildenafil (Viagra), vardenafil hydrochloride (Levitra), and tadalafil (Cialis), have only limited use in women but may be helpful in women with vascular and neuropathic loss of sensation

    2. Certain neurotransmitters (serotonin) seem to inhibit sexuality; certain neurotransmitters (dopamine, norepinephrine) may enhance sexuality, but no specific products on market; bupropion (Wellbutrin, Zyban) used off-label to enhance libido

    3. Herbal products and vaginal preparations such as Avlimil and Zestril have been reported in limited clinical trials to enhance libido and sexual response

    4. Stimulatory products such as vibrators may enhance sexual response

    5. Vaginal dilators or physical therapy stretching and relaxation exercises can reduce dyspareunia

    6. Marital and/or sexual counseling

D. Osteoporosis treatment and prevention

    1. Optimize calcium (1000–1500 mg/day) and vitamin D intake (800 IU/day)

    2. Correct other causes of bone loss (hyperparathyroidism, hyperthyroidism, overuse of steroids)

    3. Weight-bearing exercise and balance training

    4. Fall prevention—good lighting, soft carpeting, support bars, eliminating sources of tripping and slippery surfaces

    5. Bisphosphonates

      a. Long-acting pyrophosphate analogues that inhibit bone resorption

      b. Half-life up to 10 years

      c. Excreted by kidney

      d. Alendronate (Fosamax), risedronate (Actonel) PO, ibandronate (Boniva) PO and IV, zoledronic acid (Reclast) IV; various other injectable and oral bisphosphonates available and in clinical trials

6. Raloxifene (Evista) antiresorptive selective estrogen receptor modulator) reduces spinal fractures

7. Salmon calcitonin (salcatonin) 40–50 times more potent than human calcitonin with longer half-life; available in nasal spray or injection

8. Teriparatide (Forteo) recombinant human parathyroid hormone, administered chronic low dosing (daily subcutaneous injections); has anabolic affect on skeleton with reduced risk of vertebral and hip fractures[12]

9. Tamoxifen increases bone density but no specific indication for osteoporosis management

10. Tibolone synthetic hormone structurally related to norethisterone in in vivo estrogenic, progestogenic, and androgenic activities; reduced vertebral fractures by 50% in one trial with an increased stroke risk[13]

E. Cardiovascular disease

    1. Smoking cessation

    2. Weight reduction, weight optimization

    3. Decrease saturated fats

    4. Aerobic exercise

    5. Lipid level optimization per American Heart Association guidelines

    6. Low-dose aspirin for women with risk factors for cardiovascular disease or over age 65 years with no contraindications

    7. Fish consumption, oatmeal, yeast extract, flaxseed, omega 3 supplements, red wine

F. Neurodegenerative disease

    1. Acetylcholinesterase inhibitors increase availability of acetylcholine in synaptic nerves

    2. Tacrine (Cognex), donepezil (Aricept), and rivastigmine tartrate (Exelon) currently approved

G. Breast cancer risk reduction

    1. SERMs tamoxifen and raloxifene reduce estrogen receptor–positive breast cancer by 50% in high risk women[14,15]

    2. Weight loss

    3. Avoid alcohol

MENTOR TIPS

- Obtain hCG in an amenorrheic woman if remotely possible she could be pregnant.
- Menopause is not a disease.
- Premature and surgical menopause are pathologic states.
- Estrogen therapy, androgen therapy, and hormone therapy in general are like any pharmacologic intervention: the known risks and benefits need to be weighed in terms of the individual's health status, indications, and risk factors.
- Transdermal estrogen does not affect triglycerides or clotting factors at modest doses; transdermal or transvaginal rather than PO is preferred route of administration of estrogen over PO estrogen for women with cardiovascular risk factors.
- Transdermal estrogen does not raise sex hormone–binding globulin; perhaps would have less effect on testoterone bioavailability and hence libido.
- SSRIs, neurontin, and to a lesser extent phytoestrogens may address menopause symptoms in women who cannot or choose not to take estrogen.
- Be proactive in asking about vaginal dryness, sexuality, and domestic violence issues. Midlife women will often not volunteer this information.

References

1. LeBlanc ES, Janowsky J, Chan BKS, et al: Hormone replacement therapy and cognition: Systematic review and meta-analysis. Journal of the American Medical Association 285:1489–1499, 2001.
2. Shumaker SA, Legault C, Rapp SR, et al: Estrogen plus progestin and the incidence of dementia and mild cognitive impairment in post-menopausal women: The Women's Health Initiative memory study: A randomized controlled trial. Journal of the American Medical Association 289:2651–2662, 2003.
3. Shumaker SA, Legault C, Kuller L, et al: Conjugated equine estrogens and incidence of probable dementia and mild cognitive impairment in postmenopausal women: Women's Health Initiative memory study. Journal of the American Medical Association 291:2947–2958, 2004.

4. Varma TR: Effect of long-term therapy with estrogen and progesterone on the endometrium of postmenopausal women. ACTA Obstetricia et Gynecologica Scandinavica 64:41, 1985.
5. Writing Group for the PEPI Trial: Effects of estrogen or estrogen/progestin regimens on heart disease risk factors in postmenopausal women. Journal of the American Medical Association 273:199–208, 1995.
6. Writing Group for the Women's Health Initiative Investigators: Risks and benefits of estrogen plus progestin in healthy menopausal women: Principal results from the Women's Health Initiative randomized controlled trial. Journal of the American Medical Association 288:321–323, 2002.
7. Women's Health Initiative Steering Committee: Effects of conjugated equine estrogen in postmenopausal women with hysterectomy: The Women's Health Initiative randomized controlled trial. Journal of the American Medical Association 291:1701–1712, 2004.
8. Grodstein F, Martinez ME, Platz EA, et al: Postmenopausal hormone use and the risk for colorectal cancer and adenoma. Annals of Internal Medicine 128:705–771, 1998.
9. Grodstein F, Stampfer MJ, Goldhaber SZ, et al: Prospective study of exogenous hormones and risk of pulmonary embolism in women. Lancet 348:983–987, 1996.
10. Scarabin P, Oger E, PluBureau G: Differential association of oral and transdermal oestrogen-replacement therapy with venous thromboembolism risk. Lancet 362:428–432, 2003.
11. Watts NB, Notelovitz M, Timmons MD: Comparison of oral estrogens and estrogens plus androgen on bone mineral density, menopausal symptoms and lipid-lipoprotein profiles in surgical menopause. Obstetrics and Gynecology 85:529, 1995
12. Neer RM, Arnaud CD, Zanchetta JR, et al: Effect of parathyroid hormone (1–34) on fractures and bone mineral density in postmenopausal women with osteoporosis. New England Journal of Medicine 344:1434–1441, 2001.
13. Cummings SR: LIFT study is discontinued. British Journal of Medcine 332:667, 2006.
14. Fisher B, Costantino JP, Wickerham DL, et al: Tamoxifen for prevention of breast cancer: Report of the National Surgical Adjuvant Breast and Bowel Project P-1 Study. Journal of the National Cancer Institute 90:1371–1388, 1998.

15. Cummings SR, Eckert S, Krueger KA, et al: The effect of raloxifene on risk of breast cancer in postmenopausal women: Results from the MORE randomized trial. Journal of the American Medical Association 281:2189–2197, 1999.

Resources

Liu JH, Gass MLS: Management of the perimenopause: Practical pathways in obstetrics and gynecology. New York, McGraw-Hill, 2006.
Lobo RA: Treatment of the postmenopausal woman: Basic and clinical aspects. Burlington, Mass., Elsevier, 2007.
North American Menopause Society Web site: www.menopause.org
Studd J, ed: The management of the menopause, 3rd ed. London, Parthenon, 2003.

Chapter Self-Test Questions

Circle the correct answer. After you have responded to the questions, check your answers in Appendix A.

1. What is the likeliest cause of death in a postmenopausal woman?

   a. Motor vehicle accidents

   b. Heart disease

   c. Breast cancer

   d. Osteoporotic fractures

2. What tests might be done to evaluate abnormal perimenopausal bleeding?

   a. CT scan

   b. IVP

   c. Endometrial ablation

   d. Endometrial biopsy

3. What is (are) the indication(s) for testosterone in women?

   a. Vasomotor symptoms

   b. Decreased libido

   c. Hirsutism

   d. Osteopenia

4. What impact does estrogen therapy have on cancer risk?

    a. Increases colon cancer risk, decreases ovarian cancer risk

    b. Increases breast cancer risk, increases colon cancer risk

    c. Decreases endometrial cancer risk, decreases breast cancer risks

    d. Decreases colon cancer risk, increases breast cancer risks

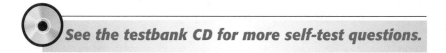

See the testbank CD for more self-test questions.

7

CONTRACEPTION

Michael D. Benson, MD

I. Factors Affecting Use

A. Safety: risk of death or serious injury

   1. Compare this risk with the risks of pregnancy: pregnancy not perfectly safe

      a. Generally 1 death per 10,000 pregnancies in the United States

      b. Mortalilty may be higher with cesarean section although cesarean occasionally performed for pregnant women with additional significant risk (such as hemorrhage)

   2. Direct risks: spermicides and barrier methods have no risk of death or serious injury; hormonal contraceptives can increase risk of thromboembolic disease particularly if other risk factors present (especially smoking)

   3. Effect on sexually transmitted diseases: barrier methods, hormonal contraceptives can reduce risk of transmission or injury of some sexually transmitted diseases

B. Efficacy (Table 7.1)

   1. How measured

      a. Pearl Index: Used to measure efficacy in contraception studies

         i. Method: number of pregnancies divided by number of women-months multiplied by 1200

         ii. Alternative: number of pregnancies divided by number of women-cycles multiplied by 1300

         iii. Problems: pregnancy risk not constant over time—studies of different lengths cannot be compared

      b. More sophisticated life tables probably more useful: pregnancy rate over time measured

   2. Perfect use assumes no user failures

TABLE 7.1

Contraceptive Efficacy 33B

Method	Percentage of Women Experiencing an Unintended Pregnancy Within First Year of Use		Percentage of Women Continuing Use at 1 Year[3]
	Typical Use[1]	Perfect Use[2]	
No method[4]	85	85	
Spermicides[5]	29	18	42
Withdrawal	27	4	43
Periodic abstinence	25		51
Calendar		9	
Ovulation method		3	
Sympto-thermal[6]		2	
Post ovulation		1	
Cap[7]			
Parous women	32	26	46
Nulliparous women	16	9	57
Sponge			
Parous women	32	20	46
Nulliparous women	16	9	57
Diaphragm[7]	16	6	57
Condom[8]			
Female (reality)	21	5	49
Male	15	2	53
Combined pill and minipill	8	0.3	68
Ortho Evra patch	8	0.3	68
NuvaRing	8	0.3	68
Depo-Provera	3	0.3	56
Lunelle	3	0.05	56
IUD			
ParaGard (copper T)	0.8	0.6	78
Mirena (LNG-IUS)	0.1	0.1	81
Norplant and Norplant-2	0.05	0.05	84

Contraceptive Efficacy 33B (continued)

Method	Percentage of Women Experiencing an Unintended Pregnancy Within First Year of Use		Percentage of Women Continuing Use at 1 Year[3]
Female sterilization	0.5	0.5	100
Male sterilization	0.15	0.10	100

Emergency contraceptive pills: Treatment initiated within 72 hours after unprotected intercourse reduces risk of pregnancy by at least 75%.[9]

Lactational amenorrhea method: Highly effective, *temporary* method of contraception.[10]

1. Among *typical* couples who initiate use of a method (not necessarily for the first time), the percentage who experience an accidental pregnancy during the first year if they do not stop use for any other reason. Estimates of the probability of pregnancy during the first year of typical use for spermicides, withdrawal, periodic abstinence, the diaphragm, the male condom, the pill, and Depo-Provera are taken from the 1995 *National Survey of Family Growth* corrected for underreporting of abortion.

2. Among couples who initiate use of a method (not necessarily for the first time) and who use it *perfectly* (both consistently and correctly), the percentage who experience an accidental pregnancy during the first year if they do not stop use for any other reason.

3. Among couples attempting to avoid pregnancy, the percentage who continue to use a method for 1 year.

4. The percentages becoming pregnant in columns (2) and (3) are based on data from populations where contraception is not used and from women who cease using contraception in order to become pregnant. Among such populations, about 89% become pregnant within 1 year. This estimate was lowered slightly (to 85%) to represent the percentage who would become pregnant within 1 year among women now relying on reversible methods of contraception if they abandoned contraception altogether.

5. Foams, creams, gels, vaginal suppositories, and vaginal film.

6. Cervical mucus (ovulation) method supplemented by calendar in the pre-ovulatory phase and basal body temperature in the post-ovulatory phase.

7. With spermicidal cream or jelly.

8. Without spermicides.

9. The treatment schedule is one dose within 120 hours after unprotected intercourse and the second dose 12 hours after the first dose. Both doses of Plan B can be taken at the same time. Plan B (one dose is one white pill) is the only dedicated product specifically marketed for emergency contraception. The Food and Drug Administration has declared the following 18 brands of oral contraceptives to be safe and effective for emergency contraception: Ogestrel or Ovral (one dose is 2 white pills); Alesse, Lessina, or Levlite (one dose is 5 pink pills); Levlen or Nordette (one dose is 4 light orange pills); Cryselle, Levora, Low-Ogestrel, or Lo/Ovral (one dose is 4 white pills); Tri-Levlen or Triphasil (one dose is 4 yellow pills); Portia, Seasonale, or Trivora (one dose is 4 pink pills); Aviane (one dose is 5 orange pills); and Empresse (one dose is 4 orange pills).

10. To maintain effective protection against pregnancy, another method of contraception must be used as soon as menstruation resumes, the frequency or duration of breast-feeding is reduced, bottle feeds are introduced, or the baby reaches 6 months of age.

Adapted from Hatcher RA, Trussell J, Steward F, et al: Contraceptive technology, 18th rev. ed. New York: Ardent Media, 2004.

3. Usual or typical use
   a. Can vary considerably depending on user—motivation is very important
   b. Perfect-use failure rate with combined oral contraceptives approximately 3/1000; typical-use efficacy is 80/1000 for first year of use
C. Ease of use, personal preference, privacy
D. Non-contraceptive benefits can be significant; for example, combined hormonal contraceptives can reduce bleeding and pain of menses, risk of ovarian/uterine cancer, and acne
E. Aside from cost per use, the initial expense, particularly with intrauterine devices (IUDs), can be barrier to utilization (Table 7.2)

TABLE 7.2

Expense of Contraception 33D

Method	Prescription Required	Specific Clinician-Associated Expense (Variable)	Cost of Prescription or Device (Average or Typical)
Combined hormonal contraceptives (pills, ring, patch)	Yes	None	$35–$40 per month (generics cheaper)
Morning-after pill	Yes (may change)	None	$30 (Plan B)
Diaphragm, cap	Yes	Initial fitting—$150	$30–$50
Condoms	No	None	$0.50/piece
IUD—Mirena	Yes	Insertion—$200	$500 (up to 5 years)
Spermicides	No	None	$0.50–$1.00/ dose
Progestin: quarterly injection	Yes	Injection fee—$10 (varies)	$50–$70 for 3-month dose
Natural family planning	No	No	Free
Withdrawal	No	No	Free

F. Reversibility: contraception generally implies reversibility; sterilization does not (see Chapter 8)

G. Availability

  1. Requirement to obtain a prescription can serve as a barrier to use

  2. Beyond prescription, specific procedure by clinician may be required (expense, time, pain)

II. Combined Hormonal Contraception

A. The mechanism results in elevated exogenous synthetic estrogen and progestin levels, which inhibit cyclic release of gonadotropins (luteinizing hormone [LH] and follicle-stimulating hormone [FSH]) and thereby prevent ovulation ; also thicken cervical mucus to impair fertility, slow tubal motility, and inhibit sperm capacitation; also render endometrium inhospitable to implantation 33A

B. Combined hormonal preparations generally have a synthetic estrogen and progestin administered at the same time; monophasic pills have the same content throughout the cycle, whereas triphasic pills typically use three different ratios of the hormones (Tables 7.3 and 7.4)

C. Common estrogens

  1. Ethinyl estradiol (EE): by far the most common estrogen

  2. Mestranol: metabolized by liver into EE (50 mcg mestranol equivalent to 35 mcg of EE)

D. Common progestins

  1. Those derived from androgens

   a. Norethindrone

   b. Norethindrone acetate (twice as potent for given weight as norethindrone)

   c. Norgestrel

   d. Levo-Norgestrel

   e. Ethynodiol diacetate

   f. Norethynodrel

   g. Desogestrel ("third-generation pill")

     i. Metabolite is etonogestrol

     ii. Metabolite utilized in vaginal ring

   h. Norgestimate ("third-generation pill")

     i. Metabolized to norelgestromin

TABLE	7.3	Common Oral Contraceptive Formulations Classified by Dose		

Daily Dose of Ethinyl Estradiol (mcg)	Progestin Type and Daily Dose (mg)	Brand Names	Total Monthly Estrogen (mcg)/ Progestin (mg)
Pills With 21 Days of Active Ingredients and 7 Days of No Active Agent			
50	Norethindrone acetate 1.0	Norlestrin 1/50	1050/21
	Norethindrone 1.0	Ovcon 50	1050/21
	Norgestrel 0.5	Ovral, Ogestrel	1050/10.5
	Ethynodial di-acetate 1.0	Demulen 1/50 Zovia 1/50	1050/21
35	Norethindrone 1.0	Ortho Novum 1/35 Norinyl 1/35 Necon 1/35, Nortrel 1/35	735/21
	Norethindrone 0.5	Brevicon, Modicon, Necon 0.5/35 Nortrel 0.5/35 Jenest 28	735/10.5
	Norethindrone 0.4	Ovcon 35	735/8.4 735/21
	Ethynodial di-acetate 1.0	Demulen 1/35 Zovia 1/35	
	Norgestimate 0.25	Orthocyclen, Sprintec	735/5.25
30	Norethindrone 1.5	Loestrin 1.5/30	630/31.5
	Norethindrone acetate 1.5	Microgestin 1.5/30	630/31.5
	Levonorgestrel 0.15	Levlen, Nordette, Levora, Portia	630/3.15
	Norgestrel 0.3	Lo/Ovral, Low-Orgestrel, Cryselle	630/6.30

Common Oral Contraceptive Formulations Classified by Dose (continued)

Daily Dose of Ethinyl Estradiol (mcg)	Progestin Type and Daily Dose (mg)	Brand Names	Total Monthly Estrogen (mcg)/ Progestin (mg)
	Drospirenone 3.0	Yasmin	630/630
	Desogestrel 0.15	Desogen, Orthocept	630/3.15
20	Norethindrone 1.0	Loestrin 1/20	420/21
	Norethindrone acetate 1	Microgestin 1/20	420/21
	Levonorgestrel 0.10	Alesse, Aviane, Levlite, Lessina	420/2.10
	Desogestrel 1.5	Mircette, Kariva, Apri	440/3.15

Pills With Active Ingredients for More Than 21 Days of Each 28-Day Cycle

20	Drospirenone 3.0	Yas	480/72
	Norethindrone acetate 1.0	LoEstrin 24 FE	480/24

Cycle Variable Pills

25	Norgestimate 0.18–7 days Norgestimate 0.215–7 days Norgestimate 0.25–7 days	Ortho Tricyclen Lo	525/4.515
35	Norethindrone 0.5–10 days Norethindrone 1.0–11 days	Ortho Novum 10/11	735/16

(continued on page 98)

Common Oral Contraceptive Formulations Classified by Dose (continued)

Daily Dose of Ethinyl Estradiol (mcg)	Progestin Type and Daily Dose (mg)	Brand Names	Total Monthly Estrogen (mcg)/ Progestin (mg)
35	Norgestimate 0.18–7 days Norgestimate 0.215–7 days Norgestimate 0.25–7days	Ortho Tri-Cyclen	735/4.515
30–6 days 40–5 days 30–10 days	Levonorgestrel 0.05–6 days Levonogestrel 0.075–5 days Levonogestrel 0.125–10 days Norethindrone 1.0	Tri-Levlen, Triphasil, Trivora, Empresse	680/1.925
20–5 days 30–7 days 35–9 days 25	Desogestrel 0.100–7 days Desogestrel 0.125–7 days Desogestrel 0.150–7 days	Estrostep Cyclessa	625/21 525/2.625

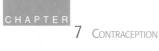

Common Oral Contraceptive Formulations Classified by Dose (continued)

Daily Dose of Ethinyl Estradiol (mcg)	Progestin Type and Daily Dose (mg)	Brand Names	Total Monthly Estrogen (mcg)/ Progestin (mg)
12-Week Cycle			
These formulations have roughly a 25% higher dose than the same formulation pill given on a 4-week cycle.			
30–84 days	Levonorgestrel 0.15–84 days	Seasonale	840/4.2 (for 4 weeks)
30–84 days 10–7 days	Levonorgestrel 0.15–84 days	Seasonique	910/4.2 (for 4 weeks)
Progestin-Only ("Minipills")			
	Norethindrone 0.30 Norgestrel 0.075	Micornor, Nor-QD, Camilla, Errin, Jo-livette, Nora-BE Ovrette, Agystin	7.35
50-mcg Mestranol (equivalent to 35-mcg EE)			
50-mcg Mestranol	Norethindrone 1.0	Ortho Novum-1/50 Necon 1/50 Nelova 1/50 M Norinyl 1/50	1050/21

TABLE **7.4**

Common Oral Contraceptive Formulations Classified Alphabetically by Brand

Brand Name	Daily Dose of Ethinyl Estradiol (mcg)	Progestin Type and Daily Dose (mg)	Total Monthly Estrogen (mcg)/ Progestin (mg)
Pills With 21 Days of Active Ingredients and 7 Days of No Active Agent			
Alesse	20	Levonorgestrel 0.10	420/2.10
Apri	20	Desogestrel 1.5	440/3.15
Aviane	20	Levonorgestrel 0.10	420/2.10
Brevicon 0.5/35	35	Norethindrone 0.5	735/10.5
Cryselle	30	Norgestrel 0.3	630/6.30
Demulen 1/35	35	Ethynodial diacetate 1.0	735/21
Demulen 1/50	50	Ethynodial diacetate 1.0	1050/21
Desogen	30	Desogestrel 0.15	630/3.15
Jenest 28	35	Norethindrone 0.5	735/10.5
Kariva	20	Desogestrel 1.5	440/3.15
Lessina	20	Levonorgestrel 0.10	420/2.10
Levlen	30	Levonorgestrel 0.15	630/3.15
Levlite	20	Levonorgestrel 0.10	420/2.10
Levora	30	Levonorgestrel 0.15	630/3.15
Loestrin 1/20	20	Norethindrone 1.0	420/21
Loestrin 1.5/30	30	Norethindrone 1.5	630/31.5
Lo/Ovral, Low-Ogestrel	30	Norgestrel 0.3	630/6.30
Microgestin 1/20	20	Norethindrone acetate 1	420/21
Microgestin 1.5/30	30	Norethindrone acetate 1.5	630/31.5

Common Oral Contraceptive Formulations Classified Alphabetically by Brand (continued)

Brand Name	Daily Dose of Ethinyl Estradiol (mcg)	Progestin Type and Daily Dose (mg)	Total Monthly Estrogen (mcg)/ Progestin (mg)
Mircette	20	Desogestrel 1.5	440/3.15
Modicon	35	Norethindrone 0.5	735/10.5
Necon 0.5/35	35	Norethindrone 0.5	735/10.5
Necon 1/35	35	Norethindrone 1.0	735/21
Nordette	30	Levonorgestrel 0.15	630/3.15
Norinyl 1/35	35	Norethindrone 1.0	735/21
Norlestrin 1/50	50	Norethindrone acetate 1.0	1050/21
Nortrel 0.5/35	35	Norethindrone 0.5	735/10.5
Nortrel 1/35	35	Norethindrone 1.0	735/21
Ogestrel	50	Norgestrel 0.5	1050/10.5
Orthocept	30	Desogestrel 0.15	630/3.15
Orthocyclen	35	Norgestimate 0.25	735/5.15
Ortho Novum 1/35	35	Norethindrone 1.0	735/21
Ovcon 35	35	Norethindrone 0.4	735/8.4
Ovcon 50	50	Norethindrone 1.0	1050/21
Ovral	50	Norgestrel 0.5	1050/10.5
Portia	30	Levonorgestrel 0.15	630/3.15
Sprintec	35	Norgestimate 0.25	735/5.25
Yasmin	30	Drospirenone 3.0	630/630
Zovia 1/35	35	Ethynodial diacetate 1.0	735/21
Zovia 1/50	50	Ethynodial diacetate 1.0	1050/21

Pills With Active Ingredients for More Than 21 Days of Each 28-Day Cycle

LoEstrin 24 FE	20	Norethindrone acetate 1.0	480/24
Yas	20	Drospirenone 3.0	480/72

(continued on page 102)

Common Oral Contraceptive Formulations Classified Alphabetically by Brand (continued)

Brand Name	Daily Dose of Ethinyl Estradiol (mcg)	Progestin Type and Daily Dose (mg)	Total Monthly Estrogen (mcg)/ Progestin (mg)
Cycle Variable Pills			
Cyclessa	25	Desogestrel 0.100–7 days Desogestrel 0.125–7 days Desogestrel 0.150–7 days	525/2.625
Empresse	30–6 days 40–5 days 30–10 days	Levonorgestrel 0.05–6 days Levonorgestrel 0.075–7 days Levonorgestrel 0.125–10 days	680/1.925
Estrostep	20–5 days 30–7 days 35–9 days	Norethindrone 1.0	625/21
Ortho Novum 10/11	35	Norethindrone 0.5–10 days Norethindrone 1.0–11 days	735/16
Ortho Tri-Cyclen Lo	25	Norgestimate 0.18–7 days Norgestimate 0.215–7 days Norgestimate 0.25–days	525/4.515
Ortho Tri-Cyclen	35	Norgestimate 0.18–7 days Norgestimate 0.215–7 days Norgestimate 0.25–7 days	735/4.515

Common Oral Contraceptive Formulations Classified Alphabetically by Brand (continued)

Brand Name	Daily Dose of Ethinyl Estradiol (mcg)	Progestin Type and Daily Dose (mg)	Total Monthly Estrogen (mcg)/ Progestin (mg)
Tri-Levlen, Triphasil, Trivora	30–6 days 40–5 days 30–10 days	Levonorgestrel 0.05–6 days Levonorgestrel 0.075–5 days Levonorgestrel 0.125–10 days	680/1.925

12-Week Cycle

These formulations have roughly a 25% higher dose than the same formulation pill given on a 4-week cycle.

Seasonale	30–84 days	Levonorgestrel 0.15–84 days	840/4.2 (for 4 weeks)
Seasonique	30–84 days 10–7 days	Levonorgestrel 0.15–84 days	910/4.2 (for 4 weeks)

Progestin Only ("Minipills")

Agystin Camilla		Norethindrone 0.30	7.35
Errin		Norethindrone 0.30	7.35
Jolivette		Norethindrone 0.30	7.35
Micronor		Norethindrone 0.30	7.35
Nora-BE		Norethindrone 0.30	7.35
Nor-QD		Norethindrone 0.30	7.35
Orvette		Norgestrel 0.075	

50-mcg Mestranol (equivalent to 35-mcg EE)

Necon 1/50	50-mcg Mestranol	Norethindrone 1.0	1050/21
Nelova 1/50 M	50-mcg Mestranol	Norethindrone 1.0	1050/21
Norinyl 1/50	50-mcg Mestranol	Norethindrone 1.0	1050/21
Ortho Novum 1/50	50-mcg Mestranol	Norethindrone 1.0	1050/21

ii. Metabolite found in patch

i. Gestodene (not available in United States)

2. Derived from spironolactone: drosprirenone (has antiadrogenic and antimineralocorticoid activity)

   a. Can elevate serum potassium, particularly in women with other risk factors (renal, hepatic, adrenal disease)

   b. Drugs that can increase risk of hyperkalemia include potassium-sparing diuretics, heparin, nonsteroidal anti-inflammatory drugs (NSAIDs) (used daily), and antihypertension agents (angiotensin-converting enzyme (ACE) inhibitors, angiotensin II inhibitors)

   c. In high-risk patients (see above), check serum potassium during first cycle

3. With one estrogen and a variety of progestins, the specific characteristics of these agents differentiate combination pills (typically these differences are small and variable in clinical practice)

   a. Classification of biologic activity (Table 7.5)

   b. Side effects from hormonal type

      i. Estrogenic (menorrhagia, dysmenorrhea, mastalgia, nausea)

      ii. Progestational (edema; depression, moodiness, irritability; headache; bloating)

      iii. Androgenic (weight gain, increase in appetite; hypertension; fatigue)

E. Route of administration and directions for use of estrogen-progestin agents

   1. Oral

      a. All pill formulations come with or without placebos included in the package: if no placebos, a 21-day pack; with placebos, a 28-day pack

         i. Patients need to be clear about days of active ingredients—this can vary depending on the pill preparation

         ii. New package needs to be started every 4 weeks on the same day of the week

         iii. Once started, the pill regimen does not change regardless of bleeding pattern

TABLE 7.5	Classification of Biologic Activity of Oral Contraceptives					
Class of Compound	Progestational Activity[1]	Estrogenic Activity[2]	Androgenic Activity[3]	Endometrial Activity[4]	Androgen:Progestin Activity Ratio[5]	
Progestins[6]						
19 Nor-Testosterone Progestins						
Estrane						
Norethindrone	1.0	1.0	1.0	1.0	1.0	
Norethindrone acetate	1.2	1.5	1.6	0.4	1.3	
Ethynodiol diacetate	1.4	3.4	0.6	0.4	0.4	
5(10) Estrane						
Norethynodrel	0.3	8.3	0	0	0	
Gonane						
Norgestimate	1.3	0	1.9	1.2	1.5	
DL-Norgestrel	2.6	0	4.2	2.6	1.6	
Levonorgestrel	5.3	0	8.3	5.1	1.6	
Desogestrel	9.0	0	3.4	8.7	0.4	
Gestodene	12.6	0	8.6	12.6	0.7	
Pregnane Progestins						
Medroxyprogesterone acetate	0.3	0	0	NA	0	

(continued on page 106)

Classification of Biologic Activity of Oral Contraceptives (continued)

Class of Compound	Progestational Activity[1]	Estrogenic Activity[2]	Androgenic Activity[3]	Endometrial Activity[4]	Androgen:Progestin Activity Ratio[5]
Other					
Drospirenone	0.5	0	0	NA	0
Estrogens[7]					
Ethinyl estradiol	0	100	0	0	0
Mestranol	0	67	0	0	0

1. Based on amount required to induce vacuoles in human endometrium [Cook CL, et al: Pregnancy prophylaxis: Parenteral postcoital estrogen. Obstet Gynecol 1986;67:331]. Desogestrel, gestodene, levonorgestrel, and norgestimate based on oral stimulation of endometrium in immature estrogen-primed rabbits relative to levonorgestrel = 5.3 [Phillips A, et al: Progestational and androgenic receptor-binding affinities and in vitro activities of norgestimate and other progestins. Contraception 1990;41:399–410].

2. Comparative potency based on oral rat vaginal epithelium assay. (norethindrone = 0.2 when ethinyl estradiol = 100 [Jones RC, Edgren RA: The effects of various steroids on vaginal histology in the rat. Fertil Steril 1973;24:284–291].)

3. Comparative potency (oral) based on rat ventral prostate assay (Norethindrone = 1.0 when methyltestosterone = 50 [Tausk M, deVisser J: International encyclopedia of pharmacology and therapeutics, Chapter 28, Section 48, Vol. II. Elmsford, NY: Pergamon Press, 1972]. Levonorgestrel and desogestrel relative to norethindrone = 1.0, norgestimate relative to levonorgestrel = 8.3 [Phillips A, et al: Progestational and androgenic receptor-binding affinities and in vitro activities of norgestimate and other progestins. Contraception 1990;41:399–410], and gestodene relative to levonorgestrel = 8.3 [Elger WH, et al: Endocrine pharmacological profile of gestodene. Adv Contracept Delivery Systems 1986;2:182–197].)

4. Based on estimation of amount required to suppress bleeding for 20 days in 50% of women [Swyer GIM, Little V: Potency of progestogens and oral contraceptives: Further delay-of-menses data. Contraception 1982;26:23].

5. Androgenic + progestational activity, based on oral animal assays. Actual activity in women may be different and will be modified by the dose of estrogen.

6. Calculated on the basis of norethindrone = 1.0 in activity.

7. Calculated on the basis of ethinyl estradiol = 100 in activity.

Reprinted with permission from EMIS, Inc. Medical Publishers, Dallas, TX. Adapted from Managing Contraceptive Pill Patients, 12th ed. 2004.

    b. Four methods of starting the first cycle relative to first day of menstrual cycle (first day of any bleeding)

        i. First Sunday

        ii. First day

        iii. Fifth day

        iv. Quick start: pills can be started in midcycle (period will usually be delayed until end of package)

    c. Start-up contraception—second method of contraception necessary for minimum of first 7 days of pill

    d. Missed pills

        i. 1 day: take two immediately, and use backup contraception through end of cycle

        ii. 2 days: take two immediately, and use backup contraception through end of cycle

        iii. 3 or more: start new package, and use backup method for 7 days

    e. Discontinuation—finishing package tends to reduce unpredictable bleeding

2. Transcutaneous (Ortho Evra)

    a. Content (for 7-day release): ethinyl estradiol (0.75 mg) and norelgestromin (6 mg)

    b. 3 weeks on; 1 week off—change patch every week; if patch loosens or falls off, replace with spare patch

    c. If patch is off for 24 hours or more, contraceptive benefit lost—use back-up contraception through first 7 days of re-start cycle

3. Vaginal ring (NuvaRing)

    a. Delivers daily (21 days): ethinyl estradiol (0.015 mg) and etonogestrol (0.120 mg)

    b. Wear ring for 3 weeks—remove for 1 week (may remove during sex but generally discouraged because of the risk of forgetting to replace in vagina)

4. Serum levels as function of administration route

    a. Patch delivers 60% more total ethinyl estradiol than does 35-mcg oral contraceptive (ring delivers less)

    b. Several warnings

        i. Efficacy more closely related to user reliability than dose, which in turn is related to remembering to take the pill, change the patch, or place the ring

ii. Safety and side effects probably diminish as dose increases, although the practical/observable effects have not been noticed clinically (few data; do not show consistent increased risk)

F. Noncontraceptive benefits

1. Those related to cycle control
   a. Reduction of menstrual bleeding and iron deficiency anemia
   b. Reduction of dysmenorrhea
   c. Reduction or elimination of ovulatory pain
   d. Increased cycle regularity
   e. Few ovarian cysts
   f. Suppression of endometriosis, possibly due to decreased retrograde menses and progestin-mediated atrophy of pelvic lesions
2. Cancer reduction/protection: endometrial and ovarian (does not increase breast cancer risk); may reduce benign breast disease
3. Suppression of ovarian androgen production
   a. Acne reduction (some pills have specific U.S. Food and Drug Administration (FDA)–granted indication for acne, but all probably work via suppression of ovarian production of testosterone)
   b. Treatment of hirsutism (chiefly in minority of patients with disordered androgen production, such as with polycystic ovary syndrome)
4. Reduction of risk for hospitalization from gonorrheal infection: reduced risk of pelvic inflammatory disease
5. May reduce disability from rheumatoid arthritis

G. Side effects
1. Nausea: more common in first month
2. Mastalgia: more common in first month
3. Menstrual irregularities: breakthrough bleeding in midcycle or amenorrhea—both typically arise from progestin-mediated thinning of endometrium
   a. More common with 20-mcg pills
   b. Can also be addressed by changing to progestin with less progestational activity

  c. More common in first three cycles but can occur anytime including after years of use
 4. Discontinue for true migraine (typically unilateral, temporal) associated with any other neurologic symptoms
 5. Cloasma, also known as the "mask of pregnancy"; darkening of facial pigmentation or any pigmented area can occur due to estrogen stimulation of melanocytes

H. Risks
 1. Myocardial infarction risk not increased in nonsmokers
  a. Risk does rise slightly with age; always less than risk of pregnancy in normotensive nonsmokers
  b. Risk rises considerably with smokers and hypertensive patients; do not prescribe to smokers over age 35 years nor to patients with uncontrolled or poorly controlled hypertension
 2. Stroke not increased in normotensive, nonsmokers, without migraine
  a. Risk of hemorrhagic stroke increased in smokers and in patients with hypertension
  b. Risk of ischemic stroke increased among those with migraine and aura
 3. Venous thromboembolism
  a. Can occur in variety of organs with variety of symptoms
  b. Estrogen dose–related
  c. Risk highest in first 2 years
  d. Special populations with thrombophilias (not often recognized prospectively) at highest risk
 4. Hypertension occurs in 1%–3% of population particularly sensitive to increased angiotensin II levels from oral contraceptives
 5. Hepatic adenomas, although benign, on rupture can cause hemorrhage; uncommon, work-up indicated for hepatomegaly on examination
 6. Possibly reduced efficacy in women over 90 kg; they may have a higher risk of pregnancy. although data not completely consistent (higher rate of pregnancies observed in heavy Ortho Evra users but not in Ortho Tri-Cyclen Lo users)

I. Drug interactions (not all-inclusive; always check specific pre-scribing information)

1. Drugs that can decrease hormonal activity and may therefore decrease contraceptive efficacy
   a. Anticonvulsants (avoid using simultaneously): increase liver metabolism of estrogens and increase binding of hormones to sex hormone–binding globulin
   b. Antibiotics (use backup for short course)
      i. Penicillin, rifampin, griseofulvin, minocycline, cotrimoxazole, metronidazole, chloramphenicol, nitrofuratoin, sulfonamide, tetracycline
   c. Migraine headache medication, benzodiazepines (use backup for short course)
2. Drugs (or drug effects) that can be affected by hormonal contraception
   a. Anticoagulants (do not prescribe hormonal contraception)—estrogen increases clotting factors
   b. Antidiabetic agents—estrogen increases serum glucose
   c. Steroids—increase serum levels
   d. Beta blockers—increase drug effects
J. Metabolic changes (list not inclusive)
   1. Increase serum glucose
   2. Increase serum levels of sex hormone–binding globulin
   3. Cause small, transient (usually) increase in blood pressure
   4. Suppress ovarian production of androgens
   5. Progestins can increase serum triglycerides and low-density lipoprotein cholesterol

III. Progestin-Only Contraception

A. Route of administration and directions for use of progestin-only preparations (sometimes called the "mini-pill")
   1. Oral: taken daily throughout the month (no rest or placebo periods) (see Table 7.3)
   2. Subdermal: Implanon
      a. Single 4-cm-long, 2-mm-wide etonogestrel-containing sterile rod implant for subdermal use; not radiopaque; contains no latex
      b. Contains 68 mg of etonogestrel—daily release rate
         i. First 6 weeks: 60–70 mcg
         ii. End 1st year: 35–46 mcg
         iii. End 2nd year: 30–40 mcg
         iv. End 3rd year: 25–30 mcg

    c. Special manufacturer training required
      i. Inserted under local anesthesia through small incision on inside of upper arm, 8 cm above elbow crease
      ii. May be placed within 7 days of last day of hormonal contraception or first 5 days of menses
      iii. Removed under local, small incision at tip of device, grasped with hemostat; if not palpable may be detected with ultrasound or magnetic resonance imaging
  3. Subcutaneous: Depo-SubQ Provera 104–104 mg of medroxyprogesterone acetate suspension injected subcutaneously in abdomen or anterior thigh every 12–14 weeks
  4. Intramuscular: Depo-Provera—150 mg intramuscular injection of medroxyprogesterone acetate every 12–14 weeks

B. Side effects, precautions, and contraindications similar to those of combined oral contraceptives with following precautions 33C
  1. Weight gain, depression, and irritability more common
  2. Amenorrhea, breakthrough bleeding more common
  3. Implants and injections associated with much higher efficacy, approaching that of sterilization, largely due to elimination of noncompliance
  4. May be used during nursing, although estrogen can diminish milk production
  5. While estrogen-containing contraceptives clearly contraindicated in smokers 35 and over, progestin-only contraception may be safer in this group as most of the risk is thought to be related to estrogen
  6. With the injectable progestins, osteoporosis due to estrogen suppression is a concern that increases with time
    a. More than 2 years of consecutive use is not recommended unless the patient has specific reasons for this form of contraception
    b. For those with more than 2 years of use, bone density studies are suggested
    c. Bone loss might not be completely reversible

IV. Emergency Contraception

A. Probably inhibits ovulation, impairs embryo transport, and blocks implantation 33A
B. Common hormonal preparations

1. Plan B: two 0.75-mg levonorgestrel tablets taken 12 hours apart within 72 hours of unprotected intercourse
2. Yuzpe method: four combined oral contraceptives pills
   a. Levonorgestrel is preferred progestin—slightly more effective than norethindrone (other progestins have not been studied for this purpose and should probably not be used)
   b. Typically two pills are taken twice—separated by 12 hours (to minimize nausea from the estrogen)
   c. Should be started within 120 hours of unprotected intercourse
   d. Cumulative desired dose—ethinyl estradiol, 100 mcg; levonorgestrel, 0.5 mg
      i. Examples: Ogestrel, Ovral, Levora, Lo/Ovral Levlen, Nordette, Alesse

C. Efficacy
   1. Plan B reduces risk of pregnancy from single unprotected act of intercourse from 8% to 1%
   2. Yuzpe method might be slightly less effective
   3. Requires prescription; will not interrupt already established pregnancy

D. Mechanisms (postulated)—prevention of ovulation, fertilization, implantation

E. Side effects, precautions, and contraindications 33C
   1. Efficacy substantially reduced with repeated use (not as effective as daily hormonal contraception)
   2. Irregular bleeding and delayed menses common
   3. Nausea is real issue for Yuzpe method—simultaneous prescription of antiemetic often appropriate
   4. Does not appear to increase risk of ectopic pregnancy

F. IUD can be used as emergency postcoital contraception if placed within 72 hours of unprotected sex
   1. Limited due to logistical difficulty of obtaining clinician appointment on short notice and disadvantages of not placing the IUD during menses (increased discomfort, risk of established pregnancy)

V. Barrier Methods

A. Provides physical barrier against sperm entering cervical canal and uterus 33A

B. Condom (male)

1. May or may not contain spermicide

2. Instructions for use

a. Must be placed over penis before any direct penis-to-vagina contact because sperm can leak out unnoticed before ejaculation

b. An extra $\frac{1}{2}$ to 1 inch of material should be present at tip of penis to prevent semen from rupturing condom

c. Penis should be withdrawn while holding onto the base of the condom immediately after ejaculation to prevent condom from slipping off as erection is lost

d. Condoms must be used only once

e. One size generally fits all, although a large size is available

3. Condoms are effective in preventing spread of STDs 33C

4. Animal skin condoms available for those allergic to latex, although efficacy is probably less; STD protection probably substantially less due to increased permeability

C. Diaphragm (must be used with spermicide)

1. Rubber that fits over cervix

a. Serves as barrier, preventing sperm from getting near cervical opening

b. Spermicide used with diaphragm kills the few sperm that get past diaphragm rim

2. Must be fitted by health-care professional

a. Largest that will fit comfortably

b. Held in place in front by resting against pubic bone and in back by far wall of vagina

c. Sizes range 50–95 mm in 5-mm increments

d. Four types related to comfort

i. Arcing spring: most memory; best for lax muscle

ii. Coil spring: intermediate memory—suitable for average tone

iii. Flat spring: least memory—best for firm tone

iv. Wide seal rim: has extra flange around inside; available as arcing or coil spring

v. Specific diaphragm inserter can be used for coil- or flat-spring diaphragms

    e. Instructions for use

        i. Place tablespoon of spermicide around diaphragm prior to insertion

        ii. Insert within 2 hours of intercourse

        iii. Leave in place for 6–8 hours after intercourse

        iv. If intercourse occurs more than once with diaphragm in place, be sure to place an applicator full of spermicide inside vagina in advance

        v. Resize with each 20-pound change in weight and after each pregnancy

        vi. Wash with soap and water, and store dry—no expiration date on diaphragm as long as it is physically intact

        vii. Insertion

          (1) Hold dome side down

          (2) Three positions for insertion: lying flat on back with knees bent and flexed outward, squatting, or raising one leg up on a chair or the side of the bathtub

          (3) After insertion confirm that diaphragm is covering cervix

D. Sponge

    1. Polyurethane sponge with polyester loop for removal containing 1 g of nonoxynol-9

    2. Must be left in place for 6 hours after intercourse and not longer than 30 hours due to increasing risk of toxic shock syndrome

E. Cervical cap

    1. Requires clinician to prescribe as size needs to be assessed to fit precisely over cervix

    2. Can be left in place for up to 2 days after intercourse although odor can be an issue with prolonged use; spermicide placed in cap prior to insertion

    3. Three brands available in United States: Prentif Cavity Rim Cervical Cap, Lea Shield, Femcap

F. Female condom

    1. Two polyurethane rings enclosed by a thin sheath of the same material and open at one end

    2. Does not contain spermicide but is coated with a silicone-based lubricant

    3. Can be inserted into vagina up to 8 hours before intercourse

4. Stronger than latex condoms, it should not be used in combination with them because the two devices might adhere to each other and become dislodged

5. Best protection against STDs because it partially covers female perineum beyond vaginal introitus

G. Noncontraceptive benefits, side effects, precautions, and contraindications 33C

1. Do not use for those with allergy or sensitivity to either latex or spermicides

2. With female barrier methods, risks of infection increase (urinary tract infections, bacterial vaginosis, toxic shock syndrome [latter very rare])

3. Important to use care in selection of vaginal lubricants—petroleum jelly can dissolve rubber

4. Condoms effective in preventing spread of STDs

5. Can be used as hygiene measure to facilitate sex during menses (do not leave in place for more than a few hours)

6. Barrier methods other than condoms slightly less effective in parous women (particularly true for sponge)

7. Male condoms may provide some benefit in reducing premature ejaculation; they also assist female hygiene

VI. Spermicide

A. Detergent breaks down sperm cell membrane 33A

B. Available as gel, foam, cream, suppository, film; all carriers of nonoxynol-9 (only spermicide available in United States)

C. Film and suppository should be placed 10 minutes before intercourse to permit dissolution

D. Should not be placed more than 1 hour in advance

E. Reapply with each act of sex

F. No douching for 8 hours

G. Can serve as sexual lubricant

H. Bactericidal in vitro—not in vivo

VII. IUDs

A. May inhibit sperm motility and may prevent implantation of embryo 33A

B. Types

1. Copper (Paragard): good for up to 10 years; often associated with increase in menstrual flow and discomfort

2. Progestin (Mirena): good for up to 5 years; addition of progestin in the IUD causes a net decrease in menstrual bleeding and pain and is a significant noncontraceptive benefit (may also inhibit ovulation)

C. Insertion and removal

1. Typically inserted during menses (this practice not specifically supported by scientific study but rather for pragmatic reasons)

   a. Dilation of cervical canal results in less discomfort

   b. Increased assurance that there is no pre-existing pregnancy

2. Method varies by device; package insert contains specific instructions

   a. Both types require sounding of the uterus

   b. Uterine abnormalities such as fibroids and congenital anomalies are contraindications to method

3. Removal can be done anytime—fertility immediately restored

4. Can be inserted immediately postpartum, although there is a higher expulsion rate (rarely done in United States)

D. Special considerations

1. Nulligravidity: insertion can be more difficult in those who have never been pregnant

2. Sexually transmitted diseases: IUDs do not offer protection; historically, an IUD with a defective design (the Dalkon Shield) was associated with an increased risk of pelvic inflammatory disease (PID); Paragard and Mirena have not been associated with an increased risk of either PID or infertility

3. Actinomyces-like organism on Pap smear:

   a. Asymptomatic: no intervention required

   b. Symptomatic: remove and treat with oral antibiotics (IUD should probably be removed in any patient with symptoms of endometritis or PID)

4. Pregnancy:

   a. IUD does not increase risk of ectopic pregnancy but is more effective in preventing intrauterine pregnancy; therefore if pregnancy occurs, higher chance that it is ectopic

   b. In early pregnancy, remove promptly—reduces risk of miscarriage and preterm labor (and endometritis if patient chooses abortion)

5. Checking the string post menses: ideally, IUD users should check for the string after each menses to ensure IUD has not been expelled (in practice, few patients do this)

VIII. Fertility Awareness Methods

A. Prevent fertilization of ovum by avoiding non-barrier intercourse during fertile time periods 33A
   1. Best estimate of fertility is 5 days before ovulation and the day of ovulation (historically this was thought to be the day of ovulation plus or minus 2 days)
   2. All methods contingent on predictability of ovulation; this assumption not valid for some women (nursing mothers, women with irregular cycles, or women who discontinued hormonal contraception fewer than 3 months ago)
   3. During this 6-day fertile time, abstinence or barrier methods of birth control must be used
   4. Although overall rate of miscarriage and birth defects not affected by this method, the subpopulation of women with prior miscarriages does have an increased risk of subsequent miscarriage if conception occurs at the extremes of the fertile period
B. Methods of predicting ovulation
   1. Calendar
      a. Keep record of menstrual cycle for 6–12 months
      b. Subtract 18 from shortest cycle and 11 from longest cycle to determine the potential fertility interval
   2. Standard days
      a. For women with cycle lengths of 26–32 days
      b. Fertile time assume to be days 8–19
   3. Ovulation
      a. Ovulation occurs at time of most abundant and "stretchy" secretions (cervical mucus) plus or minus 1 day (douching, infection, and intercourse can greatly confuse this determination)
      b. Avoid intercourse when secretions start appearing
   4. Sympto-thermal method
      a. Combination of ovulation and basal body temperature (BBT) observations
      b. BBT taken immediately on awakening before getting out of bed and (ideally) at the same time daily throughout the cycle

    c. Ovulation thought to occur the first day of sustained temperature elevation of at least 0.4°F (occasionally some women will notice a temperature drop the day before temperature rise)

    5. Ovulation detection kits can detect the gonadotropin surge 12–24 hours before ovulation occurs; fertility calculations can be applied with this information

IX. Withdrawal and Abstinence

A. Withdrawal: removal of the penis from the vagina before ejaculation

    1. Classically considered ineffective, the method works to an extent and may have an effectiveness approaching that of barrier contraception

    2. Highly dependent on user motivation

    3. May afford some protection against STDs because many pathogens are transmitted directly in the ejaculate (although they can be transmitted in the pre-ejaculate; this generally will have a much lower microbial load)

B. Abstinence: although the most effective in pregnancy prevention and STD prevention, it requires overcoming the strong biologic compulsion to copulate; some couples use variations of sexual contact such as oral sex to navigate between their needs for contraception and for a sexual outlet

---

 MENTOR TIPS

- Women over 198 pounds have two issues: fewer data on efficacy and what data there are suggest that efficacy is reduced for all hormonal contraceptives. Generally, efficacy is only slightly diminished, but this raises the question as to if and when backup contraception should be used. There is no consensus on this issue.
- Nursing mothers should use progestin-only hormonal contraception ("mini-pill").
- Choosing a pill formulation: although there is some scientific basis for minimizing side effects (see Table 7.5), this remains a bit arbitrary and empirical for a particular patient. The consistent clinical differences among different formulations are not all that great.

- Perhaps the greatest consistent effect is the reduction of breast tenderness and nausea with decreasing estrogen doses. This is offset by a rather consistent increase in the percentage of the population experiencing unpredicted bleeding.
- Although progestins may vary somewhat in their biologic effects, they are progestins in much of their activity.
- Individual patient variation is substantial (response to drugs, pre-existing outlook, medical status).
- Do not prescribe combined hormonal contraception for women 35 years and older who smoke.
- Mirena is a particularly good option for mothers who do not desire sterilization. With minimal discomfort of insertion due to cervical canal dilation, the progestin can serve to decrease dysmenorrheal and menstrual bleeding with minimal systemic effects. There is nothing to remember to do.

Resources

Two books stand out in their popularity and depth of coverage. Material from both provides some of the verbiage in the FDA-approved prescribing information for specific hormonal contraceptives and IUDs.

Dickey RP: Managing contraceptive pill patients, 12th ed. Dallas, EMIS Medical Publishers, 2004.

Hatcher RA, Trussell J, Stewart F, et al: Contraceptive technology, 18th rev. ed. New York, Advent Media, 2004.

Chapter Self-Test Questions

Circle the correct answer. After you have responded to the questions, check your answers in Appendix A.

1. 25-year-old gravid 1 para 0 LMP 5 weeks ago with an IUD in place presents with a positive pregnancy test. You should:

   a. Remove the IUD only if she desires pregnancy termination

   b. Remove the IUD only if she desires to continue the pregnancy

   c. Remove the IUD regardless of her pregnancy plans

   d. Leave the IUD in place regardless of her pregnancy plans

2. A patient on low-dose glucocorticoids for rheumatoid arthritis on Yasmin presents as a new patient. Special concerns that you might have for this patient include:

   a. The possibility of hyperkalemia due to the potassium-sparing effects of Yasmin

   b. The possibility of elevated glucose levels due to both drugs

   c. The deleterious effect of oral contraceptives on rheumatoid arthritis

   d. Both a and b

3. Estrogenic side effects include the following *except:*

   a. Nausea

   b. Menorrhagia

   c. Breast tenderness

   d. Weight gain

4. The most effective contraceptive method among typical users is:

   a. Condoms

   b. Depo-Provera

   c. Oral contraceptives

   d. IUDs

See the testbank CD for more self-test questions.

ABORTION AND STERILIZATION

Michael D. Benson, MD

I. Abortion

A. Term *abortion* applies equally to elective pregnancy termination as to spontaneous abortion (more often called *miscarriage* among the general population) 34C

B. Terminology for spontaneous abortion

    1. *Missed abortion:* embryonic or fetal demise with all the pregnancy tissue remaining inside patient

    2. *Incomplete abortion:* passage of some but not all of the products of conception from the body

    3. *Threatened abortion:* vaginal bleeding in the first 20 weeks of pregnancy

C. Diagnostic testing before abortion

    1. Ultrasound to establish gestational age and viability of pregnancy

    2. Blood type and antibody screen (anti–Rho-D immunoglobulin post procedure for Rh-negative patients)

    3. Screening for gonorrhea, *Chlamydia*, and bacterial vaginosis (depending on population and facility)

D. Surgical methods of abortion—dilation and evacuation 34A, 41E

    1. Preoperative preparation—placement of cervical osmotic dilators

        a. Hydrophylic cylinders (comprising various materials) that absorb water over hours or days and swell, thereby gradually dilating cervix

            i. Laminaria: dried seaweed (Laminaria genus)

            ii. Lamicel: magnesium-containing sponge

            iii. Dilapan: polyacrylonitrile

      b. Typically placed a few hours or a day before dilation and evacuation

      c. Not always used in first-trimester abortions, particularly those before 9 weeks

      d. Technique

         i. 5-minute office procedure

         ii. Cleanse vagina, visualize cervix with sterile speculum

         iii. Place tenaculum on anterior lip of cervix to stabilize it; patient might experience cramp or pain

         iv. One or more laminaria placed into cervix, typically by grasping the end of the removal string with a ring forceps

         v. Antiseptic-soaked gauze sponges are gently inserted into vagina (much like a tampon) to help keep laminaria in place

         vi. Patient to be counseled

            (1) May experience cramping—nonsteroidal anti-inflammatory drugs (NSAIDs) appropriate

            (2) Sponge and/or laminaria may be expelled (typically, procedure can proceed because at least partial dilation has occurred)

            (3) Nothing to be placed inside vagina (tampons, etc.)

  2. Alternative cervical preparation—misoprostol 400 mcg vaginally 4 hours before the procedure can cause cervical dilation (600 mcg for second trimester)

  3. Technique of dilation and evacuation

      a. Cervix visualized and mechanically dilated with metal rods of increasing diameter

      b. Suction curette (hollow tube), typically 7–12 mm in diameter, inserted into uterus and attached to a vacuum machine, which suctions out contents of uterus

         i. Vacuum needs to maintain pressure

         ii. Size of tube in millimeters roughly corresponds to weeks of pregnancy for first trimester

      c. Grasping instruments are introduced into the uterus to remove any part of the pregnancy that might have been left behind

      d. Uterine walls are curetted: gently scraped with a sharp instrument to be sure that the uterus is empty

    e. For pregnancies 11 weeks and beyond, special steps are taken to ensure uterus has been successfully evacuated

      i. The surgeon typically identifies major fetal bony structures—clavarium, spine, and all four extremities

      ii. Intraoperative ultrasound can also be used

4. Follow-up

    a. First-trimester tissue without obvious skeleton formation (most) should be sent for microscopic confirmation of embryonic material

      i. Decidua (thickened endometrium of pregnancy) might be difficult to distinguish on gross examination from true embryonic tissue

      ii. Absence of embryonic tissue on microscopic evaluation might signify ectopic pregnancy

    b. Rh-negative patients should receive anti–Rho-D immunoglobulin

      i. Dose for first trimester typically smaller—30 mg rather than usual 300 mg

      ii. Antibody screen should be negative before administration of anti–Rho-D immunoglobulin

    c. Common medications

      i. Depending on patient population, some patients receive intraoperative prophylactic antibiotics (cephalosporin) and postoperative treatment with tetracycline for several days

      ii. Methergine (0.2 mg), an ergot alkaloid that causes uterine smooth muscle to contract, may be given orally three to four times a day; might also be prescribed to minimize bleeding

      iii. Oral contraceptives or Depo-Provera occasionally started the same day

    d. Post-abortion instructions

      i. Nothing per vagina for 2 weeks (sometimes less or more depending on gestational age and nature of procedure)

      ii. Notify physician about increased pain, heavy bleeding, or fever of 100.4°F or higher.

      iii. Follow-up visit in 2 weeks

E. Medical methods of abortion `34A`

1. First trimester
   a. Combination of two drugs
      i. Mifepristone (RU-486; brand name Mifeprex); progesterone antagonist—high affinity for progesterone receptors; blocks progesterone binding
      ii. Misoprostol (Cytotec); prostaglandin E1 analogue that initiates uterine contractions; side effects are fever, diarrhea, nausea
   b. FDA-approved approach
      i. Mifepristone 600 mg orally
      ii. Misoprostol 400 mcg orally 48 hours later
      iii. Must be within 49 days of last menstrual period (LMP)
   c. Alternative
      i. Mifipristone 200 mg
      ii. Misoprostol 800 mcg vaginally 1–3 days later
      iii. Must be within 63 days of LMP
   d. Management/outcome
      i. Cramping and bleeding somewhat heavier than normal menses to be expected
      ii. Median bleeding 13 days
      iii. Heaviest bleeding lasts up to 4 hours during tissue expulsion—patient to call for bleeding filling two large pads for 2 consecutive hours
      iv. 1% need uterine aspiration; 0.1% need transfusion
2. Second trimester—laminaria sometimes placed 6–24 hours in advance 34A
   a. Hypertonic saline (3%) or urea injected directly into uterus in procedure similar to amniocentesis
      i. Typically done under ultrasound guidance
      ii. May take 12 hours to initiate contractions
      iii. Vary rarely done
   b. Vaginal medication
      i. Prostaglandin E (Cytotec) 200 mcg every 4–6 hours; contractions typically begin within 12 hours
         (1) Prostaglandin E vaginally
         (2) Side effects include low blood pressure, nausea, diarrhea, and fever; antiemetics and antidiarrheal often given prophylactically
         (3) Contractions typically begin in 12–24 hours

      ii. Misoprostol
         (1) Can be used as preoperative treatment to dilate
            cervix (400 mcg vaginally 3–4 hours before
            procedure)
         (2) Can be used with prostaglandin E beyond
            15 weeks (provided access to prostaglandin D and
            E available)

c. Delivery of fetus
    i. Very little manipulation required and little or no
      expulsive effort on part of patient
    ii. For intrauterine fetal demise, fetus often sent directly to
      pathology laboratory for further study
    iii. Handling of human tissue (fetus and placenta) may be
      regulated by state
    iv. Depending on circumstances, mothers may wish to see
      fetus or have photographs taken to help with grieving

d. Delivery of placenta
    i. Usually follows within 4 hours of delivery of fetus
    ii. Oxytocin at 25 units (not milliunits) per hour
      intravenously occasionally prescribed
    iii. Formal dilation and evacuation might be required for
      placentas that do not deliver in 4 hours
    iv. Placental tissue good source of fetal cells for
      karyotype; many laboratories ask that it be sent fresh
      for processing (no formalin or saline)

F. Safety of abortion `34B`
  1. Risk of death from continued pregnancy (United States):
    a. Vaginal birth: 10 in 100,000 (highest common estimate)
    b. Cesarean birth: 50 in 100,000 (highest common estimate)
  2. Risk of death from first-trimester abortion
    a. 1 in 100,000 to 1 in 400,000
    b. 10 to 40 times *safer* than carrying pregnancy to term
  3. Risk of death from second-trimester abortion: 18 in 100,000
  4. Complications
    a. Standard risks of any surgery—rare
      i. Hemorrhage
      ii. Infection—to reduce risk
         (1) Gonorrhea and *Chlamydia* screening often done in
            advance

(2) Prophylactic antibiotics can be given (doxycycline 100 mg twice daily for 5–7 days)

iii. Perforation of uterus

(1) Often requires no special treatment beyond prophylactic antibiotic treatment

(2) Can damage uterus or large and small intestine

b. Unique to pregnancy termination

i. Incomplete procedure

(1) Characterized by continued bleeding and cramping

(2) Incidence: perhaps 1 in 100

(3) Treated by repeat procedure

(4) Can be confused with postabortal syndrome in which uterus has significant cramping in an effort to expel a blood clot; treated with methergine 0.2 mg every 6 hours for 3 days; occasionally requires repeat uterine aspiration

ii. Asherman syndrome

(1) Uterine scarring resulting in amenorrhea (or greatly reduced menstruation)

(2) Treated by follow-up dilation and curettage (and occasional hysteroscopic lysis of adhesions) after preoperative preparation with 1–2 months of estrogen and occasional preoperative steroids

(3) Relatively uncommon—less than 1 in 100

iii. Continuing pregnancy—rare but can occur

G. Cost of abortion

1. First trimester: a few hundred dollars (including intravenous sedation); medical abortion slightly less expensive than surgical procedure, especially with intravenous sedation

2. Second trimester: more than $1000

3. Private physician in hospital is two to three times more expensive than at abortion clinic (yet complication rate at clinic actually tends to be lower, due to experience of surgeons)

H. Alternatives to abortion—generally these are well-known to the patient and have already been considered by her. 34©

1. Carrying pregnancy until term and caring for baby herself or with aid of relatives

2. Carrying pregnancy until term and putting baby up for adoption

II. Female Sterilization

A. Overview

1. All operations specifically intended for female sterilization result in some type of damage to fallopian tubes and prevent fertilization

2. Sterilization is not intended to be reversible—a key point of confusion for many patients `33A`

3. Because of irreversibility, regret can be a problem later; risk of regret increases with age less than 30 and with single status

B. Transabdominal approaches—all "tubal ligations"

1. General notes

   a. For all surgical transabdominal approaches, tube should be distinguished from adjacent (and very similar-appearing) round ligament by virtue of identifying its fimbriated end—both before and after the surgical interruption

   b. Can be done in conjunction with other procedures such as abortion but generally delayed until 8 weeks after term gestation

2. Laparoscopic tubal ligation `33E`

   a. Performed via two incisions—one infra-umbilical for laparoscope and second suprapubic for instrument port

   b. Three common methods—all roughly comparable in terms of safety and efficacy (failure rate 1–2 per 1000 per lifetime) `33B`

      i. Fallope ring: medical-grade elastic ring should not be left on the applicator for more than a minute or so to avoid stretching; the tube should be brought into the applicator very slowly and deliberately to avoid tearing the tube

      ii. Electrocoagulation: typically done with specially designed bipolar cautery forceps; 2–3 cm of the midportion of the tube is cauterized—tube turns white, and water vapor stops being released when cautery complete

      iii. Clips: Fische or Hulka clips placed over tube via specially designed applicator to occlude tube

3. Mini-laparotomy: typically done at level of pubic hair line; the smaller the incision, the more difficult the procedure; technique identical to postpartum tubal ligation

4. Postpartum tubal ligation

   a. Done on same hospitalization as birth—often with epidural catheter left in place postpartum

   b. Efficacy slightly less than that of laparoscopic approaches—failure rate perhaps 5 in 1000 in first year, rising to 20 per 1000 over decade (2%) 33B

   c. Technique

   i. 2–3 cm infra-umbilical incision (can also be done at time of cesarean section)

   ii. Midportion knuckle of tube grasped with Babcock clamp and ligated with rapidly dissolving suture (0-plain) so that cut portions of tube fall apart

   iii. Common variations (formal efficacy data lacking)

   (1) Placement of second ligature around cut portions of tube (if single suture fails, patient typically experiences hemorrhagic shock and requires reoperation and transfusion)

   (2) Cautery of tubal ostia to promote scarring and prevent fertility promoting fistula formation

5. Safety of transabdominal approaches 33C

   a. Death rate from laparoscopic tubal ligation estimated 1–10 per 100,000

   b. Death rate from mini-laparatomy and postpartum tubal ligation not established but probably similar or slightly lower

   c. General risks of abdominal surgery and/or laparoscopy apply

   d. Ectopic pregnancy risk

   i. Absolute risk reduced

   ii. For those few who do conceive after tubal ligation, ectopic rate might be as high as 50%

   iii. Patients should be reminded prior to surgery that procedure might fail and that should pregnancy be suspected, it might be life-threatening tubal pregnancy—seek medical attention

6. Expense of transabdominal approaches: done on outpatient basis and with general anesthesia 33D

   a. Hospital typically more expensive than ambulatory surgery center

   b. Expense is higher than with Essure procedure, which can be done in office (all are typically covered by insurance)

C. Essure procedure

1. Titanium alloy wire coiled around core of inflammation-provoking synthetic fibers

2. Placed via hysteroscopy (formal mentoring by manufacturer required)

a. Must be done immediately after patient menses or while on hormonal contraception to keep endometrium thin so that tubal ostia can be visualized

b. Both ostia must be clearly easily visualized before proceeding

c. Special-placement catheter threaded through 5 French operating port in hysteroscope sheath under direct visualization and inserted into tube up to a "notch" on the coil

d. Placement catheter outer sheath is retracted while coil held in place and allowed to expand

e. Catheter separated from coil by rotating it counterclockwise; next implant placed

3. Patient must use contraception until hysterosalpingogram (HSG) (fallopian tube x-ray) confirms occlusion at 3 months

a. If tubes still patent, almost all will be occluded by 6 months

b. HSG performed with low-contrast pressure; distinctly different (and less painful) from infertility HSGs

4. Safety and efficacy 33F

a. No deaths in 60,000 procedures

b. 95% success rate in implant placement on first procedure

c. 1% have tubal perforation—patient injury does not typically result but procedure is failure because tube usually still patent

d. One year failure rate is 3 per 1000

5. Typical medication involved

a. Paracervical block with local anesthetic

b. Preoperative NSAID such as Toradol 30 mg IM

c. Preoperative oral Xanax 1.0 mg (patient cannot drive if given oral anxiolytic)

6. Pros and con versus other methods

a. Pro: only female sterilization that can be done in office

b. Con: requires specialized equipment

c. Pro: typically lower cost

     i. The cost of tubal ligations done in hospital is typically $5000–$10,000; insurance usually covers procedure, although out-of-pocket expenses vary considerably

     ii. Cost of Essure procedure usually less: $3000–$5000 (implants cost over $1000)

III. Male Sterilization (Vasectomy)

A. Involves destruction of the vas deferens, thus preventing sperm from entering semen `33A`

B. Technique `33E`

   1. Local anesthetic injected into scrotal skin after preparation

   2. Small incision made in scrotum

   3. Vas deferens identified, tied off, cut, and sometimes burned

   4. Skin sutured closed with dissolving stitches

   5. Procedure repeated on other side

   6. Takes 15–30 minutes and can be done in physician's office without intravenous sedation or anesthesia

   7. Incision-less procedure utilizes placement of large-bore needle to destroy vas deferens

   8. Sterility not immediate because sperm stored beyond point of damage to vas deferens; after 10 ejaculations, semen should be examined microscopically to confirm azospermia

C. Safety and efficacy `33F`

   1. Lifetime failure rate 1 per 1000 procedures (difficult to directly assess because studies focus on azospermia, not pregnancy rate in partners)

   2. Death rate so low it may be less than one per million

   3. Not readily reversible; microsurgical repair associated with 50%–80% chance of success

D. Costs typically less than $1000 and usually covered by insurance `33D`

E. Less expensive than female sterilization because it can be done in the office, under local anesthetic, and no expensive surgical device involved

MENTOR TIPS

- Patients should be given referral to health-care providers who are comfortable discussing abortion. Certainly, the alternatives of keeping the pregnancy or adoption can be discussed, but women are generally well aware of these options and are not seeking this type of advice from their medical professionals. 34C
- Mifeprisone and misoprostol give patients option of avoiding surgical procedure at the cost of inducing a heavy bleeding episode.
- Patients receiving health care through Medicaid (or Medicare) typically have to sign a government consent form more than 30 days but fewer than 180 days in advance of any sterilization procedure to obtain financial coverage.
- Abortion almost always safer than carrying pregnancy to term; if safety (i.e., risk of death or serious injury) were the only consideration for pregnant women, the species would end.
- Pregnancy in a patient who has had a sterilization procedure must be regarded as an ectopic pregnancy until proved otherwise.
- Do a pregnancy test the day of the procedure (urine is fine). Sterilization procedures will not protect against an already established pregnancy.
- All patients should be counseled that sterilization is permanent and nonreversible and has a small chance of failure as well as a small surgical risk. 34C

Resources

Hatcher RA, Trussell J, Stewart F, et al: Contraceptive technology, 18th rev. ed. New York, Advent Media, 2004.

Chapter Self-Test Questions

Circle the correct answer. After you have responded to the questions, check your answers in Appendix A.

1. Most methods of female sterilization result in an efficacy of:

   a. 99.5% at 1 year, 98% at 10 years

   b. 99.9 % at 1 year, 99% at 10 years

   c. 99.99% at 1 year, 99.9% at 10 years

   d. 98% at 1 year, 95% at 10 years

2. Which method of abortion has largely fallen out of favor in the past 10 years?

   a. First-trimester surgical abortion

   b. First-trimester medical abortion

   c. Second-trimester surgical abortion

   d. Second-trimester medical abortion with vaginal or oral prostaglandin

   e. Second-trimester medical abortion with intrauterine installation of medication

3. What anatomic structure is commonly confused with the fallopian tube during sterilization procedures?

   a. Ovarian suspensory ligament

   b. Infundibulopelvic ligament

   c. Round ligament

   d. Uterosacral ligament

4. Which procedure can be performed in the physician's office without intravenous sedation?

   a. Essure

   b. Postpartum tubal ligation

   c. Laparoscopic tubal ligation

   d. Mini-laparotomy

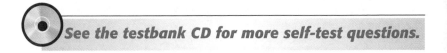

See the testbank CD for more self-test questions.

9

Sexually Transmitted Infections

Michael D. Benson, MD

I. Screening, Reporting, and Treatment of Partners 36i

A. The Centers for Disease Control and Prevention (CDC) recommend HIV screening for all patients in health-care settings.

1. This is particularly important for pregnant women to maximize strategies for prevention of transmission to the fetus.

2. Any person seeking care for a sexually transmitted infection (STI) or screening should receive an HIV test.

3. Informed consent should be obtained on an opt-out basis—patients should be told they will be tested unless they decline.

4. Universal screening is recommended because earlier detection:

a. Facilitates treatment and improves long-term survival.

b. Helps reduce the pool of undiagnosed carriers.

c. Helps prevent vertical transmission to the fetus.

B. The CDC also recommends regular gonorrhea and chlamydia screening on all sexually active females 25 years and younger.

C. Obtaining a sexual history to assess STI risk has to be done with care and discretion and must be individualized. The approach to a married patient is necessarily different from that to a young single woman. It is appropriate to ask a single patient about her number of partners in the last year, whereas this might be an inappropriate question with a married women unless a specific concern, symptom, or sign makes it relevant.

D. Women who have sex with women are probably at somewhat less risk than the general population (data sparse) but are not at no risk because infected vaginal secretions can be transferred via fingers or fomites (inanimate objects).

E. Sexually transmitted infections are, by definition, sexually transmitted.

   1. Many of these diseases can also be transmitted by nonsexual means, such as vertically (mother to fetus) or needlestick transmission.

   2. Transmission via contact with fomites such as doorknobs or toilet seats is exceptional because these microbes need warmth or moisture for communicability.

   3. Sexual transmission does not necessarily imply infidelity in the current relationship; some diseases have a substantial latent period before detection.

   4. Hepatitis A and C can and probably are occasionally transmitted by sexual contact.

      a. Neither is traditionally considered a sexually transmitted infection, and sex is not a common route of transmission.

      b. Hepatitis A is typically transmitted by oral-fecal contamination although transmission through sexual contact can occur.

      c. Hepatitis C transmission probably occurs through a break in the skin or in mucous membranes associated with bleeding and resulting from sexual activity.

F. Some STIs have to be reported to the local health department; the reporting laboratory generally does this, and the health department may make inquiries; confidentiality requirements are generally waived, although this can vary by state.

G. Partners should be treated; debate exists about the particulars.

   1. Partner notification has not been established to reduce STI prevalence or incidence (few data; data not supportive).

   2. Ideally, partners would benefit from an individualized physician assessment to check for other diseases, comorbidities, and drug interactions before receiving treatment.

   3. "Expedited partner therapy," whereby a prescription is delivered by the patient to her partner, has been associated with a higher probability of partner notification and reduced reinfection for chlamydia and gonorrhea.

H. Public health campaigns have the following profile.

   1. Public education to change behavior has been a key feature of efforts to control the spread of STIs since the 1300s when the King of England closed the public baths in an effort to stem the spread of syphilis.

2. Data on efforts are mixed—the urge for sexual contact is deeply ingrained and human behavior remains poorly understood.

3. Condom use, reduction of number of sexual partners over lifetime, early disease detection, and screening are keystones of public health campaigns.

II. Diseases Characterized by Cervicitis

A. Definition: cervicitis is a mucopurulent cervical discharge or friable cervix (not terribly sensitive or specific finding for STIs)

B. Chlamydia 36A–D

1. Microbe: *Chlamydia trachomatis* (gram-negative, aerobic, intracellular pathogens that are difficult to stain; coccoid or rod-shaped and require growing cells to remain viable)

2. Epidemiology

   a. Most frequently reported STI in United States with 3 million new cases annually

   b. Prevalence highest in those 25 years and younger; CDC recommends annual screening for this population

3. Symptoms/diagnosis

   a. Usually asymptomatic

   b. Vaginal discharge from purulent cervicitis

   c. Can cause urethritis (dysuria, frequency, urgency, purulent urethral discharge [rare])

   d. Variety of biotechnology tests available; generally more sensitive than culture and highly specific

     i. Endocervical swabs

      (1) Chlamydia antigen tests: enzyme-linked immunosorbent assay (ELISA) or direct fluorescent antibody tests detect chlamydia antigen

      (2) DNA tests: nucleic acid amplification test (NAAT) and nucleic acid hybridization test (somewhat less sensitive)

     ii. Urine tests: NAAT (nucleic acid amplification test)

     iii. DNA tests: can remain positive for up to 3 weeks after successful treatment due to presence of dead organisms

   e. Test for cure (after 3 weeks): recommended only for pregnant women in special circumstances, such as suspected noncompliance

   f. Treatment: Table 9.1

TABLE 9.1	Treatment of Sexually Transmitted Infections	
Disease	Treatment	Treatment in Pregnancy
Chlamydia	Azithromycin 1 g orally once OR Doxycycline 100 mg orally twice a day for 7 days **Alternatives** Erythromycin base 500 mg orally four times a day for 7 days OR Erythromycin ethylsuccinate 800 mg orally four times a day for 7 days OR Ofloxacin 300 mg orally twice a day for 7 days OR Levofloxacin 500 mg orally once a day for 7 days	Azithromycin 1 g orally once OR Amoxicillin 500 mg orally three times a day for 7 days **Alternatives** Erythromycin base 500 mg orally four times a day for 7 days (also 250 mg orally four times a day for 14 days) OR Erythromycin ethylsuccinate 800 mg orally four times a day for 7 days (also 500 mg orally four times a day for 14 days)
Gonorrhea (cervix, urethra, and rectum— pharynx where specified)	Ceftriaxone 125 mg) OR Cefixime 400 mg orally (not for pharynx) Also—treat for *Chlamydia* unless ruled out (Alternative treatment of spectinomycin 2 g IM not available in U.S.) **Gonorrhea treatment above PLUS**	Same
Chlamydia and gonorrhea	Azithromycin 1 g orally once OR Doxycycline 100 mg orally twice a day for 7 days	**Gonorrhea treatment above PLUS** Azithromycin 1 g orally once

(continued on page 138)

Genital herpes		
First episode	Acyclovir 400 mg orally three times a day for 7–10 days OR 200 mg orally five times a day for 7–10 days OR	See text
	Famciclovir 250 mg orally three times a day for 7–10 days OR	
	Valacyclovir 1 g orally twice a day for 7–10 days	
Recurrence/ episodic	Acyclovir 400 mg orally three times a day for 5 days OR 800 mg orally twice a day for 5 days OR 800 mg orally three times a day for 2 days	See text
	Famciclovir 125 mg orally twice a day for 5 days OR 10,000 mg orally twice a day for 1 day	
	Valacyclovir 500 mg orally twice a day for 3 days OR 1 g orally once a day for 5 days	
Suppression	Acyclovir 400 mg orally twice a day	See text
	Famiciclovir 250 mg orally twice a day	
	Valacyclovir 500 mg or 1 g orally once a day	
Syphilis		
Primary and secondary	Benzathine penicillin G 2.4 million units IM once	Same
Latent early	Benzathine penicillin G 2.4 million units IM once	Same
Latent late	Benzathine penicillin G 2.4 million units IM each at 1-week intervals × three doses	Same

Treatment of Sexually Transmitted Infections (continued)

Disease	Treatment	Treatment in Pregnancy
Tertiary	Benzathine penicillin G 2.4 million units IM each at 1-week intervals × three doses	Same
Neurosyphilis	Aqueous crystalline penicillin G 3–4 million units IV every 4 hr for 10–14 days OR Procaine penicillin 2.4 million units IM once a day for 10–14 days plus probenecid 500 mg orally four times a day	Same
Chancroid	Azithromycin 1 g orally once OR ceftriaxone 250 mg IM once OR ciprofloxacin 500 mg orally twice a day for 3 days OR erythromycin base 500 mg orally three times a day for 7 days	Same (do not use ciprofloxacin)
Granuloma inguinale	Doxycycline 100 mg orally twice a day 1) Until all lesions completely healed 2) No fewer than 3 weeks OR Ciprofloxacin 750 mg orally twice a day OR Erythromycin base 500 mg orally four times a day OR	Erythromycin base 500 mg orally four times a day 1) Until all lesions completely healed 2) No fewer than 3 weeks IV gentamicin may be helpful

Lymphogranuloma venereum	Trimethoprim–sulfamethoxazole 160/800 mg twice a day
	Doxycycline 100 mg orally twice a day for 3 weeks
	OR
	Erythromycin base orally four times a day for 3 weeks
	Erythromycin base orally four times a day for 3 weeks
Outpatient treatment PID	**Single IM injection + doxycycline** orally 100 mg twice a day for 14 days
	a. Ceftriaxone 250 mg IM
	b. Cefoxitin 2 g IM and probenecid 1 g orally
	c. Ceftizoxime or cefotaxime IM
	Note: outpatient treatments suggest additional use of metronidazole 500 mg orally for 14 days
	If pregnant, patient should be hospitalized and receive parenteral treatment
Inpatient treatment PID	**Regimen A:** Cefotetan 2 g IV every 12 hr
	OR
	Cefoxitin 2 g IV every 6 hr
	PLUS
	Doxycycline 100 mg orally or IV every 2 hr
	Regimen B Clindamycin 900 mg IV every 8 hr
	PLUS
	Gentamicin 2 mg/kg loading dose followed by 1.5 mg/kg every 8 hr
	Clindamycin 900 mg IV every 8 hr
	PLUS
	Gentamicin 2 mg/kg loading dose followed by 1.5 mg/kg every 8 hr
	Alternative Ampicillin/sulbactam 3 g IV every 6 hr
	PLUS

(continued on page 140)

Treatment of Sexually Transmitted Infections (continued)

Disease	Treatment	Treatment in Pregnancy
	Doxycycline 100 mg orally or IV every 12 hr **Note:** oral treatment may begin within 24–48 hr of clinical improvement and should be continued for 14 days	
HIV/AIDS	See text	See text
Pediculosis pubis	Permethrin 1% cream to affected areas for 10 min OR Pyrethrins with piperonyl butoxide for 10 min **Alternatives** Malathion 0.5% applies for 8–12 hr OR Ivermectin 250 mcg/kg once and repeated in 2 weeks **Note:** medications to be washed off thoroughly after prescribed application—they can cause neurotoxicity	Permethrin 1% cream to affected areas for 10 min OR Pyrethrins with piperonyl butoxide for 10 min
Scabies	Permethrin cream 5% applied from neck down for 8–14 hr OR Ivermectin 200 mcg/kg orally; repeat in 2 weeks **Note:** medications to be washed off thoroughly after prescribed application	Permethrin cream 5% applied from neck down for 8–14 hr

C. Gonorrhea `36A-D`

    1. Microbe: *Neisseria gonorrhoeae,* gram-negative diplococci with their adjacent sides flattened

    2. Epidemiology: second most common STI in United States; 600,000 new cases each year

    3. Symptoms/diagnosis

        a. Asymptomatic in 50% of women

        b. Symptoms (often 2–5 days after infection) include purulent discharge from vagina or urethra, postcoital bleeding, dysuria, pelvic pain or dyspareunia, and sore throat in oral infection

        c. Diagnostic tests same as for chlamydia

        d. Cultures useful for sensitivity testing in recurrent gonorrhea

        e. Large number of women with gonorrhea also infected with chlamydia; if DNA test for chlamydia negative, treatment for both not indicated

    4. Test for cure: not recommended although follow-up testing for re-infection recommended after 3 months

    5. Treatment: see Table 9.1

D. Pelvic inflammatory disease (PID) (salpingitis) `36E-H`

    1. Microbes: most often a polymicrobial infection

        a. Sexually transmitted: complication of gonorrhea and chlamydia infections

        b. Anaerobes of normal vaginal flora: *Gardnerella vaginalis, Haemophilus influenzae, Streptococcus agalactiae*

        c. Intestinal tract gram-negative rods: *Escherichia coli*

        d. Miscellaneous: cytomegalovirus, *Mycoplasma hominis* and *M. genitalium, Ureaplasma urealyticum*

    2. Diagnosis

        a. Problems with diagnosis

            i. No single set of clinical or laboratory criteria highly specific and sensitive; as criteria for diagnosis increase, specificity improves but with corresponding loss of sensitivity

            ii. Sensitivity and specificity also affected by disease prevalence in population; PID diagnosis much more likely correct in young sexually active woman than in middle-aged married female for given set of clinical findings

b. Clinical criteria
  i. Minimal criteria suggested by CDC (one or more sufficient to warrant treatment in woman at risk for STIs): cervical motion tenderness, uterine tenderness, adnexal tenderness
  ii. Additional criteria (improve specificity): fever (>38°C although authorities differ on minimum elevation), purulent cervical discharge

c. Laboratory and diagnostic tests
  i. Cervical assay for *N. gonorrhoeae* or *C. trachomatis;* often negative
  ii. Laparoscopy is most specific; may show tubal erythema; reddened, dilated small vessels; and purulent discharge
  iii. Imaging (magnetic resonance imaging [MRI] or ultra-sound), which may suggest thickened tubes, fluid-filled tubes, and tubo-ovarian complex; Doppler may show increased blood flow to tubes
  iv. Endometrial biopsy
    (1) Can have isolated endometritis; biopsy might be warranted if laparoscopy negative
    (2) Infiltration of endometrium with plasma cells and neutrophils suggest infection
  v. Wet mount—white blood cells (WBCs) abundant
  vi. Blood tests (WBC count, erythrocyte sedimentation rate, C-reactive protein) nondiagnostic but may indicate inflammatory process
  vii. Practical issues
    (1) Laparoscopy invasive; rarely performed unless differential diagnosis suggest other surgical conditions
    (2) Endometrial biopsy result takes 1–2 days
    (3) Absence of cervical pus or WBCs on wet mount call diagnosis into question

3. Complications: from tubal damage
  a. Few data regarding efficacy of treatment in preventing long-term complications; treatment does improve short-term outcomes

    b. Infertility 6%–15% with one episode and increases subsequently

    c. Ectopic pregnancy several-fold increase (up to 10-fold)

    d. Chronic pelvic pain (presumably due to adhesions)

4. Treatment: see Table 9.1

    a. Often initiated with empiric diagnosis only; morbidity rate of overtreatment generally less than that of undertreatment

    b. Indications for in-patient treatment with parenteral antibiotics and close observation

        i. Uncertain diagnosis in patient with significant illness

        ii. Pregnancy

        iii. Failure to respond to oral medication

        iv. Poor compliance

        v. Inability to tolerate oral medication

        vi. Nausea and vomiting precluding oral medication

        vii. High fever or other indications of serious illness (e.g., pain)

        viii. Tubo-ovarian abscess

    c. Surgery

        i. Increasingly drainage by interventional radiology used and may avoid necessity of surgery

        ii. Removal of infected organ(s), up to and including hysterectomy and bilateral salpingo-oophorectomy; may be required for those with serious abscess

        iii. Patients with severe infections and/or ruptured abscesses often have adhesions and inflammatory attachments of tissues and bowel that might make laparoscopic procedures particularly difficult

III. Diseases Characterized by Genital Ulcers

A. Genital herpes `36A-D`

    1. Microbe: herpes simplex virus (HSV) is a double-stranded DNA virus

    a. Two types: HSV-1 and HSV-2; share approximately 50% homology of their genetic materials

    b. HSV-1 typical oral infection; can cause up to 50% of new cases of genital herpes; much less likely to recur and cause asymptomatic shedding than HSV-2

    c. HSV-2 causes majority of current genital infections

    d. Genital infection with one type does not prevent infection with the other type

  2. Epidemiology: 50 million people in United states are estimated to have genital HSV; 200,000 new cases annually

    a. Asymptomatic shedding of virus most common form of transmission, although individuals most contagious during presence of genital sores when viral shedding is highest

    b. Daily suppression medication reduces chance of transmission to partner

  3. Diagnosis

    a. Clinical course

      i. The first infection with either viral type can be entirely asymptomatic

      ii. Initial episode (typically within 1 week of inoculation)

        (1) Single or multiple vesicles with clear fluid that itch or burn; cause extremely tender ulcers when rupture

        (2) Fever can result, particularly with first episode

        (3) On occasion, lesions in or near urethra can result in urinary retention (can be treated by having patient void in bathtub; on occasion, placement of Foley catheter necessary for a few days)

        (4) Mean duration of first episode 12 days

      iii. Recurrent episodes

        (1) Pain and itching tend to be less severe

        (2) Mean duration 4.5 days

        (3) Fever, urinary retention exceptionally rare

        (4) Classical vesicle/ulceration pattern may not appear; simple localized erythema with linear cracks in skin may be only evidence

    b. Tests

      i. Polymerase chain reaction (PCR) tests for viral DNA more sensitive than culture but not United States Food and Drug Administration (FDA)–approved

      ii. Culture has low sensitivity (good specificity) and further diminished with recurrent episodes

      iii. Serologic test can distinguish type 1 from type 2 and aid with prognosis (type 2 almost always sexually transmitted, more contagious, and more likely to recur); oral type 1 infection very common

    iv. Among U.S. adults 26% positive serology for HSV-2; 67% positive for HSV-1

4. Pregnancy

  a. Vertical transmission to newborn

    i. Neonatal herpes associated with high mortality rate and neurologic injury among survivors

    ii. Greatest risk is with initial infection close to term (can be as high as 30%–50%)

    iii. Some increased risk with genital ulcers at time of labor or ruptured membranes (<1%) although, in general, passive transfer of maternal antibodies across placenta protects fetuses of mothers with known HSV infection; cesarean section may reduce risk of vertical transmission

  b. Risk of recurrence may be reduced with suppressive therapy close to term (at 36 weeks); some human experience with acyclovir suggests no increased risk of birth defects (data lacking for famciclovir and valacyclovir)

5. Treatment: see Table 9.1

  a. Speeds healing and symptom resolution by a few days in primary and recurrent episodes

  b. Can reduce frequency of recurrence; whereas some patients have single lifetime episode, those with frequent outbreaks (five per year or more) might benefit from daily prophylaxis

  c. Daily prophylaxis can substantially reduce risk of transmission to partners (by up to 70%)

  d. HSV-1 infections much less likely to require chronic suppressive therapy than HSV-2 infections

B. Syphilis `36A-D`

  1. Microbe: *Treponema pallidum* gram-negative spirochete bacterium with a relatively small genome and limited metabolic capacity; relies on its host for many needs; three other *T. pallidum* species: *T. pallidum pertenue,* which causes yaws; *T. pallidum carateum,* which causes pinta; and *T. pallidum endemicum,* which causes bejel

  2. Serologic testing

    a. Non-treponemal tests

      i. Titers correlate with disease reactivity

      ii. Fourfold change in titer required for clinical significance

iii. Titers become nonreactive over time but can be weakly positive for life

iv. Two common tests are Venereal Disease Research Laboratory (VDRL) and rapid plasma reagin (RPR); equally valid but cannot be compared

b. Treponemal tests

i. Titers do not correlate with disease activity—commonly positive lifelong

ii. Fluorescent treponemal antibody absorbed (FTA-ABS)

iii. *T. pallidum* particle agglutination (TP-PA)

c. Dark-field microscopic examination of lesions (primary and secondary syphilis)—spirochetes visible

3. Clinical course

a. Primary syphilis

i. Incubation period 10–90 days; average 21 days

ii. Chancre appears; firm, painless ulcer with sharp borders located at point of entry (may not always be visible); local lymph node swelling possible

iii. Chancre persists for 4–6 weeks, then heals

b. Secondary syphilis

i. Characterized by skin rash that appears 1–6 months (commonly 6–8 weeks) after primary infection

(1) Symmetrical reddish-pink nonpruritic rash

(2) Involves trunk and extremities

(3) Can occur on palms of hands and soles of feet

(4) In moist areas of body, skin lesions become flat, broad, and whitish; called condylomata lata

(5) Mucous patches may also appear on genitals or in mouth

(6) Most contagious stage

(7) Other symptoms are fever, sore throat, malaise, weight loss, headache, meningismus, enlarged lymph nodes

(8) Acute meningitis occurs in about 2% of patients; hepatitis; renal disease; gastrointestinal problems (gastritis, proctitis, ulcerative colitis); arthritis; ophthalmic problems (optic neuritis, iritis, uveitis)

c. Tertiary syphilis

i. 1–10 years after initial infection (can occur decades later)

    ii. Occurs in up to a third of those with initial infection (not inevitable sequelae even without treatment)

    iii. Gummas—soft, tumor-like growths in skin and mucous membranes or in skeleton

    iv. Charcot joints—degeneration of joint surfaces resulting from loss of proprioception

    v. Clutton joints—bilateral knee effusions

    vi. Neurosyphilis—four clinical types

        (1) Asymptomatic neurosyphilis

            (A) Approximately 35%–40% of patients

            (B) Demonstrated by cerebrospinal fluid (CSF) examination

                (i) Abnormal cell count, protein level, or glucose level

                (ii) Reactivity to VDRL antibody test

                (iii) Negative CSF FTA-ABS test result excludes neurosyphilis

        (2) Acute syphilitic meningitis

            (A) Occurs within first 2 years of infection

            (B) Headache, meningeal irritation, and cranial nerve abnormalities typically involving cranial nerves at base of brain

            (C) Prodromal symptoms lasting weeks to months before focal deficits of vascular syndrome identifiable

                (i) Symptoms include unilateral numbness, paresthesias, extremity weakness, headache, vertigo, insomnia, and psychiatric abnormalities such as personality changes

                (ii) Focal deficits initially are intermittent or progress slowly over a few days

        (3) Tabes dorsalis (locomotor ataxia)—disorder of the spinal cord; results in a characteristic shuffling gait

            (A) General paresis

                (i) Personality changes, changes in emotional affect, hyperactive reflexes

                (ii) Argyll-Robertson pupils—small and irregular pupils constrict in response to focusing the eyes, but not to light

        vii. Cardiovascular complications commonly involve aorta, resulting in inflammation, aneurysm, regurgitation

    d. Latent syphilis: serologic proof of infection without signs or symptoms of disease

        i. Early latent syphilis: for 1 year or less from time of initial infection without signs or symptoms of disease

           (1) Very contagious

           (2) Treatment: single intramuscular (IM) injection of long-acting penicillin

        ii. Late latent syphilis: infection for more than 1 year but having no clinical evidence of disease

           (1) Not contagious

           (2) Treatment: three weekly IM injections of long-acting penicillin

        iii. Because stage is "latent," initial time of infection usually not known—patients presumed to be contagious (early) but also treated with three antibiotic doses (late)

  4. Syphilis in pregnancy

    a. Can result in miscarriage, intrauterine fetal demise, and newborn death

    b. Surviving neonates may have congenital syphilis (paralysis, deafness, blindness, facial deformities)

    c. Risk related to length of time fetus has been exposed to untreated syphilis in the mother

  5. Treatment: see Table 9.1

C. Chancroid

  1. Microbe: *Haemophilus ducreyi*

  2. Diagnosis

    a. Clinical: painful genital ulcer with tender, suppurative inguinal lymphadenopathy

    b. PCR tests available with individual commercial laboratories

    c. Diagnosis probable if:

        i. One or more painful genital ulcers

        ii. Syphilis and herpes excluded:

           (1) Negative dark-field examination of ulcer exudates

           (2) Negative serologic test done at least 7 days after onset

           (3) Herpes test on exudates negative

3. Other considerations:
  a. Facilitates HIV transmission
  b. 10% of patients also have HIV or syphilis
  c. Patients should be tested for HIV and syphilis and rechecked 3 months later if initially negative
4. Treatment: see Table 9.1
D. Granuloma inguinale (donovanosis)
  1. Microbe: *Klebsiella granulomatis,* intracellular gram-negative; rare in United States
  2. Diagnosis
    a. Clinical presentation: painless beefy red ulcer; progressive; no lymphadenopathy
    b. Laboratory tests: Donovan bodies on biopsy; PCR available with some commercial laboratories
  3. Disease course: ulcers heal from outside in; can recur 6–18 months after treatment
  4. Treatment: see Table 9.1
E. Lymphogranuloma venereum
  1. *Chlamydia trachomatis*
  2. Diagnosis
    a. Tender, unilateral groin lymphadenopathy
    b. Genital ulcer or papule may occur at entry site—often resolves before patient receives care
    c. Laboratory testing of ulcer or lymph node samples (via aspiration) for *C. trachomatis* (culture; direct immunofluorescence; nucleic acid amplification; chlamydia serology >1:64)
  3. Clinical course includes proctitis in patients who have had anal receptive sex; may see blood per rectum; pain; fever; tenesmus; invasive, systemic infection; can result in colorectal fissures and strictures
  4. Treatment: see Table 9.1

IV. Human Immunodeficiency Virus 36A–D
A. Overview
  1. Microbe: human immunodeficiency virus (HIV)
    a. HIV closely related to the human T-cell leukemia virus, the first virus ever to be clearly demonstrated to be a cause of human cancer (leukemia); is a retrovirus—has an enzyme, reverse transcriptase, that codes DNA from RNA

b. Not described in United States before 1981

c. HIV impairs immune system; patients experience unusual or opportunistic infections and malignancies not normally seen in otherwise healthy people

B. Screening

1. Two subtypes: HIV-1 (most common type in United States) and HIV-2 (endemic in West African countries); in United States, usual screen is chiefly for antibodies to HIV-1

   a. Enzyme immunoassay—can be done in 30 minutes

   b. HIV antibodies detectable in 95% of population infected within 3 months

   c. Negative test cannot preclude recent infection

2. Confirmation and follow-up testing—positive screen needs to be confirmed (Western blot, immunofluorescent assay)

C. Clinical course

1. Asymptomatic period: in one study 20% of patients remained asymptomatic after 7.5 years of infection; with more widespread screening, most common presentation is asymptomatic

2. Acute retroviral syndrome: this includes fever, malaise, lymphadenopathy, and skin rash; occurs in first weeks after infection—often before serology positive; highly contagious

3. *Pneumocystis carinii* pneumonia

   a. Occurs in up to 60% of those with clinically recognized HIV

   b. Patients complain of shortness of breath and a productive cough for 2–4 weeks before they invariably become severely ill and require hospitalization

   c. May require transbronchial lung biopsy to distinguish from other lung illness

4. Kaposi sarcoma

   a. 25% of those who do not receive treatment develop clinical AIDS

   b. Reddish purple to dark blue flat or raised sores that first commonly appear on the legs; lesions may resemble insect bites or bruises, but they often spread over much of the body; occasionally, sores can first develop in gastrointestinal tract

D. Diagnosis

1. Screening for other diseases (other STIs, tuberculosis, toxoplasmosis, hepatitis B and C)

2. HIV-specific testing

    a. Serum HIV p24 antigen: can be used to diagnose HIV infection before seroconversion; as antibody levels go up, immune complexes are formed, and p24 antigen levels drop

    b. HIV RNA or branched DNA PCR: primarily used to follow the disease course by measuring viral load; some patients receiving combination antiretroviral therapy actually have no detectable viral genomes in their serum, leading to serious speculation about whether this therapy represents a "cure"

    c. CD4+ and CD8+ lymphocyte subsets: although HIV affects diverse aspects of the immune system, it seems to have a predilection for CD4 (T4) receptor lymphocytes; CD8 (T8) lymphocytes rebound faster after the initial infection so the T4/T8 ratio is inverted

    d. Absolute CD4 levels are often used to guide treatment decisions; cell counts less than 200 suggest aggressive disease, even in an asymptomatic patient

E. Treatment

    1. Two classes of drugs commonly used

        a. Reverse transcriptase inhibitors (RTIs)

            i. Inhibit the action of viral reverse transcriptase in converting viral RNA into DNA

            ii. Examples include zidovudine, azidothymidine, didanosine, zalcitabine, stavudine, and lamivudine

        b. Protease inhibitors (PIs)

            i. Block the action of HIV protease, responsible for cleavage of viral protein precursors; prevent production of infectious virions

            ii. Examples include saquinavir (Invirase), ritonavir (Norvir), and indinavir (Crixivan)

    2. Objective is to eliminate any evidence of virus from bloodstream

    3. Treatment almost always involves use of multiple drugs

    4. Current debate whether HIV can be "cured"—evidence that virus can be eliminated from bloodstream for years

    5. Mortality rate in first-world countries has plummeted—still highly lethal in countries with poor medical infrastructure and those that cannot afford to provide polydrug treatment

F. Prevention of transmission to newborn
1. Screening of all pregnant women in early pregnancy
2. Use of antiretrovirals during pregnancy
3. Elective cesarean at 38 weeks
4. Avoidance of breastfeeding

V. Hepatitis B 36A-D
A. Microbe: hepatitis B virus
1. Virus is spherical and consists of three distinctly identifiable proteins or antigens
   a. Surface antigen in the outer coat of the virus and recognized in blood testing
   b. Inner core antigen: coat surrounds an inner protein
   c. e-antigen: also associated with the inner core
2. Appearance of e-antigen denotes significant liver disease and a highly infectious state; individuals without evidence of surface antigen and with anticore antibody only rarely infectious
B. Routes of transmission
1. Direct contact with infected blood (blood transfusions, dirty needles, childbirth, sexual contact)
2. Transplacental (?)
3. Saliva (?)
C. Diagnosis
1. Symptoms
   a. Most people acquiring hepatitis B infection probably remain free of symptoms and develop permanent immunity
   b. Only 20% of infected individuals develop symptoms
      i. Incubation period for symptomatic patients typically lasts 40–110 days but can vary with number of viral particles initially introduced into the body and method and site of exposure
      ii. Transient symptoms include fever, malaise, loss of appetite, nausea, vomiting, rash (flat, red areas that itch), arthritis (affects hands and larger joints of arms and legs), and jaundice
      iii. Course of jaundice
         (A) 3–10 days after onset
         (B) Worsens over a 2-week period, although patient begins to feel better

(C) Fades during recovery phase of 2–4 weeks

c. Laboratory testing

    i. Serum markers of hepatitis B infection

       (1) Hepatitis B surface antigen—patient infectious

       (2) Hepatitis B surface antibody—patient immune and not infectious

       (3) Hepatitis B e antigen—patient highly infectious, liver disease probable

    ii. Serum markers of liver inflammation—bilirubin and liver transaminases can be temporarily or chronically elevated

    iii. Liver biopsy—occasionally needed to help with differential diagnosis or establish presence of other liver disease

D. Disease course

  1. Long-term disease: 2%–6% of those infected by hepatitis B (approximately half the symptomatic group) not able to eradicate surface antigen

  2. Asymptomatic long-term carriers: contagious but experience no liver damage

  3. Chronic persistent hepatitis: mild chronic liver inflammation that eventually resolves

  4. Chronic active hepatitis

    a. Recurrent symptoms of hepatitis for several years

    b. Patients may develop cirrhosis or liver cancer

    c. 1% of patients infected with hepatitis B die

  5. Risk of chronic infection inversely related to age of infection—90% of infected infants develop chronic infection; these individuals are at increased risk for a variety of diseases including cirrhosis and liver cancer; a small fraction of this group dies from the disease

E. Prevention

  1. Hepatitis B immune globulin (HBIG): provides 3–6 months of protection; typically used for postexposure prophylaxis

  2. Hepatitis B vaccine

    a. Contains surface antigen produced in yeast by recombinant DNA technology

    b. Provides postexposure protection and pre-exposure immunity

   c. Recommended for:
   - i. All adolescents
   - ii. All adults at risk (including health-care workers)
   - iii. Any adult who requests it
   - iv. Newborns whose mothers are carriers (should also receive HBIG)

   d. Vaccination schedule depends on age and brand; typically two to four doses

   e. Vaccination screening
   - i. Pre-vaccination screening not generally recommended except for those in close contact with infected individuals
   - ii. Post-vaccination screening not recommended for general population (exception of health-care workers, HIV patients, and those in close contact with infected individuals)

VI. Parasitic Infections

A. Pediculosis pubis (pubic lice)

1. Microbe: *Phthirus pubis,* a parasitic organism
2. Can be transmitted via fomites (inanimate objects) such as towels and linen
3. Diagnosis based entirely on history (description by patient) or physical examination
   a. Pruritus in groin; visible lice (black motile specks) or nits (white eggs)
   b. Pubic lice can grasp wider hair shafts than head lice; public lice can move to head, but head lice cannot move to groin
4. Thoroughly wash clothing and bedding at high temperature or dry-clean
5. Lice on eyelashes require occlusive ophthalmic ointment twice a day for 10 days
6. Treatment: see Table 9.1

B. Scabies

1. Microbe: *Sarcoptes scabiei*
2. Diagnosis
   a. Symptoms (pruritus) result from sensitivity reaction to mites

   b. Examination: burrows visible as fine wavy lines up to
       1 cm long
   c. Laboratory: scrapings from burrows mixed with clear
       solution; mite can be seen through microscope
   3. Thoroughly wash clothing and bedding at high temperature or
       dry-clean
   4. Symptoms may persist for up to 2 weeks after treatment
   5. Crusted scabies occur in immunocompromised or
       malnourished—more difficult to treat
   6. Treatment: see Table 9.1

VII. Molluscum Contagiosum
   A. Virus infects skin; may be transmitted by fomites
   B. Diagnosis
       1. Umbilicated, non-tender papules <5 mm with pearly
           white centers
       2. May biopsy if in doubt
   C. Treatment: cryotherapy; often resolves without treatment

---

 MENTOR TIPS

- Pregnant women should be routinely screened for three sexually transmitted infections: syphilis, HIV, and hepatitis B. Early detection and treatment can greatly reduce transmission to fetus and the substantial morbidity that can result.
- Sexually active young women should be checked regularly for chlamydia and gonorrhea because the prevalence in this age group is quite high.
- The diagnosis of PID is often difficult to establish with certainty. The morbidity rate from overtreatment is generally less than the morbidity rate from undertreatment.
- When one sexually transmitted infection is diagnosed, look for others.
- Although laws vary from state to state, gonorrhea, chlamydia, HIV, and syphilis generally require reporting to the state health department. Although the laboratories will do this routinely, physician compliance with health department inquiries is specifically permitted by the federal privacy laws (such as HIPAA).

Resources

Centers for Disease Control and Prevention (CDC): Update to CDC's sexually transmitted infections treatment guidelines, 2006: Fluoroquinolones no longer recommended for treatment of gonococcal infections. Morbidity and Mortality Weekly Report 56(14):332–336, 2007.

Centers for Disease Control and Prevention (CDC), Workowski KA, Berman SM: Sexually transmitted infections treatment guidelines, 2006. Morbidity and Mortality Weekly Report 55(RR–11):1–94, 2006.

Chapter Self-Test Questions

Circle the correct answer. After you have responded to the questions, check your answers in Appendix A.

1. Which STI does not typically result in ulcers?

   a. Syphilis

   b. Chancroid

   c. Herpes

   d. Molluscum contagiosum

2. Which disease is *not* transmitted by fomites?

   a. Herpes

   b. Molluscum contagiosum

   c. Pediculosis pubis

   d. Scabies

3. A 17-year-old female presents with dulling, aching lower abdominal pain. On physical examination, she is afebrile; her abdomen is soft and nontender; there is no purulent discharge in the vagina; and she has no cervical motion tenderness. She does have bilateral adnexal tenderness and abundant white cells on wet mount of her cervical secretions but no other pathogens. The appropriate clinical management for this patient is to:

   a. Obtain gonorrhea and chlamydia assays and wait for results before treatment

   b. Obtain a white blood cell count, sedimentation rate, and C-reactive protein to help establish the diagnosis

    c. Recommend laparoscopy in the next 24–48 hours to aid in establishing a diagnosis

    d. Begin treatment with levofloxacin 500 mg orally once daily for 14 days and metronidazole 500 mg bid for 14 days while awaiting laboratory results

4. Appropriate drugs for the treatment of gonorrhea and/ or chlamydia during pregnancy include:

    a. Ciprofloxacin

    b. Doxycycline

    c. Azithromycin

    d. Levofloxacin

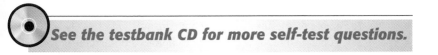

See the testbank CD for more self-test questions.

10

INFERTILITY, ENDOMETRIOSIS, AND CHRONIC PELVIC PAIN

Sigal Klipstein, MD

I. Definition of Infertility 48A

A. Primary infertility

1. Female partner has never been pregnant
2. Couple unable to conceive after unprotected intercourse for at least 1 year

B. Secondary infertility

1. Female partner has had at least one prior conception
2. Couple unable to conceive after unprotected intercourse for at least 1 year

II. Scope of Problem

A. Approximately 15% of couples unable to achieve a pregnancy within 1 year of attempting conception

B. Fecundability is the probability that a single cycle will result in a pregnancy and is approximately 20%–25% per month. After 1 year of infertility, the fecundability decreases to 2%–3% per month. The chance of conception among reproductive-age couples is:

1. 57% within 3 months
2. 72% within 6 months
3. 85% within 1 year

C. Ovarian aging

1. Loss of oocytes occurs before birth and continues even in absence of ovulation (i.e., in women on hormonal contraception, during pregnancy, in prepubertal life).

2. Most rapid loss occurs between 20 weeks of intrauterine gestation and birth.

3. Each woman undergoes follicular atresia at a different rate.

4. Fertility begins to decrease at approximately age 27 years and accelerates after age 35 years; significant losses of fertility in population studies occur between ages 38 and 40 years and with each year at age 40 and beyond.

5. Menopause occurs on average at age 51 years; it occurs earlier in smokers.

6. Fertility declines are evident at least a decade prior to the menopausal transition.

III. Etiology of Infertility 48B

A. 40% male factor; various types

  1. Azoospermia: no sperm in ejaculate

  2. Oligospermia: low sperm count

  3. Asthenospermia: low sperm motility

  4. Teratospermia: high percentage of abnormal forms

  5. Cryptorchidism

    a. Failure of descent of testes into scrotum (may be unilateral or bilateral)

    b. A common finding, occurring in 3% of full-term and 30% of preterm boys

    c. Testes usually located somewhere along inguinal canal and descend into scrotum within first few weeks after birth

    d. In virtually all physiologic cases cryptorchidism is unilateral

    e. Bilateral cryptorchidism requires further analysis as it may represent such life-threatening conditions as a virilized female with severe, salt-wasting congenital adrenal hyperplasia

    f. Prolonged cryptorchidism may lead to abnormal sperm parameters

  6. Congenital absence of the vas deferens

    a. Sperm form but unable to leave testes and be ejaculated with seminal fluid

    b. Often associated with cystic fibrosis in men (may be the only finding, so check for cystic fibrosis (CF) gene mutations)

    c. Responsible for 1%–2% of cases of male infertility

7. Klinefelter syndrome (47,XXY)
   a. Individuals often tall
   b. Low/no sperm in ejaculate
   c. May be able to obtain sperm with testicular biopsy
   d. Often undermasculinized
   e. Testicular failure common
   f. May need androgen replacement
8. Hypogonadotropic hypogonadism
   a. Low luteinizing hormone (LH) and follicle-stimulating hormone (FSH) levels
   b. Small testicular volumes
   c. Low androgen levels
   d. Treat with gonadotropins or gonadotropin-releasing hormone (GnRH) pulses
9. Varicocele
   a. Dilated veins of spermatic cord
   b. Increased scrotal temperature may affect spermatogenesis
   c. May require varicocelectomy
   d. Treatment of varicoceles (especially if small or detected only by ultrasound) remains controversial
10. Obstruction (i.e., status post vasectomy)
11. Retrograde ejaculation
12. Y-chromosome microdeletions
    a. Found on *AZF* genes, which are involved in spermatogenesis
    b. Often severely oligospermic/azoospermic
    c. Sperm sometimes obtainable from testicular biopsy
    d. If men with these microdeletions have male offspring, offspring may inherit the defect and have infertility
13. Chromosomal translocations
14. Idiopathic
15. Infections (i.e., mumps, orchitis)
16. Endocrinopathies
17. Sertoli cell–only syndrome
    a. Only Sertoli cells line the seminiferous tubules (no Leydig cells)
    b. Present with azoospermia
    c. Diagnosis is made by testicular biopsy
    d. Most cases are idiopathic
    e. No known treatment (except sperm donation)

18. Erectile dysfunction
   a. May be physiologic or psychogenic
   b. Physiologic causes ruled out if nocturnal tumescence is detected
   c. Physiologic often a sequel of chronic disease (i.e., diabetes mellitus, neurologic disorders, endocrine disorders)
   d. May be drug-induced
   e. Treat with sex therapy, phosphodiesterase inhibiting agents (i.e., Viagra, Cialis), correction of underlying medical disorder (not always possible), electroejaculation

B. 40% female factor
   1. Ovulatory dysfunction (40%)
      a. Polycystic ovarian syndrome (PCOS)
         i. Anovulation: no spontaneous ovulation
         ii. Oligo-ovulation: infrequent ovulation
         iii. Incidence: 5%–8% of women
         iv. Mechanism: dysregulation between FSH/LH secretion and local ovarian effects (mediated by insulin-like growth factor-1 [IGF-1]), increased testosterone, ovaries appear polycystic (>10 follicles per ovary)
      b. Congenital adrenal hyperplasia
         i. Check 17-hydroxyprogesterone levels at 8 a.m. (>200 ng/dL requires further evaluation with adrenocorticotropin hormone (ACTH) stimulation)
      c. Streak ovaries (hypogonadism)
         i. Turner syndrome (45,X)
         ii. Hermaphrodite
         iii. Gonadal dysgenesis
      d. Absence of ovaries in women with a female phenotype and a male karyotype (46,XY) are a finding in testicular feminization; also known as androgen insensitivity syndrome
      e. Hypothalamic amenorrhea
         i. Kallman syndrome
            (1) Hypogonadotropic hypogonadism
            (2) Often associated with anosmia
            (3) Failure of migration of GnRH neurons through cribiform plate
         ii. Exercise-induced amenorrhea
         iii. Anorexia nervosa

(1) Caloric restriction, often with a psychological component

(2) May suppress hypothalamic pituitary access and lead to anovulation (FSH and LH levels low)

  iv. Concern about bone health as hypothalamic amenorrhea is associated with hypoestrogenism, and estrogen is necessary for development of peak bone mass

2. Tubal/pelvic pathology (i.e., tubal blockage) (40%)

  a. Often a sequelae of pelvic inflammatory disease (PID)

  b. May be associated with diethylstilbestrol (DES) exposure

  c. Look for hydrosalpinx (fluid-filled tube) on ultrasound or hysterosalpingogram

  d. Tubal agenesis is a rare, isolated finding

  e. Endometriosis

    i. May cause tubal infertility

    ii. Associated with decreased fecundity

3. Uterine factors (10%)

  a. Fibroids

    i. Submucosal fibroids may interfere with implantation, fetal development

    ii. Intramural and subserosal fibroids generally do not need to be removed, unless they are very large

  b. Asherman syndrome

    i. Adhesions within endometrial cavity

    ii. Greatest risk following postpartum instrumentation (i.e., dilation and curettage [D&C] for retained placenta)

  c. Meyer-Rokitansky-Kuster-Hauser syndrome

    i. Also known as congenital absence of uterus and vagina

    ii. Due to complete müllerian agenesis, leading to an absence of the uterus and upper two thirds of vagina (and often fallopian tubes)

    iii. Incidence: 1/5,000 female births

  d. Other müllerian anomalies (bicornuate, didelphys, unicornuate, septum)

    i. Incidence: approximately 5% of females

    ii. Associated with recurrent pregnancy loss, endometriosis, preterm labor, malpresentations (i.e., breech)

    iii. T-shaped uterus associated with DES exposure

4. Unexplained (10%)

C. Many couples have multiple causes or components of both male- and female-factor infertility

D. Factors that influence fertility include:

    1. Age of couple (decreased fecundity with age)

        a. In couples with a female age >35 years, initiate evaluation after 6 months of infertility

    2. Coital frequency (also decreases with age)

    3. Cigarette smoking (longer time to conception)

IV. Evaluation of the Infertile Couple 48C

A. History and physical

    1. Menstrual cycle frequency and length

    2. Gravidity, parity, pregnancy outcomes

    3. Coital frequency and sexual dysfunction

    4. Duration of infertility

    5. Surgical history, particularly pelvic/abdominal

    6. Medications, allergies

    7. Tobacco, alcohol, drug history

    8. History of sexually transmitted diseases

    9. Family history of birth defects, reproductive difficulties, spontaneous abortions, early menopause, mental retardation

    10. Symptoms of thyroid disease, pelvic pain, galactorrhea, hirsutism, dyspareunia

    11. Physical examination includes weight, body mass index (BMI), thyroid and breast examinations, signs of hyperandrogenism/hirsutism, pelvic tenderness, and vaginal/uterine/cervical abnormalities

B. Male infertility evaluation—semen analysis

    1. Volume: 15–5.0 mL

    2. pH: >7.2

    3. Concentration: >20 million sperm/mL

    4. Percent motility: at least 50%

    5. Morphology by strict criteria: at least 4% normal

    6. Physical examination looking for varicocele, hypospadias, cryptorchidism, testicular volume, penile length, extent of virilization

C. Female infertility evaluation

    1. Hysterosalpingogram to evaluate the uterus and tubal patency 411

2. Cycle day 3 FSH and LH level to evaluate ovarian reserve
   a. Released by anterior pituitary
   b. >10 mIU/mL abnormal
   c. Elevated levels indicate diminished ovarian reserve and predict poorer response to treatment, increased spontaneous abortion rate, lower fecundity
3. Confirmation of ovulation
   a. Mid-luteal (cycle day 21) progesterone level >5 ng/mL confirms ovulation
   b. Basal body temperature rises by approximately 1°F above baseline at ovulation; temperature best taken prior to any morning activity
   c. LH surge: best indicator of ovulation; occurs around day 13–14 in a 28-day menstrual cycle; lasts 48–50 hours; ovulation occurs 10–12 hours after peak LH levels achieved
4. Thyroid-stimulating hormone (TSH) and prolactin levels (released by anterior pituitary)
5. Ultrasound to rule out uterine (i.e., fibroids) and ovarian pathologies (i.e., cysts, endometriomas)
6. Laparoscopy if pelvic pain, endometrioma, or suspicion for endometriosis or pelvic adhesions (no longer performed as part of routine infertility evaluation)

V. Treatment of Infertility

A. Male factor infertility
   1. Urology consult
      a. If azoospermia on semen analysis, there may be sperm in reproductive tract; requires testicular or epididymal sperm extraction
      b. If oligo- or asthenospermia, and varicocele, varicocelectomy may be an option
      c. Vasectomy reversal if previous history of vasectomy
      d. If hypogonadotropic hypogonadism, treat with pulsatile gonadotropins or GnRH
   2. Intrauterine insemination (IUI)
      a. Appropriate if total motile sperm count is >10 million/mL (mL of ejaculate × percent motile × total sperm/mL)
      b. May be used as an adjunct to ovulation induction
   3. In vitro fertilization (IVF) with intracytoplasmic sperm injection (ICSI)

      a. Used in cases when total motile sperm count <10 million
      b. Used in cases of severe teratospermia (<4% normal forms)
   4. Donor sperm insemination
      a. Used in cases of azoospermia
      b. Used when IVF not an option due to cost constraints
      c. Used by single women
      d. Used when male carriers have a heritable genetic disorder (i.e., cystic fibrosis, Tay-Sachs)

B. Female factor infertility
   1. Anovulation
      a. If due to PCOS
         i. Ovulation induction with clomiphene citrate or gonadotropins
         ii. If associated with hyperinsulinemia, consider metformin (may induce ovulation)
         iii. In severe cases where assisted reproductive technology not an option, ovarian drilling has some efficacy
         iv. Aromatase inhibitors may be as effective as clomiphene but are not FDA-approved for this indication
         v. Some women do not ovulate with clomiphene citrate and require gonadotropin therapy
      b. If due to hypothalamic hypogonadism, pulsatile exogenous GnRH therapy may be used (but gonadotropins easier and more readily available)
      c. If due to hyperprolactinemia, bromocriptine or cabergoline are appropriate
   2. Tubal disease (blockage, absence)
      a. Tubal reversal if s/p tubal ligation
      b. Tubal reconstruction if segmental blockage or localized damage
      c. Lysis of peritubal adhesions
      d. For blockage or absence, IVF most common treatment modality
   3. Uterine factor
      a. Fibroids
         i. Submucosal fibroids should be removed via hysteroscopy
         ii. Intramural fibroids should be removed if large, but controversy exists regarding effect of such fibroids on fertility

   iii. Subserosal fibroids should generally not be removed unless symptomatic
  b. Endometrial polyps
  c. Hysteroscopic resection is standard of care but impact on fertility is controversial
4. Endometriosis
  a. Mild or minimal endometriosis should be treated with surgery in women with infertility as it improves chance of spontaneous conception
  b. Severe endometriosis can be treated surgically or with gonadotropins or IVF
  c. Autoimmune premature ovarian failure
5. Premature ovarian failure
  a. Menopause prior to age 40 years
  b. Diagnosed by cessation of menses and elevated gonadotropin levels
  c. Often associated with detection of ovarian antibodies
  d. Should check for other autoimmune diseases, including systemic lupus erythematosus (SLE), thyroid disorders, pernicious anemia, adrenal insufficiency, and hypoparathyroidism
  e. Treat with hormone replacement therapy
  f. Donor egg for fertility
6. Unexplained infertility
  a. Treat empirically
  b. In women >35 years, clomiphene citrate is acceptable first step; <35 years it is less effective
     i. Overall success rate approximately 8% per cycle (if used with IUIs); 5% if used alone)
     ii. IUI: sperm washed and centrifuged to allow only viable sperm to remain in a small pellet; pellet reconstituted and sperm injected into uterus via transvaginal approach
     iii. Diminishing returns after three to six cycles
  c. If clomiphene citrate not successful, consider gonadotropin therapy; overall success rate 10%–15%; use with caution as it carries a 25% risk of twins and a 10% risk of high-order multiples.

      d. IVF treatment of choice if ovulation induction fails to achieve pregnancy and in women older than 40 years

C. Fertility drugs

  1. Clomiphene citrate

     a. Estrogenic compound with mixed agonist/antagonist effects

     b. Used for ovulation induction

     c. Particularly effective in women with PCOS and its associated anovulation

       i. Low risk of multiple pregnancy (5%–8%)

       ii. Rarely causes visual changes and must be discontinued

       iii. May cause irritability, breast tenderness, thickening of cervical mucus

  2. Gonadotropins

     a. Formulated as pure FSH, pure LH, or a combination of both (FSH is necessary to stimulate ovarian follicles; LH used as an adjunct)

     b. Used for ovulation induction

     c. Associated with development of ovarian hyperstimulation syndrome (OHSS)

       i. Large ovaries (often abdominally palpable)

       ii. Ascites (transudate), thought to be mediated by vasoactive endothelial growth factor (VEGF)

       iii. Associated with hemoconcentration and risk of deep vein thrombosis and pulmonary embolism (DVT/PE)

       iv. Treat with paracentesis, anticoagulation

     d. Monitor estrogen levels and ovarian response to prevent OHSS and multiple gestation

     e. Risk of multiple gestation 25%

     f. Risk of high-order multiples (triplets +) 10%

  3. Dopamine agonists (bromocriptine, cabergoline)

     a. Used for women with hyperprolactinemia

     b. Inhibit prolactin release at level of the pituitary

     c. Should be discontinued once pregnancy is confirmed

     d. Side effects: orthostatic hypotension, headaches

D. Assisted reproductive technology (ART)

  1. IVF with embryo transfer (ET)

   a. Downregulation of hypothalamic-pituitary-ovarian axis (ovulation must not occur until it is triggered as oocytes can be retrieved only from ovarian follicles)

     i. GnRH agonists (leuprolide acetate, naferelin) lead to FSH/LH surge, followed by downregulation; GnRH agonists must be taken 10–14 days for full effect

     ii. GnRH antagonists (ganirelix, cetrorelix) have no FSH/LH surge; work within hours

   b. Controlled ovarian hyperstimulation with gonadotropins: FSH is the primary gonadotropin; LH often also used

     i. Recombinant FSH (follitropin α and β)

     ii. Recombinant LH (lutropin α)

     iii. Purified human menopausal gonadotropins (hMG) derived from urine of postmenopausal women

   c. Trigger of ovulation with human chorionic gonadotropin (hCG)

     i. Mimics the LH surge

     ii. May use recombinant or urinary hCG

   d. Retrieval of oocytes

     i. Performed approximately 36 hours after hCG administration

     ii. Utilizes transvaginal ultrasound guidance

     iii. Performed under intravenous sedation

   e. IVF of oocytes

     i. Oocytes mixed with sperm or injected directly with sperm (ICSI)

     ii. Performed in embryology laboratory in a strictly controlled environment (temperature, carbon dioxide levels)

   f. Embryos mature in the laboratory for 2–6 days (days 1–3: morula; days 5–6: blastocyst)

   g. Embryo transfer into uterus via transcervical approach under ultrasound guidance

   h. Supernumerary embryos may be cryopreserved for future use

     i. Typically, transfer involves one to three embryos at a time, but many more embryos may be available for transfer

     ii. Embryos can be cryopreserved for many years

    i. Unfertilized oocytes may also be cryopreserved, but many do not survive the thaw process, do not fertilize, do not develop, and do not result in pregnancy

        i. Oocyte cryopreservation requires further development

        ii. There have been live births from oocyte cryopreservation

        iii. Used prior to chemotherapy or radiation in women who are undergoing treatment for cancer and wish to preserve their fertility

        iv. Being marketed to single women as a way of extending their fertile life span

2. Gamete intrafallopian transfer (GIFT)

    a. Controlled ovarian hyperstimulation and oocyte retrieval identical to IVF

    b. Upon retrieval, oocytes mixed with sperm in a test tube

    c. Egg and sperm mixture placed into fallopian tubes *prior to fertilization* via laparoscopy

    d. Widely used in the past, as initially success rate was higher than with IVF

    e. As better culture conditions have been developed, has become a much less important assisted reproduction modality

    f. Used in cases of severe cervical stenosis

    g. Used by couples who wish to avoid extracorporeal fertilization (e.g., for religious reasons)

3. Zygote intrafallopian transfer (ZIFT)

    a. Like GIFT, but *fertilized* oocytes are transferred into fallopian tubes

    b. Rarely used in contemporary ART

VI. Psychological Impact of Infertility 48D

A. Infertility is often an isolating experience.

B. Couples frequently do not share their infertility with others.

C. Depression is common in couples undergoing treatment.

D. Depression and despair worsen with each failed treatment cycle.

E. Counseling is an important component of caring for the infertile couple and should be offered multiple times throughout the process.

VII. Endometriosis

A. Growth of endometrial tissue in sites other than uterine cavity (usually within pelvic cavity)

B. Common sites of implants: 38C ovaries, uterosacral ligaments, pouch of Douglas, pelvic peritoneum, rectosigmoid colon and bowel, fallopian tube

C. Prevalence

1. Asymptomatic women: 2%–50% (depends on diagnostic criteria used and population studied)
2. Dysmenorrhea: 40%–60%
3. Infertility: 20%–30%

D. Risk factors

1. Menstrual history (early menarche, late menopause)
2. Lack of hormonal exposure (higher in those who never use OCPs)
3. Müllerian anomalies (bicornuate, unicornuate)

E. Theories of pathogenesis 38A

1. Retrograde menstruation of endometrial tissue sloughed through patent fallopian tubes into peritoneal cavity (most women experience this to some extent)
2. Immune defect/altered cellular immunity (failure of immunologic mechanisms to eradicate endometrial glands that find their way into peritoneal cavity)
3. Coelomic metaplasia (transformation of peritoneum into endometriotic tissue)
4. Ectopic transplantation of endometrium
5. Vascular and lymphatic distribution
6. Metastasis
7. Multifactorial (interaction between genetic and environmental factors)

F. Symptoms include pelvic pain, cyclical dysmenorrheal (often just before/during menses), dyspareunia, infertility, and painful micturation and defecation; 38B some women have widespread endometriosis and no pain; others have multiple symptoms and very minimal endometriosis

G. Physical findings (there may be none) 38B

1. Tenderness in the posterior fornix or adnexa
2. Nodularity of the posterior cul-de-sac on rectovaginal examination
3. Uterosacral nodularity
4. Adnexal mass (endometrioma)

5. Retroverted uterus (due to pelvic adhesions secondary to endometriosis)

H. Diagnosis 38D

1. History and physical (often inconclusive)
2. Transvaginal ultrasound: only useful if ovarian endometrioma visualized; retroversion of uterus is suggestive of disease
3. Magnetic resonance image (MRI): may detect subperitoneal deposits
4. CA-125: may be slightly elevated (not diagnostic)
5. Laparoscopy: gold standard; only modality that can effectively *rule out* endometriosis
6. Biopsy (from laparoscopy)
   a. Glands and stroma
   b. Hemosiderin-laden macrophages

I. Treatment 38E

1. Medical
   a. Danazol
      i. Inhibits the mid-cycle urinary LH surge, inducing a chronic anovulation
      ii. Increases testosterone, leading to untoward androgenic side effects
      iii. Historically, a first-line agent; now rarely used
      iv. Side effects: weight gain, fluid retention, fatigue, decreased breast size, acne, emotional lability, deepening of the voice (irreversible), adverse effects on lipid profile, liver damage
   b. Progestin (i.e., medroxyprogesterone acetate)
      i. Presumed mechanism: decidualization, leading to endometrial attenuation over time
      ii. Side effects: weight gain, depression, irregular bleeding
   c. Oral contraceptives
      i. Often taken continuously
      ii. Mechanism: amenorrhea, possibly apoptosis of eutopic endometrial tissue
      iii. Side effects: thrombosis, hypertension, headaches, breast tenderness, liver adenomas (benign)
   d. Gonadotropin-releasing hormone agonists (i.e., leuprolide acetate)

      i. Mechanism: pituitary desensitization leading to pseudomenopausal state and amenorrhea

      ii. Side effects: hot flashes, vaginal dryness, decreased libido, depression, headache

      iii. Prolonged use associated with osteopenia/osteoporosis (counteract with estrogen/progesterone add-back)

2. Surgical

   a. Objectives

      i. Restore normal anatomic relationships

      ii. Excise all visible disease to the extent possible

      iii. Prevent/delay recurrence

      iv. Endometriosis becoming more of a medically diagnosed and managed disease

         (1) Surgical confirmation of endometriosis as source of pelvic pain no longer required for treatment with GnRH agonists

         (2) Infertility attributed to endometriosis treated preferentially with assisted reproductive technology rather than surgical extirpation of scarring and endometriosis implants

   b. Approach:

      i. Fulguration of endometriotic implants

      ii. Excision of lesions

      iii. Deeply infiltrating disease may necessitate bowel/rectum resection

      iv. In recalcitrant disease where childbearing is complete, hysterectomy with bilateral salpingo-oophorectomy should be considered (hysterectomy alone associated with a six-fold risk of recurrence when ovaries are left in place)

VIII. Chronic Pelvic Pain (CPP)

A. Overview

   1. Patients with CPP require multidisciplinary approach

   2. Frequent follow-up warranted

   3. Treatment should be tailored to presumed etiology

   4. Specific diagnosis often elusive

   5. Involvement of mental health professionals should be sought early in treatment process

    6. Therapy often unsatisfying and patients may not respond

    7. Relapse of pain is frequent

B. Definition 39A

    1. Duration of 6 or more months

    2. Non-cyclic in nature

    3. Predominantly localized to lower abdomen

    4. Causes functional disability

C. Prevalence 15%–20% of women age 18–50 years 39B

D. Etiology 39B

    1. Gynecologic

        a. Endometriosis

        b. Gynecologic malignancies

        c. Ovarian remnant syndrome

        d. Pelvic congestion syndome

        e. Tuberculous salpingitis

        f. Pelvic adhesive disease

        g. Adenomyosis

        h. Leiomyomata

        i. Atypical dysmenorrhea/ovulatory pain

        j. Adnexal cysts

        k. Endometrial/cervical polyps

        l. Chronic ectopic pregnancy

        m. Chronic endometritis

        n. Cervical stenosis

        o. Chronic ectopic pregnancy

        p. Genital prolapse

        q. Intrauterine devices

    2. Urologic

        a. Interstitial cystitis

        b. Chronic urinary tract infection (UTI)

        c. Kidney stones

        d. Urethral diverticulum

    3. Gastrointestinal

        a. Irritable bowel syndrome

        b. Constipation

        c. Cholelithiasis

        d. Chronic appendicitis

        e. Diverticulitis

        f. Peptic ulcer disease

      g. Inflammatory bowel disease

      h. Neoplasia

      i. Peritoneal inclusion cysts

   4. Psychosocial

      a. Substance abuse

      b. Depression

      c. Personality disorder

      d. Somatoform disorders

   5. Musculoskeletal

      a. Fibromyalgia

      b. Osteoporosis

      c. Herniated disc

      d. Arthritis

      e. Trauma

E. Populations at increased risk:

   1. Physical and sexual abuse: 40%–50% of women with CPP have a history of abuse

   2. PID: CPP develops in 18%–35% of women with acute PID; mechanism unclear

   3. Endometriosis

      a. Found via laparoscopy in 33% of women with CPP

      b. May cause pain directly by invading nerves

      c. May act indirectly via viscero-visceral interactions

      d. Some women may have persistent pain after eradication of endometriosis

   4. Interstitial cystitis (IC)

      a. Chronic inflammation of bladder

      b. Irritative voiding symptoms of urgency and frequency in absence of other pathology

      c. CPP reported by up to 70% of women with IC

      d. May be present in up to 85% of women presenting with CPP

   5. Irritable bowel syndrome (IBS)

      a. Etiology unknown

      b. Chronic, relapsing abdominopelvic pain and bowel dysfunction (at least 12 weeks in the previous 12 months)

      c. Constipation, diarrhea, or both

      d. Relieved with defecation

      e. Found in 50%–80% of women with CPP

6. Post pregnancy
  a. Delivering a large infant
  b. Operative delivery
  c. Lumbar lordosis
  d. Use of gynecologic stirrups for delivery
7. Previous surgery
  a. Abdominopelvic surgery
  b. Cervical surgery leading to stenosis
  c. Hysterectomy
  d. Cesarean delivery
8. Musculoskeletal disorders
  a. Peripartum pelvic pain syndrome
    i. Ligamentous strain and damage
    ii. May occur during or after pregnancy
    iii. May affect pelvic girdle and lower spine
  b. Faulty posture (lumbar lordosis, thoracic kyphosis)
  c. Fibromyalgia
F. Diagnosis `39C-D`
  1. Ask patient to fill out a pain diary
  2. Complete history
    a. Location of pain
    b. Radiation of pain
    c. Onset
    d. Cyclic versus constant
    e. Impact on lifestyle
    f. Relation to menses
    g. Aggravating/alleviating factors
    h. Dyspareunia
    i. History of pelvic infection
    j. Bowel and bladder habits
    k. Surgical history
    l. Mood disorders, depression
    m. Physical/sexual abuse history
    n. Drug history
  3. Diagnostic studies
    a. Transvaginal ultrasound rules out pelvic mass, ovarian cysts/endometriomas, leiomyomas
    b. MRI/computed tomography: only if ultrasound is abnormal
    c. Laparoscopy

    i. Rules out endometriosis

    ii. Rules out pelvic adhesive disease

    iii. May perform conscious laparoscopic pain mapping in severe cases

  d. Interstitial cystitis

    i. Check an intravesical potassium sensitivity test

    ii. Compare potassium versus saline installation

    iii. Cystoscopy (glomerulations and decreased bladder capacity)

4. Physical examination

  a. Neuromuscular

    i. Trigger points

    ii. Musculoskeletal pain

  b. Abdomen

    i. Hernias

    ii. Distention

    iii. Bowel sounds

    iv. Tenderness

  c. Pelvis

    i. Uterine mobility/fixation

    ii. Cervical motion tenderness

    iii. Adnexal masses

    iv. Rectovaginal examination to rule out endometriotic implants

    v. Uterosacral nodularity

  d. Psychosocial evaluation

    i. Mental health history

    ii. Somatic complaints (somatoform disorder)

    iii. History of physical/sexual/emotional abuse

    iv. History of substance abuse

    v. Self-image, anorexia nervosa, bulimia

    vi. Consider psychological referral

  e. Laboratory evaluation

    i. CBC, sedimentation rate

    ii. Cervical cultures for *Neisseria* gonorrhea and chlamydia

5. Clinical recommendations (depend on presumed diagnosis) `39E`

  a. Psychological intervention

    i. Counseling

ii. Psychotherapy
iii. Cognitive therapy
iv. Behavioral modification
v. Often combined with medical therapy
b. Antidepressants, e.g., tricyclics and selective serotonin reuptake inhibitors (SSRIs) (may improve pain tolerance)
c. Trigger point injection (uses local anesthesia; may be helpful at the abdominal wall, vagina, and sacrum)
d. Analgesics
  i. Nonsteroidal anti-inflammatory drugs
  ii. Opioids (must be careful to avoid addiction and dependency)
e. Combined oral contraceptives
  i. Work for primary dysmenorrhea
  ii. Suppress ovulation
  iii. Result in uterine quiescence
  iv. Stabilize prostaglandin release
  v. Reduction in pain in context of endometriosis
  vi. Continuous administration recommended
f. Progestins
  i. Effective for endometriosis-related pain
  ii. May be as effective as combined oral contraceptives
g. GnRH agonists
  i. Downregulate hypothalamic-pituitary axis
  ii. Decrease estradiol levels
  iii. Shown efficacy in relieving endometriosis-associated pain
  iv. Avoid bone loss by adding back estrogen + progesterone, or progesterone (norethindrone) alone
h. Exercise
i. Antibiotics (if PID/infectious etiology suspected)
j. Interstitial cystitis
  i. Oral: pentosan polysulfate sodium (Elmiron)
  ii. Intravesical instillation: dimethylsulfoxide (DMSO), glucocorticoids, heparin, local anesthetics, Elmiron, silver nitrate
k. Physical therapy
  i. Transcutaneous electrical nerve stimulation (TENS)

    ii. Manual therapy of myofascial trigger points in pelvic floor

l. Surgical intervention

    i. Excision or fulguration of endometriosis

    ii. Adhesiolysis

    iii. Presacral neurectomy

        (1) Most effective in central dysmenorrhea

        (2) May be effective for endometriosis-associated pain

    iv. Laparoscopic uterine nerve ablation (LUNA)

        (1) Transection of uterosacral ligaments via laparoscopy

        (2) Effective in primary dysmenorrhea

    v. Hysterectomy

        (1) Only if woman has completed childbearing

        (2) Only when medical therapy fails

        (3) Oophorectomy decreases risk of recurrence of endometriosis

m. Alternative therapies: vitamin B_1, magnesium, magnetic field therapy (magnets applied to abdominal trigger points), acupuncture

MENTOR TIPS

- Infertility is defined as unprotected intercourse for 1 year without achieving a pregnancy.
- Abnormal sperm parameters include oligospermia (low sperm count), azoospermia (no sperm in ejaculate), asthenospermia (low sperm motility), and teratospermia (low percentage of normal forms).
- Female infertility may be tubal (blocked or absent tubes), ovulatory dysfunction (most commonly due to polycystic ovarian syndrome, but consider hypothalamic amenorrhea), uterine factor (i.e., septum, fibroids, polyps), diminished ovarian reserve (i.e., aging, premature ovarian failure), or unexplained.
- The basic fertility evaluation consists of a semen analysis; hysterosalpingogram to check for tubal patency and confirm normal endometrial cavity; hormonal evaluation that includes FSH, TSH, and prolactin levels; and a sexual and reproductive history.

- Two important risks of infertility treatment are the development of OHSS and the increased rate of multiple (and high-order) pregnancies.
- The extent of disease in women with endometriosis cannot be predicted by the severity of symptoms. Some women have widespread disease and are asymptomatic, whereas women with minimal disease may experience significant pain.
- Chronic pelvic pain shows a strong association with sexual and physical abuse.
- The cause of chronic pelvic pain is often difficult to ascertain, and treatment frequently yields suboptimal results. Relapse of pain is frequent.

Resources

Chronic pelvic pain. Practice Bulletin, American College of Obstetrics and Gynecology, 2004.

Farquhar C: Endometriosis. British Medical Journal 334:249–253, 2007.

Moore KL, Persaud TVN: The developing human: Clinically oriented embryology, 7th ed. Philadelphia, WB Saunders, 2002.

Scott JR, Gibbs RS, Karlan BY, et al (eds): Danforth's obstetrics and gynecology, 9th ed. Baltimore and Philadelphia, Lippincott Williams & Wilkins, 2003.

Speroff L, Fritz MA: Clinical gynecologic endocrinology and infertility, 7th ed. Baltimore and Philadelphia, Lippincott Williams & Wilkins, 2004.

Chapter Self-Test Questions

Circle the correct answer. After you have responded to the questions, check your answers in Appendix A.

1. A 16-year-old female comes to the office complaining that she has never menstruated. She states that she has not had any breast development. Which of the following should be included in your initial evaluation?

   a. Physical examination

   b. Testing of serum FSH and LH levels

   c. Testing of serum TSH and prolactin levels

   d. All of the above

2. A 27-year-old female complains of pain with intercourse. She has never been able to achieve full penetration. Your evaluation and treatment should include all of the following *except:*

a. Psychological evaluation and questions regarding a history of sexual abuse

b. Physical examination to rule out organic causes of dyspareunia

c. Expectant management

d. Instruction on the use of vaginal dilators

e. Pelvic ultrasound

3. GIFT *differs* from IVF in that only IVF:

a. Requires ovarian hyperstimulation with gonadotropins

b. Requires that ovulation be triggered with hCG

c. Involves the transfer of embryos into the uterus via the cervix

d. May be used to overcome the effect of diminished ovarian reserve

4. Which of the following may be involved in the etiology of chronic pelvic pain?

a. History of sexual abuse

b. Endometriosis

c. History of pelvic inflammatory disease

d. All of the above

e. None of the above

See the testbank CD for more self-test questions.

FIRST-TRIMESTER BLEEDING

CHAPTER 11

Michael D. Benson, MD

I. Overview 15A, 16A

A. Any kind of bleeding may be commonly encountered during the first trimester of pregnancy:
   1. Any bleeding or no bleeding
   2. Normal periods or delayed, early, light, or heavy periods
   3. Early implantation bleeding, which may occur close to time of expected menses ("I can't be pregnant—I just had a period.")

B. Threshold for doing pregnancy test should be very low in women 50 years and under.

C. Pregnancy test should be considered for reproductive-age women who:
   1. Have any irregularity in bleeding (late, early, light, heavy, mid-cycle)
   2. Are undergoing surgery, x-rays, or other medical procedures
   3. Present to the emergency room for any condition

D. Urine pregnancy test is widely available over the counter, inexpensive, available in minutes, and very accurate.

E. Personal history of abstinence can be very misleading. Patient history about time of last intercourse often wrong (often surprisingly so). When it really matters, do a pregnancy test.

F. About a third of pregnant women experience some sort of bleeding in the first trimester—half have a viable pregnancy.

G. Differential diagnosis includes miscarriage, ectopic pregnancy, gestational trophoblastic neoplasia, lower genital tract lesion (less common), viable pregnancy, trauma, and pelvic inflammatory disease (PID) (rare).

181

II. Terminology 16B

A. *Spontaneous abortion:* loss of pregnancy before 20 weeks gestation

    1. The term *abortion* has political and emotional connotations that can be quite insensitive and distressing to a patient losing a desired pregnancy—*miscarriage* is probably a better choice of words

    2. Types of spontaneous abortion (does not imply etiology)

        a. *Threatened:* any vaginal bleeding before 20 weeks

        b. *Inevitable:* dilated cervix prior to actual passage of tissue

        c. *Incomplete:* dilated cervix with expulsion of only a portion of the products of conception

        d. *Complete:* expulsion from the uterus of all products of conception

        e. *Missed:* embryonic demise, with products of conception remaining within the uterus; in spontaneous abortion the embryo dies and then days, weeks, or months later, tissue expelled from body

        f. *Recurrent:* three or more consecutive spontaneous abortions 16C

B. *Elective abortion:* medical intervention that results in removal of pregnancy from the uterus before viability (see Chapter 8)

C. *Septic abortion:* abortion complicated by infection 16E

    1. Usually due to previous instrumentation with retained products of conception—almost never seen in United States

    2. Common complication of illicit abortion

    3. Symptoms/signs: fever, abdominal pain, uterine tenderness

    4. Diagnostic testing

        a. Cultures: cervical, uterine contents (when available), blood, urine

        b. Complete blood count (CBC)

        c. Type and crossmatch

        d. Ultrasound to check for retained products of conception

        e. Serial human chorionic gonadotropin (hCGs) as clinically appropriate

    5. Treatment

        a. Surgical: uterine curettage if tissue remains (high risk of uterine perforation)

        b. Antibiotics: penicillin, gentamicin, clindamycin

        c. ICU if septic shock

III. Diagnosis of Pregnancy

A. Embryonic development

  1. Conceptus is embryo until 12 weeks, and fetus thereafter

  2. Stages of development:

    a. Fertilized ovum—undergoes cleavage in fallopian tube into blastomere

    b. Becomes morula—solid sphere of dividing cells

    c. Morula enters uterine cavity on day 3 or 4 after fertilization

    d. Cells on surface of morula differentiate into trophoblast, which subsequently becomes placenta

    e. Blastocyst forms from morula; fluid-filled internal cavity develops

    f. Implantation: blastocyst invades endometrium at day 6 or 7; consists of 100–250 cells

    g. Endometrial changes: completely surrounds blastocyst, which collapses

      i. Endometrium during pregnancy referred to as "decidua"

      ii. Decidua basalis: between blastocyst and myometrium

      iii. Decidua capsularis: covers implanted blastocyst

      iv. Decidua vera: endometrium on wall opposite implantation site

    h. Trophoblast differentiation: approximately day 8 after fertilization

      i. Cytotrophoblast

        (1) Mononuclear cells

        (2) Germinal cells for syncytium

        (3) Form inner layer of chorionic villi

      ii. Syncytiotrophoblast

        (1) Amorphous cytoplasm; no cell borders

        (2) Multiple nuclei highly variable in size and shape

        (3) Cannot reproduce

        (4) Produces placental hormones

        (5) Forms outer layer of chorionic villi

    i. Yolk sac; early structure visible on ultrasound

      i. Begins forming in 2nd week after fertilization; fully developed by 4th week

      ii. Becomes part of digestive system

      iii. May supply nutrition to early embryo

    j. Chorionic villi cover entire embryo by 12 days after fertilization

       i. Villi near decidua basalis become placenta

       ii. Villi oriented away from decidua basalis form chorionic membrane (exterior of amnionic membranes)

       iii. By 12 weeks yolk sac disappears, and amnionic membrane fuses with chorionic membrane

B. Normal patterns of hCG elevation during pregnancy

  1. Structure of hCG—glycoprotein

    a. Alpha chain—identical with other glycoprotein hormones: TSH, LH, and FSH

    b. Beta chain—distinguishes hCG from other protein hormones

    c. Forms in serum

       i. Free alpha and beta sub-units

       ii. "Nicked" beta units: partial enzymatic degradation

       iii. Full molecule is the one that varies and is measured clinically on serum and urine hCG tests

  2. hCG levels

    a. Thought to be produced in small quantities beginning 1 day after fertilization (not detectable clinically at this time)

    b. Detectable in maternal serum as early as 7 days after fertilization

    c. Typically 100 mIU/mL at 14 days past fertilization/time of missed menses

       i. Serum hCG detectable before missed period somewhere between 7 and 10 days after implantation

       ii. Urine hCG varies by assay sensitivity, typically 25–50 mIU/mL (roughly comparable to serum levels)

    d. Early pregnancy: double every 2–3 days

    e. Peak at 8–10 weeks typically at 100,000 mIU/mL (highly variable)

    f. Steady drop until 20 weeks to 10–20 K range, where it remains for rest of pregnancy

    g. Higher in twin pregnancies

    h. Higher at term in pregnancies with female fetuses

    i. Only known function is maintenance of corpus luteum in early pregnancy

    j. Not related to nausea of pregnancy

    k. Produced by almost all tissues in both men and women; never "undetectable"; threshold for pregnancy typically 5–10 mIU/mL, depending on laboratory and assay used

C. Progesterone levels: produced by corpus luteum until roughly 6 weeks post fertilization; placental production then takes over

    1. 20 ng/mL: almost always associated with normal, viable pregnancy

    2. <5 ng/mL: almost never associated with normal, viable pregnancy (does not differentiate between nonviable intrauterine pregnancy versus ectopic pregnancy)

    3. Caveat: 70% of viable pregnancies have progesterone levels in between

D. Transvaginal ultrasound

    1. "Discriminatory zone" gestational sac should be seen with hCG level of 1500 mIU/mL

        a. Roughly 21 days post conception (1 week after missed menses)

        b. Varies somewhat between laboratories and specifics of ultrasound performance

        c. Gestational sac can be confused with:

            i. "Pseudogestational sac": fluid collection within uterus associated with ectopic pregnancy

            ii. Separation of decidua in failed intrauterine pregnancy

    2. Fetal heart motion

        a. Median hCG of 5200

        b. Almost always seen in viable pregnancies at 28 days post fertilization (6 weeks post last menstrual period [LMP])

        c. Slow initially: 85–100 when first detected

E. Symptoms of pregnancy: many women actually experience symptoms distinct enough to know or suspect they are pregnant even before missed menses

    1. Anorexia, nausea, vomiting; can occur in any combination and in any severity

    2. Hyperemesis gravidarum: severe nausea and vomiting associated with weight loss and ketonuria

        a. Associated with lower rate of miscarriage; not because of protective effect of vomiting but presumably higher hormone levels associated with healthy pregnancy and increased nausea

   b. More common with multiple gestational or gestational
   trophoblastic neoplasia (not sensitive or specific)
   c. Treatment: no large studies
      i. Over-the-counter remedies
        (1) H_1 blockers
         (A) Dimenhydrinate (Dramamine)
           (i) 50–100 mg every 4–6 hours orally
              or rectally
           (ii) Maximum daily dose 400 mg (200 mg if
              used with doxylamine)
         (B) Doxylamine (Unisom)
           (i) 12.5 mg three to four times per day
        (2) Phorphorate carbohydrate solution (Emetrol)
         (A) 15–30 mL orally every 15 minutes
         (B) Maximum of five doses without relief
        (3) Vitamin B_6
         (A) 10–25 mg three to four times per day
        (4) Ginger capsule—250 four times daily
        (5) Acupuncture, wrist bands—efficacy unknown
      ii. Prescription
        (1) Ondansetron (Zofran): 8 mg orally
         dissolving tablets
         (A) Effective; does not require passage into
           gastrointestinal (GI) tract for effect
         (B) Extremely expensive: in practice, unaffordable
           without third-party payment (covered by
           Medicaid and most insurers)
        (2) Promethazine (Phenergan): 12.5–25 mg every
         4 hours (orally, rectally, IM, or IV)
        (3) Trimethobenzamide (Tigan): 200 mg every
         6–8 hours rectally
        (4) Metoclopramide (Reglan): 10 mg orally every
         6 hours or 10 mg IV every 8 hours (facilitates
         gastric emptying)
      iii. Brief hospitalization for intravenous hydration
        occasionally appropriate, particularly for ketonuria
      iv. Total parenteral nutrition (TPN): for intractable emesis
        and prolonged weight loss, TPN via central venous
        catheter is appropriate (rare, but does happen)

3. Breast tenderness: often resolves by 12 weeks
4. Constipation or diarrhea: pregnancy more often constipating due to slowing of smooth muscle motility from progesterone (prenatal vitamins and supplemental calcium can also be source of substantial GI distress)
5. Implantation bleeding: classically occurs as spotting at time of expected period (can be mistaken for normal period)

IV. Epidemiology of Miscarriage

A. It has been estimated that majority of pregnancies are lost prior to first menstrual period
B. Among clinically recognized pregnancies, an estimated 15%–20% result in first-trimester miscarriages
C. Approximately two thirds of miscarriages have abnormal karyotype
D. Risk factors for miscarriage include advancing maternal age (particularly over 40 years), poorly controlled diabetes, smoking, poorly controlled hypertension, multiple gestation, pregnancy loss in immediate past pregnancy, and alcohol consumption (two drinks or more per day)

V. Diagnosis of Miscarriage 16F

A. With serial hCGs and improvements in ultrasound visualization and availability, embryonic demise before actual expulsion of tissue diagnosed more often than in the past
B. Often better to rely on two observations before making definitive diagnosis; e.g.:
1. Falling hCGs and absent fetal heart motion
2. Presence of fetal heart motion followed subsequently by absence
C. Diagnosis of miscarriage often source of intense (if somewhat self-limited) emotional distress to patient
1. Avoid statements such as "It was meant to be," "It was for the best," and "You can have another."
2. The diagnosis can come as a complete surprise and cause considerable upset. One way to mitigate the patient's distress is to introduce the idea that all might not be well but "further testing is needed." This allows the patient to consider the possibility that the pregnancy might not be viable. Serial hCGs or a confirmatory ultrasound in a week are legitimate confirmations.

D. General information

    1. Periods resume 4–8 weeks after tissue expelled from uterus

    2. Most physicians suggest abstinence for 1–2 weeks following miscarriage as well as contraception until at least first period arrives

VI. Evaluation of Recurrent Miscarriage

A. After thorough evaluation, over half of women have no identified cause (after only one or two miscarriages, vast majority of women have no identifiable cause)

B. Even after three consecutive miscarriages, probability of viable pregnancy with next conception still higher than 50% (this makes evaluation of treatment difficult as many pregnancies would be successful without treatment)

C. Specific problems

    1. Genetic: karyotype both parents to look for balanced translocations

    2. Anatomic: hysterosonogram or hysterosalpingogram to assess uterus for septum or significant intrauterine lesions such as submucous fibroids

    3. Immunologic:

        a. Antiphospholipid antibody syndrome

            i. Diagnosis

                (1) Lupus anticoagulant

                (2) Anticardiolipin antibodies

                (3) One or both positive on two occasions, at least 6 weeks apart

            ii. Treatment is heparin or low-dose aspirin

    4. Thombophilias: role in early pregnancy loss unclear

    5. Endocrine: luteal phase defect

        a. Postulated cause of early miscarriage in which ovary does not produce sufficient progesterone long enough to support pregnancy

        b. No compelling evidence that such a condition exists

        c. Low progesterone associated with abnormal pregnancy, not impaired ovarian function

        d. Progesterone supplementation has not been shown to be an effective treatment for miscarriage

    6. Infection (rare); workup as suggested by history

VII. Treatment of Miscarriage 16D

A. Expectant management

    1. Patient can simply wait for the natural process of expulsion to occur after the diagnosis of embryonic demise.

    2. Physical process typically involves a few hours of intense cramping and heavy bleeding that ends with the passage of the pregnancy tissue.

    3. NSAIDs can help manage the pain.

    4. Rarely, bleeding can be heavy enough to require medical treatment or even blood transfusion.

B. Schedule dilation and evacuation

    1. Benefits:

        a. Minimizes physical discomfort of expulsion

        b. Can be scheduled; eliminates uncertainty of waiting

    2. Risk:

        a. Probably not greater than that of the natural process

        b. Includes (but not limited to):

            i. Hemorrhage requiring blood transfusion

            ii. Damage to abdominal organs, requiring additional surgery to repair (uncommon and would occur chiefly through unrecognized uterine perforation)

            iii. Infection

            iv. Asherman syndrome: scarring of uterus that would prevent menses and reduce fertility (generally correctable)

            v. Incomplete procedure, necessitating a second surgery for persistent bleeding and cramping

C. Administer Rh(D) immunoglobulin to Rh-negative patients

    1. Evidence weak; isoimmunization very rare

    2. Generally given at time of tissue passage (as opposed to time of diagnosis of embryonic demise)

    3. For first-trimester pregnancies, reduced dose recommended

        a. Protects against transfusion of 2.5 mL of fetal blood

        b. Dose is 50 mg of Rh immune globulin

        c. Common U.S. brand name MICRhoGAM

        d. Also recommended for ectopic pregnancies

VIII. Diagnosis of Ectopic Pregnancy

A. Risk factors 15B

    1. Background risk: roughly 1 in 80 pregnancies

2. Prior ectopic pregnancy: risk rises 10-fold to 1 in 8
3. PID: often retrospective diagnosis at time of laparoscopy
4. Pregnancy with intrauterine device (IUD) or hormonal contraception
   a. Absolutely less likely than no contraception
   b. Intrauterine pregnancy more effectively prevented
5. Tubal ligation
   a. Half of pregnancies after tubal ligation are ectopic
   b. Absolute risk lower than without tubal ligation
6. Conception via assisted reproductive technology (risk increases with greater number of embryos transferred during in vitro fertilization [IVF])
7. Prior tubal surgery
8. Smoking: risk is actually directly dose-related

B. Symptoms 15C
   1. Bleeding
      a. Vast majority of patients with ectopic pregnancies have bleeding; typically abnormal in some way
      b. Very few patients have no bleeding since LMP by the time pregnancy diagnosed
   2. Abdominal pain and cramping
      a. Sometimes very difficult to distinguish from the normal, mild cramping often seen in early pregnancy or the tenderness associated with a large corpus luteum cyst
      b. Can be highly variable: constant, intermittent, sharp, dull, or achy
      c. Can occur on one side, both sides, in the middle, or radiate to the back
   3. Other
      a. Shoulder pain can occur with substantial intra-abdominal bleeding as result of diaphragmatic irritation
      b. GI symptoms: highly variable, as with normal pregnancy
      c. Hemorrhagic shock (ideally, most ectopic pregnancies diagnosed and treated before this time)

C. Diagnostic aids 15D
   1. hCG (slowly rising; plateauing)
   2. Progesterone <5 mg
   3. Ultrasound: no gestational sac with hCG of 1500 or greater

4. Culdocentesis: needle placed through vaginal vault behind uterus to check for intra-abdominal bleeding; largely replaced by ultrasound 〔4D〕

5. Laparoscopy: can directly visualize ectopic pregnancy, although with early or small cases diagnosis can be missed

6. Biopsy of uterine cavity (via endometrial biopsy or dilation and curettage)
   a. Can distinguish between nonviable uterine pregnancy (pregnancy tissue found on pathology) and ectopic (no pregnancy tissue found)
   b. Rarely necessary

7. If severe pain or hemorrhagic shock in presence of positive pregnancy test, proceed directly to laparoscopy or laparotomy (preferred if significant intra-abdominal bleeding suspected)

8. Location
   a. Ampullary (midportion of tube) majority (80%) of ectopic pregnancies
   b. Isthmic—12%
   c. Fimbrial—5%
   d. Other—all uncommon:
      i. Cornual and interstitial—can be particularly hard to diagnose and are disproportionately lethal (rupture here leads to more bleeding than in fallopian tube proper)
      ii. Abdominal
      iii. Cervical—gestational sac below level of internal os
      iv. Ovarian

9. Natural course
   a. Not all ectopic pregnancies end in rupture (only a minority)
   b. Many spontaneously miscarry
   c. A few go entirely unrecognized by patient or physician

10. Physical findings—almost never sensitive and specific enough to materially contribute to diagnosis
    a. Smaller than expected uterus (although still slightly enlarged)
    b. Mass and/or tenderness in one adnexa

D. Consider heterotopic pregnancy
   1. Multiple gestations in which at least one pregnancy in uterus and one outside

2. Risk estimated to be 1 in 10,000–40,000 in spontaneous conceptions

3. Higher risk in conceptions via assisted reproductive technology

4. Very difficult to diagnose

IX. Treatment of Ectopic Pregnancy 15E

A. Observation

    1. Appropriate for known or suspected ectopic with decreasing hCGs

    2. Once decline has been established, monitor hCG at least weekly until it falls to nonpregnant levels

B. Medical—treatment with methotrexate

    1. Requirements

        a. No evidence of intra-abdominal bleeding

        b. Normal pulse and blood pressure

        c. Highly compliant patient who will get follow-up testing and call for change in symptoms

        d. Absence of severe pain

    2. Use caution (success somewhat reduced) for hCG >10,000 mIU/mL or if fetal heart motion on ultrasound

    3. Contraindications to methotrexate include breastfeeding, liver disease, renal disease, hematologic abnormalities, active lung disease, peptic ulcer, and methotrexate sensitivity (unlikely to be known in advance)

    4. Laboratory evaluation (after hCG data have helped establish diagnosis): liver function tests, serum creatinine, complete blood count (CBC) with platelets

    5. Dose: methotrexate 50 mg/m^2 (need height and weight)

    6. Side effects

        a. Minor and self-limited: GI irritation (nausea, vomiting, diarrhea, stomatitis), alopecia, lung inflammation

        b. Serious (very uncommon) (leucovorin [active metabolite of folic acid] may be helpful): liver toxicity, bone marrow suppression

    7. Follow-up

        a. Pain may increase in days following treatment—pregnancy may separate from wall of tube and cause local bleeding ("tubal abortion")

b. hCG often rises in first several days after administration (not helpful to measure)

c. hCG at weekly intervals—should drop at least 15% and then steadily thereafter

d. hCG should be monitored to nonpregnant levels

C. Surgical

  1. Types of treatment:

  a. Linear salpingostomy: tube opened on antimesenteric border; pregnancy removed; bleeding cauterized; sometimes edge of opening oversewn in running "baseball" fashion

  b. Partial salpingectomy: portion of tube containing ectopic pregnancy clamped on either side and excised

  i. Indicated for intractable bleeding

  ii. Sometimes done with a second ectopic pregnancy in same location to reduce risk of recurrence on subsequent pregnancies

  iii. Also indicated for isthmic ectopic pregnancies as this portion of tube much more susceptible to obstruction (reanastomosis can take place in second procedure)

  c. Salpingectomy:

  2. All three procedures above can be done via laparoscopy or mini-laparotomy; laparotomy may be preferable with patient who has substantial intra-abdominal bleeding

  3. Persistent or chronic ectopic pregnancy is potential complication

  a. Ectopic tissue remains after surgical removal of bulk of pregnancy

  b. Can require additional or medical treatment

  c. hCGs should be monitored weekly to nonpregnant levels

  d. Some physicians give prophylactic methotrexate postoperatively to reduce chance of persistent, viable tissue

D. Subsequent fertility and ectopic risk appear similar when comparing medical and surgical treatment

MENTOR TIPS

- For women younger than age 50 years, do urine pregnancy tests.
- Most miscarriages will not have an emotionally satisfying explanation.
- Even after three miscarriages, the chance of carrying to viability exceeds 50% on the very next pregnancy with no intervention.
- Serum hCG levels separated by 2 or 3 days as well as ultrasound are key to establishing both early viability and location.
- The diagnosis and treatment of ectopic pregnancy has changed considerably in the past decade, from primarily relying on surgical intervention to primarily relying on nonsurgical diagnosis and medical treatment.

Resources

Benirschke K: Normal early development. In Creasy RK, Resnik R, Iams JD (eds): Maternal-fetal medicine: Principles and practice, 5th ed. Philadelphia, Saunders, 2004.

Management of recurrent pregnancy loss. American College of Obstetricians and Gynecologists Practice Bulletin 24. May, 2001.

Medical management of tubal pregnancy. American College of Obstetricians and Gynecologists Practice Bulletin 3. December, 1998.

Speroff L, Fritz MA: Clinical gynecologic endocrinology and infertility, 7th ed. Baltimore and Philadelphia, Lippincott Williams & Wilkins, 2004.

Chapter Self-Test Questions

Circle the correct answer. After you have responded to the questions, check your answers in Appendix A.

1. Which is generally *not* a cause of irregular vaginal bleeding in reproductive age women?

a. Ectopic pregnancy

b. Trauma

c. Gestational trophoblastic neoplasia

d. Ovarian cancer

2. Which has *not* occurred by 10 days after implantation?

    a. Trophoblast differentiation

    b. Blastocyst forms

    c. Endometrium undergoes decidual changes

    d. Chorionic villi cover entire embryo

3. Which is *not* true about symptoms of early pregnancy?

    a. Many women can tell they are pregnant before the urine pregnancy test is positive.

    b. Hyperemesis gravidarum is thought to have a psychological component reflecting the woman's ambivalence about pregnancy.

    c. Corticosteroids have been shown to be effective in treatment of hyperemesis gravidarum.

    d. The differential diagnosis of hyperemesis gravidarum includes multiple gestation and gestational trophoblastic neoplasia.

4. Which is *not* a risk factor for miscarriage?

    a. Well-controlled hypertension

    b. Diabetes

    c. Pregnancy loss in immediate past pregnancy

    d. Alcohol consumption of 21 drinks per week

See the testbank CD for more self-test questions.

BREAST DISEASE

Michael D. Benson, MD

I. Breast Cancer Epidemiology

A. Approximately 175,000 women in the United States diagnosed with breast cancer annually

B. Annual deaths from breast cancer: about 41,000

C. Lifetime risk for individual: 9%–11%

D. Mean and median age for breast cancer diagnosis: early 60s

E. Risk factors

    1. By history

        a. History of breast abnormalities (ductal carcinoma in situ [DCIS] and lobular carcinoma in situ [LCIS])

        b. Age (increasing age increases risk)

        c. Age at menarche (younger than age 12 increases risk)

        d. Age at first live birth (first-term pregnancy after 30 years or no term delivery increases risk)

        e. Race (white women at greater risk than black women)

        f. Breast cancer among first-degree relatives

        g. History of breast biopsies, regardless of actual disorder (believed that clinical decision to proceed with a biopsy identifies women at increased risk, although the precise mechanism is unclear)

        h. Alcohol use associated with increased risk; influence of obesity less clear

    2. Gail Model: published by National Institutes of Health (NIH); computer-calculated algorithm that generates 5-year risk percentage for women 35–59 years old to determine those who may benefit from prophylactic selective estrogen receptor modulators (SERMs), such as tamoxifen

        a. 5-year risk of 1.66% or greater would experience 50% reduction in breast cancer risk with prophylactic tamoxifen

 b. Historical information required
  i. Menses <12 years
  ii. First child >30 years
  iii. Childless
  iv. First-degree relative with breast cancer
  v. History of breast biopsy (fine needle or other)
  vi. Biopsy with DCIS or LCIS or atypical hyperplasia
3. Breast cancer in pregnancy
 a. Occurs roughly 1 in 3000 gestations
 b. Stage for stage, prognosis largely the same as for non-pregnant women of the same age
 c. Pregnancy continuation needs to be discussed with women in the first two trimesters who require radiation or systemic treatment

II. Breast Anatomy (Fig. 12.1)
 A. Blood supply
  1. Internal thoracic artery

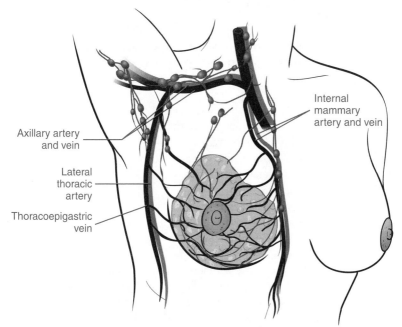

Internal mammary artery and vein

Axillary artery and vein

Lateral thoracic artery

Thoracoepigastric vein

FIGURE 12.1 **Breast vasculature and lymphatic system.**

      2. Medially: anterior intercostal arteries

      3. Laterally: axillary artery (pectoral branch, external mammary branch)

   B. Key lymph node groups for staging (see Fig. 12.1): axillary, internal mammary, infraclavicular, supraclavicular

   C. Nerves

      1. Thoracodorsal

         a. Branch of brachial plexus (C5–C7)

         b. Runs close to posterior axillary wall along ventral surface of subscapular muscle

         c. Innervated upper half of latissimus dorsi

      2. Long thoracic (descends along anterior axillary line or serratus anterior muscle)

      3. Intercostal brachial (cutaneous nerves that innervate skin of medial upper arm; pass across base of axilla)

      4. Medial and lateral pectoral (pass from axilla to lateral chest wall; supply both pectoral muscles)

III. History and Physical Examination of Breast

   A. History

      1. Lump characteristics (location, size, duration, consistency/firmness, number, tenderness, mobility)

      2. Does patient do breast self-exam regularly?

      3. Skin changes such as erythema, warmth, dimpling/retraction

      4. Related issues

         a. Family history of breast cancer

         b. Prior biopsies/mammograms

         c. History of recent trauma

         d. History of exercise/new activities

         e. Recent lactation/childbirth

      5. Nipple discharge

         a. Unilateral/bilateral

         b. Bloody or other

         c. Spontaneous or elicited

   B. Physical examination `40A`

      1. Seated upright and supine (for women under 40 years with no complaints, a supine examination may be satisfactory)

      2. Arms raised to facilitate axillary examination

      3. Press the middle three fingers of dominant hand gently against the breast tissue in a systematic fashion, moving circumferentially around the breast while stabilizing the area with the other hand

4. Follow breast tissue to axilla, and check axilla
5. Press gently; excessive pressure will encounter underlying muscles and ribs
6. Diffuse small irregularities common; nodules that stand out from the rest of breast tissue and are not symmetrical in the opposite breast merit further investigation
7. Note nipple inversion (particularly if new; often a normal, long-standing finding in many patients even if unilateral)

IV. Genetics and Preventive Surgeries

A. Two genes (*BRCA1* and *BRCA2*) strongly linked to development of breast cancer
B. Links to other gynecologic cancers have been discovered
C. Estimated that women with either of these gene mutations have up to 85% chance of developing breast cancer and increased risk (perhaps not as high) of developing ovarian cancer
D. Prophylactic mastectomies and oophorectomies are important options, although understanding of the role of these genes in development of cancer remains limited

V. Breast Cancer Screening

A. Breast self-examination 2B
    1. No evidence that it improves early detection or survival; some evidence that it does neither
    2. Benefit of discussion is that it may help reduce false-positives
        a. Emphasis on gentle pressure reduces chance patient presents for mass by palpating underlying muscle and ribs
        b. Emphasis on "new" and "persistent" lump reduces alarm over physiologic, cyclic changes in breast and breast irregularities that have not changed since adolescence
B. Mammography 41M
    1. Evidence of benefit in early detection and long-term survival weak
    2. Screening test only
        a. Substantial false-negative rate: 10% of women with biopsy-proven cancer have negative mammogram
        b. Substantial false-positive rate

       i. Significant public health issue in terms of expense of follow-up and distress caused in patients

     ii. 5%–15% of patients require additional testing

   iii. Estimated 30% of women ages 40–49 years have false-positive mammogram with annual screening; 8% require a biopsy

  c. Digital mammography might be slightly more sensitive than plain film studies

  d. Radiation dose = 0.7 mSV (annual background dose = 3 mSV); no discernible increased risk in cancer

3. Suggested regimen `7A`

  a. First screen "baseline" at age 35–40 years

  b. Annually at age 40 years

4. May be done during pregnancy and lactation, although may be more difficult to interpret

5. Primary utility is as a screening test in normal patients; not an appropriate test alone to determine whether a palpable breast lump is malignant or benign

C. Physician examination: optimal regimen or evidence for benefit not established `40A`

  1. Breast checked circumferentially, pressing lightly with three middle fingers

  2. Tail of breast extends upward under axilla and should be checked also

  3. Breast is mixture of adipose and glandular tissue; may not feel perfectly uniform, but examination focus is to find any area that feels distinctive from surrounding tissue

  4. Sometimes, examining the breast with patient seated and supine can make questionable findings more distinct

  5. For those patients complaining of discharge, nipple can be squeezed gently to confirm symptom

D. Discredited screening tests include ultrasonography (poor sensitivity and specificity), magnetic resonance imaging (MRI) (high false-positive rate), and thermal imaging

VI. Diagnostic Studies of Breast Lesion `40B`

  A. Breast aspiration

    1. Office procedure that can determine whether a dominant breast mass is solid or cystic. As cystic masses are almost never associated with malignancy, breast aspiration can be practically diagnostic.

   a. Swab the skin over the lesion with an alcohol wipe.

   b. Insert a syringe with a 21-gauge (or smaller) needle directly into the lump.

   c. Aspirate the lump.

2. The diagnosis of breast cyst is made if fluid is obtained and the lump in question shrinks substantially.

3. The fluid can range from clear to yellow, green, or brown. Clear fluid in particular is reassuring, although discolored fluid also is often associated with benign lesions.

4. Whether the aspirated fluid should be sent for cytology is controversial; test results usually provide little additional information.

5. If the fluid is to be sent, it can be spread thinly over a microscope slide and then fixed in the same way as a Pap smear.

6. Patient should return in 4 weeks for confirmation that mass has not returned.

7. Patient should be counseled to examine her breasts herself and to return for any new, persistent nodule.

B. MRI

1. Role in screening and diagnosis evolving

2. Not used for screening general population due to high false-positive rate

3. May be useful for those with *BRCA1* and *BRCA2* mutation

4. More expensive than mammography and takes longer

C. Ductal lavage/aspiration

1. Useful for attempting to localize size of bloody discharge

2. Very thin tube placed in duct opening for aspiration or lavage (typically done by general surgeons)

D. Ultrasound: chiefly used to determine if palpable lump is hollow (cystic) or solid; may be used to guide aspiration

E. Thin-needle aspiration 41N

1. Typically performed by radiologist

2. Uses specialized needle and syringe to make 10 to 20 rapid passes through the dominant mass while aspirating; three or four separate efforts are made to help ensure that the suspicious area is sampled

3. For suspicious areas that show up only on mammography, radiologist generally performs needle localization, in which a thin wire or needle is placed in breast to mark radiographically the area to be excised; after issue removed, tissue x-rayed again to ensure it was the abnormality seen in the original mammogram

4. Normal histology cannot absolutely prove that a specific area is benign because one cannot be absolutely sure that the right area is sampled; in many situations, however, the procedure can be sufficiently reassuring that a breast biopsy can be deferred

F. Core biopsy: large-gauge needle guided by palpation, ultrasound, or mammography to obtain tissue sample of sufficient size to assess tissue architecture (in contrast to thin-needle aspiration in which invasion is more difficult to assess); if done for suspicious microcalcifications, specimen x-rayed afterward to be sure proper sample was obtained

G. Open biopsy: area of concern removed under local anesthesia

VII. Clinical Approach to Dominant Mass

A. A nodule that has persisted for 4 weeks or more and is distinct from surrounding breast tissue

B. Determine whether solid or cystic: ultrasound or breast aspiration during examination

1. If cystic on scan or disappears with aspiration, malignancy possibility largely eliminated

2. If solid, tissue sample must be obtained using one of the procedures described above

C. A normal mammogram cannot prove that a palpable lump is benign

VIII. Benign Breast Disease 40C

A. "Fibrocystic breast disease"

1. No consensus on definition

2. No risk to health

3. Commonly refers to dense, nodular breasts that become painful cyclically; also a reference to breast that has "dense" appearance on mammography

4. Concept originated because patients with this designation were believed to be unusually difficult to examine

5. Probably should avoid this terminology

6. Historical link with caffeine consumption is debatable

B. Intraductal papilloma

    1. Most likely cause of bloody nipple discharge

    2. Diagnosis via fiberoptic ductaloscopy or ductal lavage (typically by a general surgeon)

    3. Treatment (if desired) is local excision

C. Fibroadenoma

    1. Smooth, mobile, nontender, solitary mass 2–3 cm although can grow quite large

    2. Requires core biopsy to confirm benign

    3. No treatment required unless patient desires; sometimes disappears spontaneously

D. Cystosarcoma phyllodes (benign phyllodes tumor)

    1. Can be benign, borderline, or malignant

IX. Medical Prevention

A. Selective estrogen receptor modulators (SERMs) can reduce risk of cancer in selected women by up to 50% in comparison with placebo

B. SERMs attach to some estrogen receptor sites and thereby reduce the effect of estrogen

C. Side effects include hot flashes and nausea

D. No benefit for vaginal dryness

E. Complications include deep venous thrombosis and endometrial cancer (more of a concern with tamoxifen than with later drugs)

X. Breast Cancer Staging 40©

A. Signs/symptoms of breast cancer

    1. Most palpable, malignant masses initially discovered by patients and brought to medical attention

    2. Most common finding is lump that is distinct from surrounding breast tissue that has persisted for more than 4 weeks

    3. Typically not painful

    4. Distribution: upper outer quadrant, 45%; nipple/areola, 25%; upper inner quadrant, 15%; lower outer quadrant, 10%; lower inner quadrant, 5%

B. Histologic types

    1. Infiltrating ductal carcinoma: 60%–70% of malignancies

    2. Medullary carcinoma: dense lymphocytic infiltration

    3. Mucinous (colloid) carcinoma: gelatinous appearance grossly

4. Infiltrating comedo carcinoma: histology—areas of necrosis
5. Inflammatory carcinoma: histologic features of infiltrating ductal carcinoma in which more than third of breast has erythema and edema
6. Paget disease: erosion of nipple in which biopsy reveals Paget cells (large cells with irregular nuclei); manifestation of underlying breast cancer
7. Carcinoma in situ (CIS): diagnosed by breast biopsy
   a. Lobular CIS
      i. Up to one third of patients develop breast cancer in either breast
      ii. Tumor usually multifocal; not a discrete mass
      iii. Close follow-up or occasionally prophylactic bilateral mastectomy appropriate
      iv. Typically occurs in premenopausal woman
      v. "Atypical lobular hyperplasia" may be precursor lesion
   b. Ductal CIS
      i. Up to two thirds of patients develop invasive cancer in the same breast
      ii. May be treated with mastectomy (within lymph node biopsy) or lumpectomy and radiation
      iii. More common in postmenopausal women
      iv. "Atypical ductal hyperplasia" may be precursor
C. Receptor determination
   1. Estrogen receptor positive: associated with better prognosis and improved responsiveness to cytotoxic and hormonal therapy
   2. Progesterone receptor positive: also associated with improved prognosis and responsiveness to therapy
   3. *Her-2/neu* growth factor receptor overexpression
      a. Determined by histologic staining of malignant tissue
      b. Receptor positive status associated with increased risk of recurrence
D. Tumor, node, metastasis (TMN): surgical/pathologic staging system
   1. Not intuitive
   2. Staging depends on very specific combinations of tumor size, status of lymph nodes, and presence or absence of distant metastases

3. Full details of staging information beyond scope of this chapter can be found in appropriate monographs
4. General principles regarding tumor, lymph node, and metastases classifications
   a. Tumor size
      i. T0 = no evidence of primary tumor
      ii. T1 = tumor less than 2 cm in greatest dimension
      iii. T2 = 2–5 cm or less in greatest dimension
      iv. T3 = >5 cm
      v. T4 = any size tumor with direct extension to skin or chest wall
   b. Lymph nodes (always ipsilateral; contralateral is metastatic disease)
      i. N0 = no lymph node metastases
      ii. N1 = cancer in movable lymph nodes
      iii. N2 =
         (1) Cancer in fixed or matted axillary nodes
         (2) Clinically apparent in internal mammary node ("clinically apparent" means palpable or detectable with mammography)
      iv. N3 =
         (1) Infraclavicular *or* supraclavicular nodes
         (2) Clinically apparent internal mammary nodes *and* axillary nodes
      v. pNX—regional lymph nodes cannot be assessed
   c. Distant metastases
      i. MX—cannot be assessed
      ii. M0—no distant metastases
      iii. M1—distant metastases
      iv. 85% go to bone, lung, liver
5. Stages 0–IV
   a. Stage 0: CIS
   b. Stage I: tumor <2 cm in diameter; no metastatic disease in lymph nodes
   c. Stage II: tumor >2 cm in diameter *or* any disease in axillary lymph nodes
   d. Stage III: tumor >5 cm *or* fixed or matted axillary nodes *or* clinically apparent internal mammary nodes

e. Stage IV: cancer outside of one breast and its contiguous lymph nodes

XI. Breast Cancer Treatment

A. Lumpectomy (segmental mastectomy) with sentinel node biopsy and follow-up radiation therapy
   1. Lumpectomy consists of removal of primary tumor with small border of normal tissue
   2. Sentinel node biopsy: dye injected into axillary lymphatics; one or two stained lymph nodes dissected
      a. If sentinel nodes negative, almost no chance of axillary metastases
      b. If positive, complete axillary lymph node dissection subsequently performed for regional control
      c. Commonly recommended for women with positive lymph nodes; may be of most benefit in those with premenopausal diagnosis
   3. Occasionally recommended for those with just local disease
   4. After a few weeks of healing from lumpectomy, treatment consists of 4500–5000 cGy of radiation in doses of 180–200 cGy per session
B. Cytotoxic therapy
   1. Cyclophosphamide, methotrexate, and 5-flourouracil for six cycles; benefits greater in younger women
   2. Alternative regimen gaining in usage is cyclophosphamide, adriamycin, and paclitaxel
   3. Usually recommended with positive lymph nodes, large tumors, or high-risk histologic types
C. Hormonal therapy
   1. Indicated for those positive for estrogen receptors, with or without positive lymph nodes
   2. Three classes of agents (Table 12.1)
      a. SERMs: block some actions of estrogen by occupying receptors
      b. Aromatase inhibitors: lower circulating estrogens in postmenopausal women
      c. Estrogen receptor downregulators: reduce or destroy estrogen receptors (have no estrogen-like actions, unlike SERMs)

TABLE 12.1	Hormonal Agents Used for the Treatment and Prevention of Breast Cancer		
Brand Name	Generic Name	Class (Mechanism)	Comments
Nolvadex	tamoxifen	SERM	Used for: 1) high risk, no CA 2) DCIS 3) invasive CA with + estrogen receptors
Evista	raloxifene	SERM	Ongoing studies; did reduce CA incidence in women being treated for osteoporosis
Fareston	toremifene	SERM	Approved in U.S. for advanced disease; does not seem to increase risk of endometrial CA
Arimidex	anastrozole	Aromatase inhibitor; type 2; nonsteroidal inhibitor (blocks aromatase temporarily)	Approved for women with early disease right after surgery
Femara	letrozole	Aromatase inhibitor; type 2; nonsteroidal inhibitor (blocks aromatase temporarily)	Approved for women with early disease right after surgery and for those who have finished 5 years of tamoxifen
Aromasin	exemestane	Aromatase inhibitor; type 2; steroidal inhibitor; blocks aromatase permanently	Approved for those with early disease and those who have completed 2–3 years of tamoxifen
Faslodex	fulvestrant	Estrogen receptor downregulator	Approved for advance hormone receptor positive breast CA

    3. Oophorectomy occasionally recommended for women with premenopausal disease (now largely replaced with tamoxifen)

    4. GnRH analogs may be followed with megestrol acetate (potent progestin) if patient experiences disease progression

D. *Her/neu-2* growth factor receptor targeting

    1. Overexpression occurs in up to 30% of population

    2. Appears to be significant response rate to intravenous monoclonal antibody against this receptor in combination with cisplatin

E. Modality choices

    1. Chemotherapy commonly recommended for those with tumors >1 cm

    2. Those with estrogen receptor–positive tumors also receive hormonal therapy

F. Mastectomy

    1. Halstead procedure: removal of breast, pectoral muscles, and axillary lymph nodes en block

    2. Extended radical mastectomy: additional removal of internal mammary lymph nodes

    3. Modified radical mastectomy: preservation of pectoral muscles

        a. Largely replaced more extensive surgeries above

        b. Is itself being replaced by segmental mastectomy, sentinel lymph node biopsy, radiation, and systemic therapy

---

 MENTOR TIPS

- Mammograms cannot prove that a solid mass is benign.
- A persistent solid breast lump requires tissue diagnosis.
- Breast cysts—fluid-filled breast lumps—are almost never associated with malignancy.
- Breast MRI is more sensitive than mammography but much less specific.

Resources

breastcancer.org

This Web site contains information about selective estrogen receptor modulators.

Chang SS, Haigh PI, Giuliano AE: Breast disease. In Berek JS, Hacker NF (eds): Practical gynecologic oncology, 4th ed. Sydney, Lippincott Williams & Wilkins, 2005.

http://www.myriadtests.com/provider

This Web site has specific information regarding risk assessment and BRCA testing indications and procedures.

Chapter Self-Test Questions

Circle the correct answer. After you have responded to the questions, check your answers in Appendix A.

1. A 40-year-old female presents with a palpable lump in her left breast that has persisted through one menstrual cycle. You are unable to aspirate fluid in the office, and a mammogram has benign findings. Your next step is to:

   a. Counsel the patient to return if the lump grows or changes.

   b. Have patient return for another examination in 3 months.

   c. Give tamoxifen for breast cancer prophylaxis.

   d. Arrange to have lump biopsy (fine-needle aspiration, core biopsy, open biopsy).

2. The most common cause for a bloody nipple discharge is:

   a. Intraductal carcinoma in situ.

   b. Intraductal papilloma.

   c. Cystosarcoma phyllodes.

   d. Fibroadenoma.

3. Which statement is *not* true about the demographics of breast cancer?

    a. Annual mortality is roughly 25% of rate of new diagnoses

    b. Median age is in early 50s

    c. Lifetime risk is roughly 10%

    d. Absence of term pregnancy associated with increased risk

4. Which risk factor does *not* apply to the Gail model?

    a. Race

    b. Weight

    c. History of prior biopsy (even if benign)

    d. History of intraductal carcinoma in situ

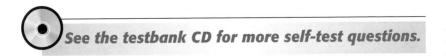

See the testbank CD for more self-test questions.

CHAPTER 13

INCONTINENCE AND PELVIC ORGAN PROLAPSE

Michael D. Benson, MD

I. Anatomy and Innervation of Urinary Tract (Fig. 13.1)
  A. Musculature
  1. Bladder: detrusor muscle is smooth muscle
     a. Capable of passive distention
     b. Contracts with voiding
  2. Urethra: consists of smooth and striated muscle
  B. Innervation: parasympathetic: void; sympathetic: hold
  1. Parasympathetic (S2–S4): cholinergic stimulation results in bladder contraction
  2. Sympathetic (T10–L2) alpha adrenergic: activation increases urethral pressure
  3. Sympathetic (T10–L2) beta adrenergic: activation decreases bladder tone
  4. Skeletal (pudendal nerve, S2–S4): voluntarily increases urethral pressure
  C. Epithelium: transitional epithelium lines bladder and urethra and is estrogen-sensitive

II. Urinary Incontinence and Other Voiding Difficulties 37B
  A. Overview
  1. Urinary incontinence
     a. Stress urinary incontinence (SUI): loss of urine with a sudden increase in abdominal pressure (such as with sneezing, laughter, or exercise); two types:
       i. Genuine stress incontinence
         (1) Urethral function and pressures normal (by far the most common)

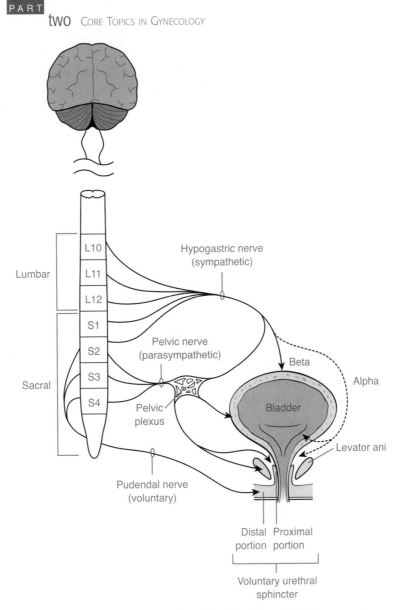

FIGURE 13.1 Innervation of the bladder and urethra.

(2) Classically attributed to urethral hypermobility

(3) Normally with Valsalva maneuver, urethra compressed behind pubis flexing the urethrovesical (UV) angle and thus promotes continence; with SUI, fibromuscular connective tissue supporting bladder and urethra compromised; bladder drops out of pelvis

(4) With increased abdominal pressure, pressure rises on top of bladder but not equally at the bladder neck

  ii. Instrinsic sphincteric deficiency ("low pressure urethra")

(1) Less common

(2) Urethra does not generate normal closing pressures; urine easier to push through with increasing pressure; also called "stovepipe urethra"

(3) Results from denervation of urethra through surgery or radiation; other causes include scarring, medication

b. Urge incontinence: also known as detrusor instability or overactive bladder (OAB)

  i. Uncontrolled contractions of bladder musculature can lead to involuntary expulsion of urine

  ii. Bladder spasms can occur randomly but can also be triggered by activity, increases in abdominal pressure, or a filling bladder

  iii. Symptoms include sudden urge to void and frequent voidings during the day and getting up to void more than once per night

c. Mixed incontinence: symptoms of both stress and urge incontinence

d. Nocturnal enuresis

e. Continuous incontinence: constant urine loss with the concomitant inability to void significant amounts

  i. Can suggest urinary tract fistula

(1) Fistulous tract can occur almost anywhere in the urinary system and most commonly exits through the vagina

(2) Fistulas can be result of malignancies, surgical injuries, or complications of radiation treatment

      ii. Can also result from neurologic conditions, particularly central nervous system (CNS) dysfunction, such as Alzheimer, and demyelinating disorders such as multiple sclerosis

    f. Overflow incontinence: classic symptoms are uncontrollable dribbling of urine and inability to generate strong urine stream

      i. Results from a chronically overfilled bladder

      ii. May be caused obstruction of the urethra (such as by a tumor) or bladder hypotonia, typically from neurologic disease either in the CNS or the peripheral nerves innervating the bladder

2. Other types of voiding difficulties, which can reduce quality of life without resulting in actual incontinence, are nocturia, urgency, frequency, and urinary hesitancy/retention

3. Epidemiology

    a. Not normal process of aging but prevalence increases with age: 20% among young adult women and perhaps 40% among older women

    b. Childbearing strongly associated with stress incontinence—particularly vaginal birth—although relationship problematic

      i. Not all parous women incontinent

      ii. Not all nulliparous women continent

      iii. Continence not always closely linked with extent of injury during childbirth in all studies

    c. Other risk factors include obesity, family history, postmenopausal estrogen use, pelvic surgeries (including hysterectomy and rectal surgery), lung disease, possibly smoking (unclear in absence of lung disease), and dietary risks (alcohol, caffeine [latter particularly with urge incontinence])

    d. Medications linked to incontinence include angiotensin-converting enzyme (ACE) inhibitors, alpha-adrenergic antagonists, benzodiazepines, calcium channel blockers, loop diuretics, opioids, and sympatholytics

B. History 37A, 37C

  1. Frequency (episodes per day/week/month)

  2. Volume lost

3. Precipitating events

4. Trend (same, better, worse)

5. Number of voids per day

6. Number of voids during sleep (nocturia)

7. Past medical history including pregnancies and pelvic or vaginal surgery and radiation

8. Current medications

9. Anal incontinence (flatus or stool)

10. Voiding diary or log for 3–7 days

   a. Prospective record of time and amount of fluid intake, voids, leaking episodes, and activities during time of the incontinent episode

   b. Can be done quantitatively

   i. Voiding volumes via collection hat in toilet

   ii. Incontinence volumes deduced from use of tarred pads stored in sealed plastic bags and reweighed after use

   iii. Rarely useful in clinical setting

C. Physical examination

1. Rarely diagnostic by itself, but like the history, it can narrow the possibilities; findings of particular interest include:

   a. Abdominal scars

   b. Abdominal masses

   c. Presence and amount of herniation into the vagina of bladder, uterus, small bowel, or rectum

   d. Pelvic masses (particularly enlargements of uterus or ovaries)

   e. Anal tone

   f. Presence of a fistula (occasionally visible or palpable)

D. Diagnostic tests

1. Office tests without special equipment

   a. Urinalysis, culture (occult urinary tract infection [UTI] can cause/aggravate incontinence)

   b. Q-tip test: Q-tip covered with 5% lidocaine gel gently inserted into urethra to the level of bladder neck (UV junction); with patient in lithotomy position, the resting angle of the Q-tip relative to the floor is then noted, followed by a measurement of straining angle; normal angle <30 degrees; greater angles suggest urethral hypermobility, which is consistent with stress incontinence

c. Witnessed incontinence episode: have patients perform a provocative maneuver such as coughing or bouncing on their heels while they have a full bladder and the urethral meatus is under direct observation; particularly good idea to witness incontinence before performing any surgical corrective procedure

d. Postvoid residual: volume of urine remaining in the bladder after voiding; measured by straight catheterization within a few minutes after a void
  i. <50 mL normal
  ii. > 200 mL suggests urinary retention; neurologic workup might be appropriate
  iii. No consensus on meaning of volumes in between (<100 mL probably normal)

2. Advanced testing: urodynamic testing (not a precise term)
  a. Cystometry—measurement of one or more pressures related to voiding as the bladder is being filled with either carbon dioxide gas or a fluid such as saline; three common pressures are measured either simultaneously or consecutively: bladder, intra-abdominal, and urethral; sensing devices can employ water manometry, intraluminal computer chips, or other technologies
    i. Terminology often associated with testing; "channel" refers to number of outputs—not the number of inputs—continuously recorded by the measuring device; typical graphic output arrayed as:
      (1) Channel 1: bladder (detrusor) pressure
      (2) Channel 2: intra-abdominal pressure (sensor in vagina or rectum)
      (3) Channel 3: urethral pressure
      (4) Channel 4: true detrusor pressure (bladder minus intra-abdominal pressure)
      (5) Channel 5: true urethral pressure (urethral minus intra-abdominal pressure)
      (6) Channel 6: true urethral pressure minus true bladder pressure (if a negative number, urine should be lost)
    ii. During cystometrogram patient asked to indicate:
      (1) First sensation: when she first senses bladder filling
      (2) Second sensation: when she would normally void

(3) Third sensation: when she can no longer tolerate further filling
  iii. No universally accepted "normals" for these values
    (1) Most can hold 500 mL of fluid
    (2) Provocative maneuvers such as coughing or dropping on heels are performed to replicate conditions in which urine is lost
    (3) Occasionally maneuvers trigger a detrusor contraction that can be measured, thereby distinguishing detrusor instability from genuine stress incontinence
  iv. Urethral pressure measurements
    (1) Obtained by having two pressure-sensing foramens in the bladder catheter or by slowly withdrawing pressure-sensing catheter along urethra
    (2) Difference between maximum urethral pressure and resting bladder pressure is maximum urethral closure pressure
    (3) Values less than 20 cm of water suggest a diagnosis of low-pressure urethra
    (4) Functional length of urethra can be measured this way
    (5) Leak point pressure: intravesical pressure at which urine leakage occurs due to increased abdominal pressure in absence of detrusor contraction
  b. Other tests
    i. Uroflowmetry consists of timing length and volume of voiding
      (1) Can be done simply with a graduated urine collection basin and a stopwatch or with electronic devices
      (2) More useful for men with prostatic hypertrophy, but occasionally helpful for women who complain of hesitancy
    ii. Urethrocystoscopy: observation of mucosal surface of urethra and bladder
      (1) Mobility of UV junction during provocative maneuvers such as coughing noted
      (2) Lack of mobility suggests "frozen" urethra (low-pressure urethra or intrinsic sphincteric deficiency)

E. Treatment

    1. Stress incontinence

        a. Nonsurgical treatment: limited efficacy and/or requires substantial patient effort

            i. Therapy to strengthen voluntary skeletal muscle

                (1) Weighted vaginal cones: commercial weights held in place for increasing length of times and amounts of weight

                (2) Pelvic floor physical therapy

                (3) Kegel exercises: repetitive voluntary isometric contraction of pelvic floor muscles (much more effective with biofeedback and pelvic floor physical therapy)

            ii. Medical treatment

                (1) Alpha-adrenergic agents

                (2) Local estrogen in postmenopausal women: thickens vaginal epithelium and lower urethra and makes more compliant

        b. Surgical treatment: more effective although few randomized studies comparing techniques; "suburethral" sling procedures recommended for subset of patients with instrinsic sphincteric deficiency

            i. Abdominal procedures

                (1) Marshall-Marchetti-Krantz: sutures attach tissue lateral to urethra to periosteum of posterior symphysis

                (2) Burch: sutures attach tissue lateral to urethra to Cooper ligament (on top of symphysis, extending laterally); laparoscopic approach probably less effective

                (3) Suburethral sling procedure: placement of sling material underneath urethra with ends fixed to abdominal site

            ii. Vaginal procedures

                (1) Anterior colporrhaphy: plication of connective tissue lateral to bladder to help support it; not very effective for incontinence

                (2) Needle urethropexy: sutures pass under urethra and fixed to Cooper ligament or abdominal fascia (Pereyra, Stamey, Raz procedures)

                (3) Sling procedures: materials include porcine collagen, cadaver fascia, patient's fascia from abdominal wall or thigh, polypropylene mesh

(4) Tension-free vaginal tape (TVT): placement of polypropylene mesh beneath urethra without displacement of urethra; ends not fixed to tissue; typically outpatient procedure

   (A) Retropubic approach: material passed beneath urethra and behind symphysis; forms U-shaped support

   (B) Obturator approach: material passed through obturator foramen and beneath urethra; forms hammock-shaped support

   (C) Simple vaginal approach: much shorter mesh positioned beneath urethra through vaginal incision; forms partial bottom portion of U-shaped or hammock support

   (D) Complications: erosion of sling into vagina, urethra, bladder; infection; perforation of pelvic viscera during placement; inflammatory response to mesh (extremely rare)

iii. Transurethral injections

  (1) Intrinsic sphincteric deficiency (low-pressure or immobile urethra)—glutaraldehyde cross-linked bovine collagen can be injected during an office procedure just distal to the bladder neck; this added bulk narrows caliber of urethra, thus promoting continence

   (A) More than one injection often required

   (B) Benefits last from months to years

  (2) Urinary stress incontinence with or without intrinsic sphincteric deficiency: ethylene vinyl alcohol copolymer

   (A) Often more than one injection required

   (B) Benefits last from months to years (relatively new product)

iv. Other

  (1) Artificial sphincters: limited utility due to high complication rate

  (2) Ureteral diversion

2. Urgency, frequency, and urge incontinence

  a. Behavior modification (fluid restriction, time voiding/bladder training, Kegel exercises)

  b. Pelvic floor physical therapy and biofeedback

  c. Medication (Table 13.1)

TABLE 13.1   **Medications for Detrusor Instability (Overactive Bladder)**

Generic Name (Brand Name)	Usual Dosage	Mechanism of Action	Side Effects	Contraindications and/or Precautions
Propantheline bromide 15 mg (Pro-Banthine)	1 tablet bid to 2 tablets four × day	Anticholinergic	Dry mouth, reduced sweating, tachycardia, blurred vision, constipation, urinary retention	Narrow-angle glaucoma, intestinal obstruction, ulcerative colitis, myasthenia gravis
Hyoscyamine 0.15 mg (extended release 0.375 mg) (Cystospaz)	1 or 2 tablets up to four × day; extended release, q12h	Anticholinergic	Dry mouth, reduced sweating, tachycardia, blurred vision, constipation, urinary retention	Narrow-angle glaucoma, intestinal obstruction, ulcerative colitis, myasthenia gravis
Tolterodine tartrate 2- and 4-mg tablets (Detrol LA)*	One tablet (2 mg) bid	Anticholinergic, muscarinic receptor antagonist	Dry mouth, reduced sweating, blurred vision, constipation	Urinary retention, narrow-angle glaucoma, gastric retention, may prolong QT interval
Oxybutynin chloride 5 mg (Ditropan, Ditropan LA, Oxytrol patch)	½ tablet bid to 1 tablet four × day; long-acting: 5, 10, or 15 mg once daily Patch—change twice weekly	Antispasmodic, anticholinergic, muscarinic receptor antagonist	Dry mouth, reduced sweating, tachycardia, blurred vision, constipation, urinary retention	Narrow-angle glaucoma, intestinal obstruction, ulcerative colitis, myasthenia gravis

Solifenacin succinate (Vesicare)	5 or 10 mg tablet once daily	Anticholinergic—muscarinic receptor antagonist	Dry mouth, reduced sweating, blurred vision, constipation	Urinary retention, gastric retention, uncontrolled narrow-angle glaucoma; may prolong QT interval
Darifenacin (Enablex)	7.5 mg or 15 mg once daily	Anticholinergic—muscarinic receptor antagonist (M3-specific)	Dry mouth, reduced sweating, blurred vision, constipation	Urinary retention, gastric retention, uncontrolled narrow-angle glaucoma
Dicyclomine hydrochloride, 10 mg (Bentyl)	1 tablet bid to 4 tablets four × day	Antispasmodic, anticholinergic	Dry mouth, reduced sweating, tachycardia, blurred vision, constipation, urinary retention	Narrow-angle glaucoma, intestinal obstruction, ulcerative colitis, myasthenia gravis
Flavoxate hydrochloride 100 mg (Urispas)	1 or 2 tablets three to four × day	Antispasmodic	Dry mouth, tachycardia, blurred vision	Intestinal obstruction, urinary retention
Nifedipine 10 mg (Procardia)	10 mg bid to 30 mg four × day	Calcium channel blocker	Edema, flushing, nausea, headache	Congestive heart failure, severe hypotension or increasing angina after starting drug
Imipramine pamoate hydrochloride 75, 100, 125, 150 mg (Tofranil-PM)	75 mg to 150 mg daily	Adrenergic agonist, anticholinergic	Palpitations, confusion, dry mouth	Concomitant use of monoamine oxidase inhibitors, arrhythmias, glaucoma

    i. Cholinergic stimulation of parasympathetic system (S2–S4) results in bladder contraction; medications typically exert anticholinergic effect

    ii. Side effects related to anticholinergic effects: blurred vision, reduced intestinal motility, dry mouth and eyes

    iii. Acetylcholine bound by muscarinic or nicotinic receptors; bladder physiology governed by muscarinic receptors

III. Pelvic Organ Prolapse (Herniation) 37D

A. Over time connective tissue supports of pelvic organs can lose their elasticity, resulting in herniation of uterus, bladder, or rectum into vagina and even through vaginal opening

  1. Urethrocele: urethral descent along anterior vaginal wall

  2. Cystocele: bladder prolapse through anterior wall of vagina

  3. Uterine prolapse: procidentia—organ has fallen through vaginal opening

  4. Rectocele: rectal herniation through posterior wall of vagina

  5. Enterocele: small intestinal herniation (behind cervix or near top of vagina); can be difficult to distinguish from rectocele preoperatively

B. International Continence Society pelvic organ prolapse grading system[1]

  1. Staging applies to maximum extent of prolapse observed with straining, whether patient is in dorsal lithotomy position, sitting, or standing

  2. Stage descriptions

    a. Stage 0: no significant prolapse (no leading edge of prolapsed organ within 2 cm of hymen)

    b. Stage I: leading edge of organ within 1–2 cm of hymen

    c. Stage II: leading edge within 1 cm proximal or distal to hymen

    d. Stage III: leading edge 1–2 cm distal to hymen

    e. Stage IV: leading edge of prolapsing organ at least 2 cm distal to hymen

  3. Staging system is simplification of pelvic organ prolapse quantification system (POP-Q) (see reference[1])

C. Symptoms of prolapse

  1. Incontinence

    a. Can be symptom of a cystocele

    b. Paradoxically, as cystocele worsens, stress incontinence may be resolved due to kinking of urethra

    c. Urge incontinence

  2. Pelvic pressure, aching (includes dyspareunia, back pain, abdominal pain)

  3. Protrusion of organ through vagina (can be intermittent or constant; can vary with activity or position)

  4. Constipation

  5. "Splinting," replacement of rectum with finger pushing vaginal bulge back through the introitus to defecate

  6. Asymptomatic

    a. Mild amounts of prolapse usually produce no symptoms

    b. Symptoms can be highly variable from patient to patient with same stage of prolapse

    c. Not a common cause of urinary retention

D. Treatment of prolapse 37E

  1. Pessary: silicone vaginal insert that provides support for pelvic organs

    a. Typically have openings to provide drainage of vaginal discharge

    b. Should be removed monthly and washed with soap and water; patients with disabilities may have difficulty doing this by themselves

    c. Estrogen cream can be used twice weekly to reduce vaginal erosions where pessary comes into contact with mucosal surfaces

    d. Many different shapes; no evidence-based data to support one type over another

      i. Ring/doughnut: commonly used for uterine prolapse and cystocele

      ii. Gelhorn (mushroom-shaped): used for severe uterine or vaginal vault prolapse

      iii. Cube: can be used for prolapse of top, anterior, and posterior walls of vagina

  2. Surgery

    a. Cystocele, rectocele: anterior or posterior colporrhaphy

      i. Dissection of vaginal mucosa off underlying rectovaginal (or vesicovaginal) fascia (often compromised tissue of poor quality and difficult to identify)

ii. Excess vaginal tissue is excised

iii. Underlying fascia brought together in midline by placing sutures as far laterally as possible and tying them together

iv. Vaginal mucosa re-approximated by sutures

v. Recurrence rate over time fairly high so new approaches include placement of nonabsorbable mesh beneath anterior or posterior vaginal mucosa supported by arms of mesh material placed into adjacent tissue

vi. Sometimes distinction made between central and lateral defects, with emphasis on repairing the specific anatomical defect (e.g., paravaginal repair); limited outcomes data so far do not show benefit from this concept

b. Enterocele: typically encountered during other vaginal surgery

i. Identify peritoneal sac containing small intestine

ii. Dissect and excise sac

iii. Close peritoneum in purse-string fashion

iv. When possible, suture uterosacral ligaments together

c. Uterine prolapse

i. Vaginal hysterectomy

ii. Vaginal vault suspension: with prolapse of vagina to hymen or behind, subsequent vaginal vault prolapse is concern:

(1) Vaginal approach: sacrospinous vault suspension anchors top of vagina to sacrospinous ligament through nonabsorbable sutures

(2) Abdominal approach: vault can be suspended either by suturing it to artificial graft material, which in turn is sutured to sacrum, or by freeing up strips of abdominal fascia and using these to suspend the vagina to the anterior abdominal wall

(3) LeFort procedure: obliteration of vagina

(A) For patients too infirm to tolerate a hysterectomy and who are no longer sexually active

(B) Partially denuded anterior and posterior walls of vagina sewn together; small canal left in middle of vagina for egress of mucus and secretions

IV. Interstitial Cystitis

A. Chronic (9 months or more) hypersensitivity condition of bladder that constitutes a clinical syndrome with no clear definition; attributed to loss of glycosaminoglycan layer (GAG)

B. Symptoms (highly variable) may include urinary frequency, urinary urgency, dysuria, bladder pain, or pelvic pain

C. Other clinical characteristics
   1. Tender urethra, bladder, vulva on palpation
   2. Most common in women in ages 30s and 40s
   3. May be associated with other chronic conditions (chronic fatigue syndrome, fibromyalgia, irritable syndrome)

D. Diagnostic testing (limited sensitivity and specificity)
   1. Sterile urine (UTI must be ruled out)
   2. Cystocscopy with bladder distention under anesthesia shows glomerulations (petechiae) or Hunner ulcers
   3. Potassium sensitivity test
      a. 40 mL sterile water instilled into bladder, held for 5 minutes, pain/urgency rated, void
      b. Process repeated with 40 mL of 0.4 molar KCl
      c. Pain or urgency score increase of 2 or greater considered positive result

E. Treatment
   1. Oral: pentosan polysulfate sodium (Elmiron)
      a. Approved by U.S. Food and Drug Adminstration for this purpose
      b. Dose is 100 mg three times daily
      c. Benefit might take 4–6 months to appear
      d. Other drugs less specific but may be helpful and include drugs for urgency, amitriptyline, hydroxyzine, and gabapentin
   2. Intravesical instillation: dimethylsulfoxide (DMSO), gluco-corticoids, heparin, local anesthetics, Elmiron, silver nitrate

V. Anal Incontinence

A. Demographics
   1. Up to 15% in women over 50[2]
   2. Significant minority of women

B. Risk factors and pathophysiology
   1. Obstetric injury (recognized or unrecognized)

   a. Direct tear or rupture of anal sphincter

   b. Pudendal neuropathy during second stage

  2. Fistulas (Crohn disease, etc.)

  3. Neurologic disorder

   a. Central nervous system (dementia, sedation, multiple sclerosis, neoplasm)

   b. Peripheral (diabetes, localized neuropathy)

  4. Illnesses causing diarrhea—irritable syndrome and inflammatory bowel disease

 C. Diagnosis

  1. History

   a. Urgency, frequency of defecation, number of times per day or week, consistency

   b. Involuntary loss of gas, liquid, or solid

  2. Physical examination

   a. Assessment of rectal tone by digital examination

   b. Voluntary contraction (concentric contraction; anal verge should be pulled inward)

   c. Anal wink: tap skin to side of rectum, anus should contract, confirms motor competence S2–S4

   d. Light-touch sensation of perineum; sensory component of S2–S4

  3. Diagnostic testing

   a. Manometry: objective measure of anal sphincter pressure during contraction

   b. Transanal ultrasound: internal anal sphincter can be visualized directly

   c. EMG: largely investigational; variety of techniques (surface, concentric needle, pudendal nerve)

 D. Treatment

  1. Early diagnosis and treatment help limit muscle atrophy

  2. Biofeedback and pelvic floor physical therapy: same principles as for urinary urge incontinence

  3. Overlapping sphincteroplasty: reconstruction of torn anal sphincter

  4. Other: artificial sphincter, fecal diversion

VI. UTIs 36J

 A. Definitions

  1. Bacteriuria: colonies of 100,000 or more of a single bacterial species in a urine culture

    a. Occasionally more than one bacteria type can be cultured

    b. In the presence of symptoms, fewer than 100,000 may be clinically significant

  2. Asymptomatic bacteriuria: presence of colonies of 100,000 or greater in absence of symptoms

  3. Lower UTI: cystitis ("bladder infection")

  4. Upper UTI: pyelonephritis ("kidney infection")

B. Pathophysiology

  1. 50 times more common in premenopausal women than in men of similar age

  2. Most cases result from direct ascension of bacteria into bladder or kidneys; rarely can occur from hematogenous spread from systemic infection

  3. Offending bacteria

    a. Community-acquired: *Escherichia coli* 75%, *Staphylococcus saprophyticus* 10%

    b. Hospital-acquired: *E. coli* 50%; gram-negative 40% (*Klebsiella, Proteus, Enterobacter,* and *Serratia* species); gram-positive 10% *Enterococcus faecalis, S. saprophyticus, Staphylococcus aureus*

C. Cystitis

  1. Symptoms: dysuria, hematuria, frequency, urgency

  2. Diagnosis

    a. Specimen collection

      i. Clean catch, midstream urine

        (1) Urethral meatus wiped from front to back with mild disinfectant

        (2) Labia separated to avoid contact with urine stream

        (3) Initial stream not collected

        (4) 10 mL or so before end of stream collected in sterile container

      ii. Catheterized specimen

        (1) Urethral meatus swabbed with disinfectant

        (2) Lubricated, disposable catheter placed through meatus into bladder

        (3) Particularly useful if patient experiencing vaginal bleeding or vaginal discharge, making clean catch difficult to obtain

    b. Urinalysis

      i. Chemical dipstick—common findings

           (1) White blood cells (WBCs)

           (2) Occult blood

           (3) Leukocyte esterase: released by lysed WBCs; corresponds to presence of WBCs in urine; not terribly sensitive or specific

           (4) Nitrites: highly specific, not very sensitive; product of bacterial metabolism

        ii. Microscopic: red blood cells (RBCs), WBCs, and bacteria; epithelial cells suggest vaginal contamination

    c. Urine culture: colonies of 100,000 in women (10,000 in men) of single bacteria species

    d. Hematuria in absence of bacteriuria warrants further investigation, typically with cystoscopy and computed tomography (CT) of pelvis and abdomen to check for stones or urologic neoplasm (microscopic hematuria is renal cell carcinoma until proved otherwise)

  3. Treatment

    a. Often empirical: patients occasionally treated without urinalysis or urine culture depending on clinical circumstances

    b. 3-day course common initial treatment

      i. Trimethoprim/sulfamethoxazole (Bactrim and Septra) (increasing resistance of *E. coli*): do not use in last 4 weeks of pregnancy (newborn kernicterus risk)

      ii. Fluoroquinolones (do not use in pregnancy)

      iii. Nitrofurantoin

      iv. Cephalosporins

      v. Many organisms resistant to penicillin

    c. Complicated cystitis: cystitis in patients with significant co-existing medical conditions (e.g., diabetes, pregnancy, immune disorders, cancer, recurrence of symptoms) can make treatment less likely to succeed

      i. Treat for 7 days (or longer)

      ii. Should usually obtain urinalysis and culture

D. Pyelonephritis

  1. Symptoms

    a. Flank, back pain

    b. Fever (>100.4°F or 38°C); fevers above 103°F not uncommon; fever is key distinguishing feature from cystitis

    c. Cystitis symptoms

    d. Nausea, vomiting

    e. Chills, rigors

2. Diagnosis

    a. Cystitis symptoms with fever (often with costovertebral angle tenderness) and positive urinalysis (followed by positive culture)

    b. Signs of sepsis common; septic shock can occur in elderly hospitalized patients

    c. Serum WBC count commonly elevated

3. Treatment: empirical until results of culture and sensitivity known

    a. Outpatient candidates are those with:

        i. No significant co-existing morbidities (pregnancy, cancer, diabetes, immune problems)

        ii. Little diagnostic uncertainty

        iii. Good compliance

        iv. No nausea/vomiting

    b. 14 days of antibiotic treatment commonly recommended; compliance for this length of time poor

    c. Inpatient treatment

        i. Continued until patient afebrile with oral antibiotics; continued as outpatient

        ii. Preferred antibiotics

            (1) Third-generation cephalosporins (Ceftrioxone)

            (2) Penicillin with beta-lactam inhibitors (Unisyn, Zosyn)

            (3) Fluoroquinolones

        iii. Symptoms usually improve within 3 days (often as soon as 24 hours)

E. Recurrent cystitis—three episodes in a year

    1. Urinalysis and culture become more important to establish that symptoms have a bacterial origin

    2. Diagnostic testing typically involves CT scan to check for stones or urinary tract anomalies

    3. Cystoscopy may be appropriate but has a low yield of diagnostic findings

4. Prophylaxis regimens

    a. Voiding immediately following intercourse (common practice anyway, not terribly effective)

    b. Single antibiotic dose immediately following intercourse

    c. Low-dose daily prophylaxis for 3–6 months

 MENTOR TIPS

- The tension-free vaginal tape (TVT) surgical procedure is gaining popularity for treatment of stress incontinence. Typically an outpatient procedure, it requires little downtime for recovery and has good efficacy.
- Urgency, frequency, and urge incontinence can be effectively treated with a variety of medications (see Table 13.1) or pelvic floor physical therapy with biofeedback.
- Surgical correction of severe cystoceles often involves an anti-incontinence procedure at the same time.
- Surgical treatment of severe uterine prolapse (to introitus and beyond) often requires a specific procedure at the time of hysterectomy to suspend the vaginal vault to prevent subsequent vaginal vault prolapse.
- Patients with three UTIs in a year would benefit from further investigation and several months of prophylactic antibiotic treatment.

References

1. Bump RC, Mattiasson A, Bø K, et al: The standardization of terminology of female pelvic organ prolapse and pelvic floor dysfunction. American Journal of Obstetric Gynecology 175:10–17, 1996.

2. Roberts RO: Prevalence of combined fecal and urinary incontinence: A community-based study. Journal of the American Geriatric Society 47:837–841, 1999.

Resources

Bend AE, Ostergard DR, Cundiff GW, et al (eds): Ostergard's urogyne-
cology and pelvic floor dysfunction, 5th ed. Philadelphia, Lippincott
Williams & Wilkins, 2003.

Feener D, Fisher JR, Moen M, et al: Clinical management of urinary
incontinence. Association of Professors of Gynecology and Obstetrics
and Medical Education Collaborative. Golden, Colo., APGO, 2004.

Chapter Self-Test Questions

Circle the correct answer. After you have responded to the questions,
check your answers in Appendix A.

1. A 40-year-old G2 P2002 patient hospitalized with community-acquired
pyelonephritis has a urine culture preliminary report showing
gram-positive cocci. Her likely organism is:

a. *E. coli.*

b. *S. saprophyticus.*

c. Group B beta-hemolytic streptococcus.

d. *Klebsiella pneumonia.*

2. A 60-year-old patient presents to your office with urgency and
frequency and occasional bouts of urine loss on her way to the
bathroom. Which is the most appropriate first step in her evaluation
and treatment?

a. Urinalysis and culture

b. Detrol LA or pelvic floor physical therapy

c. Urodynamics for diagnosis

d. Schedule a TVT on an outpatient basis

3. Which is the least common complication of TVT?

a. Infection

b. Erosion

c. Perforation of pelvic viscera

d. Immune response to mesh itself

4. A 75-year-old female complains of difficulty emptying her bladder. Her straight catheterized post-void residual is 200 mL. Possible diagnoses include all the following *except:*

a. Multiple sclerosis.

b. Diabetic neuropathy.

c. Radiation injury.

d. Mild cystocele.

See the testbank CD for more self-test questions.

14

VULVAR AND VAGINAL SYMPTOMS

Michael D. Benson, MD

I. Vaginal Infections
  A. Normal findings 35A
    1. Discharge
      a. Scant to moderate amount
      b. Clear to white
      c. Acidic pH <4.5
      d. No significant odor
    2. Bacteria
      a. Lactobacilli normal
      b. Absent: *Trichomonas,* yeast, gonorrhea, *Chlamydia*
  B. Vaginal infection findings and treatments 35B
    1. Symptoms
      a. External itching, burning "raw" feeling
      b. Dyspareunia
      c. Discharge
        i. Not clear or white: yellow, green, creamy
        ii. Increased amount
        iii. Malodorous
    2. Examination
      a. Discharge
        i. Increased quantity, odor, color (as noted above)
        ii. Cottage-cheese appearance suggests *Candida*
      b. pH evaluation
        i. <4.5: normal or *Candida*
        ii. >4.5: Bacterial vaginosis, trichomoniasis
      c. Cervical appearance
        i. Strawberry cervix

      (1) Red spots covering cervix

      (2) Suggestive of trichomoniasis

    ii. Purulent discharge: suspect gonorrhea or *Chlamydia*

d. Wet mount

    i. Discharge placed on slide

    ii. Left half: one drop normal saline

    iii. Right half: one drop 10% potassium hydroxide

    iv. Cover slip to each side

    v. Saline findings

      (1) Abundant white blood cells

      (2) Clue cells: epithelial cells covered by bacteria (coccobacilli); spotty appearance cultureand sensitivity for bacterial vaginosis

      (3) Trichomonads (moving)

      (4) Lactobacilli normal; absence suggests bacterial vaginosis

    vi. Potassium hydroxide findings

      (1) Dissolves epithelial cells

      (2) Leaves mycelia ("yeast") more easy to discern, if present

      (3) Fishy odor suggests bacterial vaginosis ("whiff" test)

e. Laboratory testing

    i. Culture: not sensitive or specific

    ii. DNA probes

      (1) Commercially available kits for vaginitis: *Candida, Trichomoniasis, Gardnerella*

      (2) Combination probes for STIs: gonorrhea, *Chlamydia*

3. Specific infections and conditions and their treatments

  a. *Candida*[1]

    i. Uncomplicated

      (1) Not pregnant, not diabetic, not immunocompromised

      (2) Mild/moderate symptoms

      (3) Sporadic episodes

    ii. Complicated

      (1) More than four episodes per year

      (2) Severe symptoms

(3) Pregnant, diabetic, or immunocompromised
iii. Uncomplicated infection treatment: outlined in Table 14.1
iv. Complicated
   (1) Acute
     (A) Fulconazole 150 mg followed 3 days later by second oral dose
     (B) Non-*Candida albicans* (determined by culture)
       (i) Azole drug
       (ii) Boric acid 600-mg gelatin suppository vaginally daily for 14 days

TABLE 14.1 Treatment for *Candida*

Brand Name	Generic Name	Dose
Vaginal Treatments		
Femstat, Gynazole (OTC)	butoconazole	2% cream 5 g daily for 3 days 2% cream 5 g sustained-release once
Mycelex, Lotrimin (OTC)	clotrimazole	1% cream 5 g daily for 7–14 days 100 mg tablet daily for 7 days 100 mg twice daily for 3 days
Monistat (OTC)	miconazole	2% cream 5 g daily for 7 days 100 mg daily for 7 days 200 mg daily for 3 days 1200 mg once
Mycostatin (OTC	nystatin	100,000 units daily for 14 days
Terazol	terconazole	6.5% ointment 5 g once 0.8% cream 5 g daily for 3 days 0.4% cream 5 g daily for 7 days
Vagistat (OTC)	tioconazole	6.5% 5 g ointment once
Oral Treatment		
Diflucan	fluconazole	150 mg orally once

From Centers for Disease Control and Prevention, Workowski KA, Berman SM: Sexually transmitted diseases treatment guidelines, 2006. MMWR Recomm Rep 2006;55(RR-11):1–94.

(2) Suppression/prophylaxis

    (A) Fulconazole 150 mg orally weekly for 6 months

    (B) Clotrimazole 500-mg vaginal suppositories weekly for 6 months

b. Bacterial vaginosis

  i. Pathogens: *Prevotella, Mobiluncus, Gardnerella, Mycoplasma*

  ii. Alteration in vaginal flora in which anaerobic bacteria replace lactobacillus

  iii. Treatment of asymptomatic pregnant women controversial and not consistently associated with improved pregnancy outcome

  iv. Pathogenesis not understood

    (1) Most common cause of vaginal odor

    (2) Associated with a new sexual partner but not clearly a sexually transmitted infection (STI); treatment of partners generally not helpful

  v. Treatment

    (1) Metronidazole (avoid alcohol)

      (A) Oral: 500 mg twice daily for 7 days

      (B) Vaginal gel, 0.75% one applicator intravaginally each night for 5 days

    (2) Clindamycin

      (A) Vaginal:

        (i) Cream 2% one applicator intravaginally each night for 7 nights

        (ii) 100-mg ovules intravaginally each night for 3 nights

      (B) Oral: 300 mg orally twice a day for 7 days

c. Trichomoniasis

  i. Symptoms include malodorous yellow-green discharge, vulvar irritation, and symptoms of urethritis

  ii. Diagnosis: trichomonads visible on wet mount; DNA probe

  iii. Treatment: oral

    (1) Metronidazole

      (A) 500 mg twice a day for 7 days

      (B) 2-g dose once

      (2) Tinidazole—2 g once

    iv. Treat sex partners

    v. Same dosages for pregnancy

  d. Retained tampon

    i. Copious, malodorous discharge: classic symptom of retained tampon for more than 1 or 2 days

    ii. Roughly half the women who present complaining of retained tampon do not actually have one

    iii. Removal of tampon results in rapid resolution of discharge; antibiotic treatment optional

    iv. Toxic shock syndrome rare

II. Vulvar Disease `35B`

  A. Inflammatory diseases

    1. Contact dermatitis

      a. Diagnosis of exclusion

      b. Erythema

      c. Treatment

        i. Avoid obvious irritants (scented deodorant soaps, chemically treated feminine hygiene products, vaginal sprays)

        ii. Use weak steroids: hydrocortisone 1%–2% cream twice daily for 1 week

    2. Psoriasis

      a. Multiple red patches without scaling

      b. Treatment: steroid creams

    3. Fungal

      a. *Candida*

        i. Edema, fissures, excoriations

        ii. Redder and wetter than tinea cruris

        iii. Treatment: see Table 14.1: these agents can be applied externally as well

      b. Tinea cruris

        i. Erythema with flaking, peeling, or cracking skin most commonly beginning in skin fold

        ii. Advancing edge is redder and raised; usually scaly and sharply demarcated

        iii. Treatment

          (1) Butenafine hydrocholride (Lotrimin Ultra) 1% cream once daily for 2 weeks

(2) Tolnaftate (Tinactin) cream twice daily for 2 weeks
B. Ulcers
  1. Sexually transmitted diseases: see Chapter 9
  2. Behçet disease
    a. Vulvar, vaginal, oral, and buccal ulcers; also iritis
    b. Treatment: oral steroids
  3. Crohn disease
    a. Rare cause of vulvar ulcers
    b. Associated with fistulas
C. Vulvar dystrophies
  1. Benign
    a. Lichen sclerosis
      i. More commonly menopausal but seen at all ages
      ii. Patches of slightly raised white epithelium with thin skin surrounding
      iii. Left untreated, causes atrophy of labia minora with vaginal introitus narrowing
      iv. Associated with itching or burning
      v. Diagnosis by biopsy (hyperkaratosis, loss of rete pegs, thin epithelium)
      vi. Clobetasol propionate 0.05%
        (1) Twice daily for at least 1 month
        (2) Tapered over time (and with periodic follow-up) to once daily
        (3) Twice weekly for long-term suppression
        (4) Overuse can cause tachyphylaxis: intractable itching and burning
    b. Squamous cell hyperplasia
      i. Gray, pink, or white thickened patches of skin
      ii. Associated with itching or burning
      iii. Treatment with medium-strength steroids such as fluocinonide (Lidex) cream twice daily for 1–2 weeks
  2. Premalignant or malignant
    a. Vulvar intraepithelial neoplasia
      i. White or pigmented lesions
      ii. May be associated with itching
      iii. Human papillomavirus (HPV) implicated
      iv. Treatment: physical destruction via CO_2 laser or excision

v. See Chapter 15 (HPV) for treatment of condyloma without premalignant change
    b. Squamous cell, basal cell, or melanoma
  D. Vulvodynia (vestibulitis)
    1. Burning, dyspareunia, pain on contact
    2. Few (or no) skin changes
    3. No effective treatments proved
      a. Pelvic floor physical therapy
      b. Tricyclic antidepressants

III. Bartholin Glands Disorders

  A. Anatomy:
    1. Located at "4:00" and "8:00" relative to vaginal introitus
    2. Just beneath vulvar skin
    3. Duct empties into just inside vagina
    4. Role unclear; not required for sexual lubrication
  B. Cyst formation: swelling just beneath skin near vaginal introitus; slightly tender
  C. Abscess formation: erythema; exquisite tenderness
  D. Treatment for either cyst or abscess:
    1. Incision and drainage with placement of Word catheter
      a. Short, non-draining, rubber tube with 3-mL balloon at end
      b. Leave in place for up to 2 weeks
      c. Typically falls out shortly after placement
      d. Permits continued drainage of gland and closure from inner layers outward
    2. Marsupialization of gland
      a. Gland incised for 1 or 2 cm
      b. Cyst wall sewn to overlying skin by dissolving suture
    3. Gland excision
      a. Generally reserved for multiple recurrences
      b. Recovery more painful than less invasive alternatives
    4. Suspect adenocarcinoma for Bartholin duct abscess occurring in menopause

MENTOR TIPS

- Liberal use of 3-mm punch biopsy is helpful for diagnosis of vulvar lesions.
- Unilateral discomfort suggests STI (such as herpes) and points away from vaginal infections (such as *Candida, Trichomonas,* or bacterial vaginosis).
- Most common cause of malodorous discharge is bacterial vaginosis.
- Odor points away from a yeast infection.
- Many patients presenting with recurrent "yeast infections" do not actually have *Candida;* DNA probe testing is helpful to exclude or establish diagnosis.

References

1. Centers for Disease Control and Prevention, Workowski KA, Berman SM: Sexually transmitted diseases treatment guidelines, 2006. Morbidity and Mortality Weekly Report 55:1–94, 2006.

Chapter Self-Test Questions

Circle the correct answer. After you have responded to the questions, check your answers in Appendix A.

1. Normal appearance and laboratory finding of vaginal secretions include all *except:*

   a. Faint, fishy odor.

   b. Acidic pH.

   c. Clear to white.

   d. Scant to moderate amount.

2. Which is true about vulvar rashes?

   a. Scaling suggests psoriasis.

   b. Contact dermatitis has specific findings on biopsy.

   c. Butenafine hydrochloride is a preferred treatment for *Candida.*

   d. Candidiasis is most commonly seen in the skin folds of the groin.

3. Vulvar ulcers can be a sign of:

   a. Herpes.

   b. Syphilis.

   c. Crohn disease.

   d. Behçet disease.

   e. All of the above.

4. A 22-year-old woman presents with an exquisitely painful vulvar lesion. On examination, it appears to be a Bartholin duct abscess. She has not had similar episodes in the past. She has no drug allergies. The most appropriate treatment for her is:

   a. One week of cephalosporins with twice-daily sitz baths.

   b. Incision, drainage, and placement of Word catheter.

   c. Marsupialization.

   d. Excision of the infected gland.

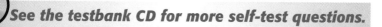

See the testbank CD for more self-test questions.

15

CERVICAL DISEASE AND HUMAN PAPILLOMAVIRUS

Michael D. Benson, MD

I. Biology of Cervical Intraepithelial Neoplasia (CIN) and Human Papillomavirus (HPV) `36A, 52A, 52C`

  A. Cervical anatomy

    1. Portio (outer portion of cervix facing vagina) covered with squamous epithelium

    2. Cervical canal lined by columnar epithelium that continues into uterine cavity and becomes endometrium—responds to estrogen and progesterone

    3. Transformation zone: place where the two cell types meet

      a. Metaplasia: columnar cells transform into squamous cells

      b. Borders of transformation zone:

        i. Original squamous-columnar junction: distal border, toward vagina

        ii. New squamous-columnar junction: proximal border, toward uterus

      c. Visible with low-power magnification

      d. Typically situated around external os

      e. Transformation zone shifts with age and childbirth

        i. Moves close to cervical canal with age—proximal border often within canal at time of menopause and not visible

        ii. Moves outward with pregnancy (mechanical, not reverse metaplasia)

        iii. Movement of columnar epithelium onto portio makes cervix look beefy red

          (1) Referred to as *ectropion*

          (2) May be mistakenly referred to as an *erosion* (*erosion* has no specific meaning and should be avoided)

(3) Now known to be physiologic process

B. CIN—cervical cancer precursors

1. Squamous cell cancer of cervix should be distinguished from the much less common adenocarcinoma of cervix, which has different biology

2. Risk factors are those for sexually transmitted diseases in general

3. Invasive cancer precursors

    a. *Dysplasia* is synonym for *CIN*

    b. CIN I

        i. Also known as *mild dysplasia* or low-grade squamous intraepithelial lesion *(LGSIL)*

        ii. Not distinguishable from HPV infection alone

        iii. Highly variable biological behavior

        iv. Majority of lesions resolve spontaneously; resolution highly affected by age; much more likely in adolescence and under age 30 years

        v. Lesions rarely progress

    c. CIN II

        i. Also known as *moderate dysplasia* or high-grade squamous intraepithelial lesion *(HGSIL)* (current terminology does not distinguish between moderate and severe dysplasia)

        ii. More likely to progress to invasive cancer than LGSIL but majority of lesions still spontaneously resolve

        iii. Inter- and intra-observer diagnosis reliability poor

        iv. Not consistently or reliably distinguished from CIN III

    d. CIN III

        i. Also known as *severe dysplasia, HGSIL* (current terminology does not distinguish between moderate and severe dysplasia) or *carcinoma in situ*

        ii. Believed to be true cancer precursor

        iii. Not all lesions progress—many (most ?) still spontaneously resolve

    e. Progression to invasive squamous cell cancer

        i. Not linear; discrete process of progression from CIN I to CIN II to CIN III

        ii. May take place as quickly as 12 months (rare)

        iii. Commonly takes several years or even decades

C. HPV
  1. Member of papillomavirus family
    a. Circular double-stranded DNA with about 7900 nucleotide base pairs
    b. Enclosed in 72-sided protein capsid
    c. Two genes, *E6 and E7*, associated with high-risk types; produce proteins that can immortalize cells
  2. Causes proliferative growth in squamous epithelial cells that is often visible to the eye on skin, including vulva
  3. While primarily associated with squamous cell lesions, may also be associated with adenocarcinoma of cervix
  4. Results in skin lesions recognized as warts
  5. Warts in genital area also known as condylomata acuminata
  6. At least 70 strains have been identified
    a. 30 or so cause genital lesions
  7. Low-risk types
    a. Types 6, 11, 26, 42, 44, 54, 70, 73
    b. Types 6 and 11 associated with vulvar condylomata
  8. Intermediate-risk types
    a. Types 31, 33, 35, 39, 51, 52, 55, 58, 59, 66, 68
    b. Included in assays for high-risk HPV
  9. High-risk types
    a. Types 16, 18, 45, 56
    b. Type 16 is associated with 50% of cervical cancers and 30% of adenocarcinomas of cervix

D. Development of cervical cancer
  1. HPV infection appears necessary but not sufficient for development of premalignant and malignant squamous cell cancer of cervix
  2. Suspected co-factors
    a. Smoking
    b. Oral contraceptives
    c. Immune compromise
    d. Other sexually transmitted diseases

E. Symptoms of CIN and cervical cancer
  1. CIN: generally none; bleeding after intercourse possible but not common
  2. Early invasive cancer: postcoital bleeding, profuse watery discharge

3. Generally no visible lesions on examination with CIN

4. Invasive cancer may not be obvious to eye although may appear as sore or ulcer on cervix that bleeds when examined

II. Pap Smear Nomenclature (Box 15.1)

III. Screening and Diagnostic Methods

A. Cervical cytology 3A, 3C-D

  1. Conventional Pap smear

    a. Broom, plastic, or wooden spatula used to swab cervical portio in a circular fashion; sample smeared thinly across slide

    b. Endocervical sample obtained with specific endocervical brush; also spread thinly across slide

    c. Slide then sprayed with fixative

  2. Liquid-based cytology

    a. Sample (typically obtained by broom) deposited in liquid transport medium (buffered alcohol) by rotating broom within the container

    b. Brand names: Thin Prep, Sure Pap

  3. Sensitivity and specificity

    a. Accuracy of cervical cytology strongly affected by:

      i. Age of population (prevalence of disease)

      ii. Endpoint: LGSIL, HGSIL, or cancer

    b. Liquid-based cytology generally shown to be more sensitive than conventional Pap

    c. LGSIL suggested by cytology not confirmed by biopsy in up to one-third of cases

    d. HGSIL cytology has much lower false-positive rate (<5%)

B. HPV DNA probe

  1. Commercially available test that identifies presence of HPV DNA from high-risk and intermediate strains

  2. Low-risk HPV viral testing not currently recommended in clinical practice

  3. Not sensitive for CIN

  4. When combined with liquid-based cytology, combination abnormal in 98%–99% of patients with CIN

C. Colposcopy: binocular-magnified view of cervix under low power (typically 7–15×) 41A

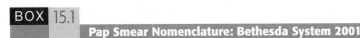

BOX 15.1

Pap Smear Nomenclature: Bethesda System 2001

Specimen Type: *Indicate conventional smear (Pap smear) versus liquid-based versus other*
Specimen Adequacy:
• Satisfactory for evaluation *(describe presence or absence of endocervical/transformation zone component and any other quality indicators, e.g., partially obscuring blood, inflammation, etc.)*
• Unsatisfactory for evaluation *(specify reason)*
Specimen rejected/not processed *(specify reason)*
Specimen processed and examined, but unsatisfactory for evaluation of epithelial abnormality because of *(specify reason)*
General Categorization *(optional)*
• Negative for intraepithelial lesion or malignancy
• Epithelial cell abnormality: see Interpretation/Result *(specify "Squamous" or "glandular" as appropriate)*
• Other: see Interpretation/Result *(e.g., endometrial cells in a woman ≥40 years of age)*
Automated Review
If case examined by automated device, specify device and result.
Ancillary Testing
Provide a brief description of the test methods and report the result so that it is easily understood by the clinician.
Interpretation/Result
Negative for Intraepithelial Lesion or Malignancy *(when there is no cellular evidence of neoplasia, state this in the General Categorization above and/or in the Interpretation/Result section of the report, whether or not there are organisms or other non-neoplastic findings)*
ORGANISMS:
• *Trichomonas vaginalis*
• Fungal organisms morphologically consistent with *Candida* spp.
• Shift in flora suggestive of bacterial vaginosis
• Bacteria morphologically consistent with *Actinomyces* spp.
• Cellular changes consistent with herpes simplex virus
OTHER NON-NEOPLASTIC FINDINGS *(Optional to report; list not inclusive):*
• Reactive cellular changes associated with:
Inflammation (includes typical repair)
Radiation
Intrauterine contraceptive device (IUD)
• Glandular cells status post hysterectomy

Pap Smear Nomenclature: Bethesda System 2001 (continued)

• Atrophy
Other
• Endometrial cells *(in a woman ≥ 40 years of age)*
(Specify if "negative for squamous intraepithelial lesion")
Epithelial Cell Abnormalities
SQUAMOUS CELL
• Atypical squamous cells
Of undetermined significance (ASC-US)
Cannot exclude HGSIL (ASC-H)
• Low-grade squamous intraepithelial lesion (LGSIL)
Encompassing: HPV/mild dysplasia/CIN 1
• High-grade squamous intraepithelial lesion (HGSIL)
Encompassing: moderate and severe dysplasia, CIS/CIN 2, and CIN 3 with
    features suspicious for invasion *(if invasion is suspected)*
• Squamous cell carcinoma
GLANDULAR CELL
• Atypical
Endocervical cells (NOS *or specify in comments*)
Endometrial cells (NOS *or specify in comments*)
Glandular cells (NOS *or specify in comments*)
• Atypical
Endocervical cells, favor neoplastic
Glandular cells, favor neoplastic
• Endocervical adenocarcinoma in situ
• Adenocarcinoma
Endocervical
Endometrial
Extrauterine
NOS
Other Malignant Neoplasms: *(specify)*
Educational Notes and Suggestions *(optional)*
Suggestions should be concise and consistent with clinical follow-up
guidelines published by professional organizations (references to relevant
publications may be included).

NOS: not otherwise specified
From U.S. National Cancer Institute (NCI) Bethesda 2001 Terminology.
    http://bethesda2001.cancer.gov/terminology.html

1. After exposure, cervix dabbed with 5% acetic acid (dilute vinegar) that highlights premalignant areas as white
2. Satisfactory
   a. Entire transformation zone seen (including new squamous-columnar junction)
   b. Entire border of any lesion fully visualized
3. Unsatisfactory
   a. Failure to meet preceding two criteria
   b. As a general rule, cone biopsy (using loop electrosurgical excision procedure [LEEP], knife, or laser cone) recommended for unsatisfactory colposcopic evaluations of abnormal cytology
      i. Procedures called diagnostic excisional procedure by American Society for Colposcopy and Cervical Pathology (ASCCP)
      ii. Recommended for evaluation of those with satisfactory colposcopy results and positive endocervical curettage (ECC) result
      iii. Pregnancy represents a special case
         (1) Unsatisfactory colposcopies are quite rare due to eversion of cervix
         (2) ECC not recommended during pregnancy
         (3) Diagnostic excisional procedure not recommended during pregnancy unless invasive cancer suspected
4. Types of abnormalities (not all-inclusive)
   a. White epithelium
   b. Punctation: red spots on background of white epithelium; pinpoint vessels (coarse suggests more severe disease)
   c. Mosaic: red lines crossing background of white epithelium; crisscrossing vessels: coarse suggests more serious disease
   d. Abnormal vessels: dilated, tortuous vessels on surface
5. Colposcopic grading of lesions
   a. Impression of CIN I, II, III, or other made at time of colposcopy
   b. Poor correlation among observers and with histology
6. Although *colposcopy* refers to examination of cervix under magnification, in practice almost always implies taking biopsies of the most abnormal-appearing areas or areas that have changed since prior colposcopy

D. Biopsies

    1. Punch biopsies: typically one or more punch biopsy samples taken of the most abnormal-appearing areas of cervix under colposcopy

        a. Local or topical anesthetic not typically required

        b. Localized bleeding controlled with $AgNO_3$ (silver nitrate) or Monsel solution (ferric subsulfate)

    2. ECC

        a. Specific instrument (Kevorkian curette) used to gently scrape cervical canal; mucus collected, then sent in formalin as separate specimen

        b. Not performed in pregnancy

        c. Particularly recommended for those with unsatisfactory colposcopy result or for those with CIN on Pap but no lesion at time of colposcopy

    3. LEEP or large loop excision of transformation zone (LLETZ) [41F]

        a. Wire loop utilizing electrocautery used to remove outer portion of cervix (entire transformation zone) intact for histology—sent in formalin

        b. Typically requires local anesthetic injections in cervix

        c. Significant bleeding can occur for up to 2–3 weeks afterward

        d. Accomplishes diagnosis and treatment

        e. Has largely taken the place of cone biopsies performed by scalpel or laser

        f. ECC typically performed immediately after sample taken and sent in separate container to pathology laboratory

        g. Generally not done in pregnancy

    4. Cone biopsy [41B]

        a. Traditional method of removing entire transformation zone for diagnosis and/or treatment

        b. Patient needs to be heavily sedated and given local anesthetic or general anesthetic

        c. Usually requires substantial suturing for hemostasis

        d. Generally not done in pregnancy

    5. Laser cone biopsy—largely replaced by LEEP

    6. Diagnostic excisional procedure

        a. Specific term defined by ASCCP

    b. Includes all methods of removing transformation zone intact for histologic evaluation (includes LEEP, knife, and laser cone biopsies)

IV. Treatment Methods
  A. LEEP
  B. Cryocautery 41C
    1. Special probe cooled by liquid nitrogen applied to cervix
    2. Ablates transformation zone
    3. Causes mild-to-moderate menstrual-type cramping during 5–10-minute procedure
    4. Results in profuse watery discharge for up to 2 weeks
    5. Can result in subsequent narrowing of cervical canal and difficulty in visualizing new squamous-columnar junction
  C. Cone biopsy
  D. Hysterectomy: never recommended for treatment of CIN

V. Cytology Screening Recommendations 7A, 52B
  A. Recommendations for screening[1]
    1. Still evolving
    2. Different organizations vary slightly in recommendations
    3. American College of Obstetricians and Gynecologists
      a. Begin 3 years after first intercourse
      b. Continue annually until age 30 years
      c. May decrease to every 2–3 years after age 30 years
    4. Stopping Pap smears
      a. American Cancer Society: discontinue after age 70 years in low-risk women
      b. U.S. Preventive Services Task Force: upper age limit 65 years
    5. Women without cervix (hysterectomy)
      a. For those with benign disease and no history of HGSIL: discontinue screening
      b. For those with history of HGSIL: screen annually until three negative Pap smear results
  B. HPV testing
    1. Combination of Pap and HPV testing much more sensitive than Pap alone
    2. Prevalence of HPV is high in women younger than 30 years
      a. Rate of regression quite high in this group

    b. HPV testing approved by U.S. Food and Drug Administration for women age 30 years and older

  3. Role of HPV testing still evolving, but normal Pap and negative HPV may not require retesting for 3 years

VI. Follow-Up of Abnormal Screening Results 52D

  A. 2006 Bethesda Consensus Conference[2]

    1. Sponsored by ASCCP

    2. Represents consensus view of 146 experts representing 29 health-care organizations

    3. Not exhaustive summary

    4. Recommendations always placed in context of patient's specific clinical circumstances such as risk factors and compliance

    5. Atypical squamous cells

      a. Atypical squamous cells of uncertain significance (ASC-US)

        i. HPV negative: repeat cytology test in 12 months

        ii. HPV positive: colposcopy with biopsies as appropriate

        iii. HPV not done: Pap smears every 6 months until two consecutive Pap smear results negative

      b. Atypical squamous cells, cannot exclude HGSIL (ASC-H)

        i. Colposcopy with biopsies as appropriate

        ii. For those without HGSIL after colposcopy: HPV testing at 12 months; Pap smears every 6 months until two consecutive normal results

    6. LGSIL

      a. Colposcopy with biopsies as appropriate

      b. Special populations

        i. Adolescents: follow-up cytology in 1 year

          (1) 12 months: HGSIL referred for colposcopy

          (2) Those with ASC-US or greater at 24 months referred for colposcopy

        ii. Postmenopausal women: three choices

          (1) HPV testing (colposcopy if positive)

          (2) Colposcopy with biopsies as appropriate

          (3) Cytology at 6 and 12 months (colposcopy for anything but negative Pap smear results)

        iii. Pregnant (nonadolescent)

          (1) Colposcopy: may defer until 6 weeks postpartum

(2) Avoid ECC

(3) Those without any evidence of HGSIL on further evaluation: do not require additional cytology or colposcopy during pregnancy

7. HGSIL

   a. Colposcopy with LEEP on same visit

   b. Special populations

     i. Adolescents

      (1) Colposcopy and biopsies as appropriate (LEEP should not be done for initial diagnosis)

      (2) LEEP appropriate for unsatisfactory colposcopy or any CIN on ECC

     ii. Pregnant women

      (1) Colposcopy and biopsies as appropriate

      (2) Avoid LEEP and ECC

8. Atypical glandular cells

   a. Colposcopy with endocervical sampling and other biopsies as necessary *and* endometrial biopsy in women 35 years and older

   b. HPV testing also recommended if not already obtained

   c. Atypical endometrial cells: endometrial biopsy and ECC and colposcopy

9. Benign-appearing endometrial cells

   a. Premenopausal: rarely associated with disease

   b. Postmenopausal: may be associated with endometrial pathology

10. Normal Pap smear result and positive HPV (only for women 30 years and older)

   a. Repeat both tests in 12 months

   b. Colposcopy if HPV positive again

VII. Treatment of Premalignant Disease of Cervix (Presumes Satisfactory Colposcopy)

A. CIN I (LGSIL)

   1. Very high rate of regression within 2 years (up to 90%)

   2. For those who progress, evidence suggests that more advanced lesions may have been present at time of initial colposcopy

   3. Risk of progression linked to antecedent history of cytology, histology, and HPV testing

4. ASCCP recommendations

 a. CIN I on biopsy preceded by ASC-US, ASC-H, or LGSIL cytology

  i. HPV testing in 12 months *or*

  ii. Cytology every 6–12 months

  iii. Further triage

   (1) If follow-up HPV result is negative or two consecutive Pap smears normal, return to routine testing

   (2) If CIN I persists for 2 years

    (A) May treat

     (i) Diagnostic excisional procedure *or*

     (ii) Ablation

    (B) May continue to monitor

 b. CIN I on biopsy preceded by HGSIL or AGC-NOS

  i. Adult population

   (1) Treatment by diagnostic excisional procedure *or*

   (2) Colposcopy and cytology every 6 months for 1 year

    (A) Diagnostic excisional treatment recommended if original findings recur

    (B) Two normal cytologies: resume routine screening

  ii. Adolescents:

   (1) Follow up with annual cytology

   (2) At 12 months, if Pap = HGSIL, perform colposcopy

   (3) At 24 months, those with ASC-US or greater should get colposcopy

  iii. Pregnant women: histology of CIN I: no treatment

B. CIN 2,3 (HGSIL)

 1. Diagnostic excisional procedure *or* ablation

 2. Special populations

  a. Adolescents

   i. Treatment *or*

   ii. Colposcopy and cytology every 6 months for 2 years

    (1) If appearance worsens or persists for 1 year: repeat biopsy

    (2) Two negative Pap smears and a normal cytology: return to routine follow-up

  b. Pregnant women

   i. Do not treat during pregnancy

PART

  ii. Colposcopy and cytology no more frequent than every 12 weeks (biopsy only if appearance worsens or cytology suggests invasive cancer)

  iii. Diagnostic excisional procedure only if invasion suspected (**caution:** heavy bleeding is real concern; should be done in hospital)

C. Adenocarcinoma in situ

 1. 30–40 times less common than CIN 3

 2. Frequently multifocal

 3. Hysterectomy treatment of choice for those who have finished childbearing

 4. Diagnostic excisional procedure acceptable for those who wish to retain fertility

  a. Repeat if margins involved or positive ECC

  b. Repeat cytology, colposcopy, and ECC at 6-month intervals for follow-up

VIII. Treatment of Vulvar and Vaginal Genital Warts

A. General principles: Centers for Disease Control and Prevention Sexually Transmitted Diseases Treatment Guidelines 2006[3]

 1. External warts do not imply cervical infection: no change in cervical cytology follow-up recommended

 2. External warts can occur in association with premalignant or malignant disease of the vulva and is a risk factor

 3. HPV testing not recommended for management of patient or assessment of sexual partner(s) with warts

 4. Patient may be infected with more than one HPV type

 5. HPV types 16, 18, 31, 33, and 35 associated with genital warts and squamous cell cancer

 6. Biopsy large lesions, lesions that look atypical, or lesions that recur

 7. Warts commonly recur within a few months of treatment

 8. Perianal warts do not imply anal-receptive intercourse in contrast to true intra-anal condyloma

 9. Can occur in mouth, urethra, cervix, vagina, anus

B. Treatment details

 1. Patient-administered

  a. Podofilox 0.5% solution or gel

   i. Apply solution with swab

ii. Apply gel with finger

iii. Apply twice a day for 3 days

iv. 4 days of no therapy

v. Repeat cycle up to four times

b. Imiquinod 5% cream

i. Apply three times a week at night for up to 16 weeks

ii. Wash off with soap and water 6–10 hours afterwards

2. Clinician-administered

a. Cryotherapy with liquid nitrogen or cryoprobe: repeat every 1–2 weeks

b. Podophyllin resin 10%–25% in compound tincture of benzoin

i. Repeat weekly if necessary

ii. Wash off after 1–4 hours

iii. Limit to <10 cm^2 to reduce toxicity

iv. Do not apply to open lesions

v. Can be toxic if absorbed systemically

c. Trichloroacetic acid (TCA) or bichloroacetic acid (BCA) 80%–90%: apply to lesion, allow to dry; repeat weekly

d. Surgical excision

e. Laser ablation

IX. HPV Vaccine

A. Directed against high-risk strains of HPV

1. Recommended even for those with CIN as vaccines protect against more than one strain

2. HPV status prior to vaccination not required or beneficial

B. Vaccination of boys not currently recommended

C. Gardasil: quadrivalent

1. Targets types 16, 18, 6, 11

2. Three doses

a. Initial dose

b. Second dose 2 months later

c. Third dose 4 months later

3. Best results if all three doses given within a year

4. Recommended for females 9–26 years old; ideally before becoming sexually active

5. Prevented 100% of premalignant changes from targeted strains at 4 years

6. Type 16 and 18 etiologic in 70% of high-grade dysplasia and cervix cancer; therefore, cervical cancer screening still required post vaccine as 30% of high-risk HPV not covered by Gardasil
7. Does not contain mercury, thimerosal, or live virus
8. Intended for prophylaxis; no therapeutic value for established infections

MENTOR TIPS

- Do not do HPV testing under age 30 years (exception is reflex testing available for ASC-US Pap smears).
- Do not treat CIN I initially.
- Unsatisfactory colposcopies are uncommon but generally need diagnostic excision procedure.
- CIN 2, 3 (HGSIL) are generally treated.
- Pregnant women do not receive treatment for CIN of any grade or endocervical curettages. They can receive colposcopy and biopsies.
- External warts do not change or modify cervical cytology follow-up.
- Partners of women with cervical HPV generally are not evaluated or treated.

References

1. ACOG Practice Bulletin 45. Cervical cytology screening. Washington, DC, American College of Obstetricians and Gynecologists, August 2003.
2. Wright TC, Massad LS, Dunton CJ, et al: 2006 consensus guidelines for the management of women with abnormal cervical cancer screening tests. American Journal of Obstetrics and Gynecology 197:346–355, 2007.
3. Centers for Disease Control and Prevention, Workowski KA, Berman SM: Sexually transmitted diseases treatment guidelines, 2006. Morbidity and Mortality Weekly Report 55 (RR-11):1–94, 2006.

Chapter Self-Test Questions

Circle the correct answer. After you have responded to the questions, check your answers in Appendix A.

1. Which is true about the transformation zone?

   a. Squamous cells mature into columnar epithelium.

   b. The original squamous-columnar junction is the boundary of the transformation zone closest to the endometrium.

   c. It shifts outward with pregnancy.

   d. Beefy red–appearing cervix (ectropion) is a sign of cervical dysplasia.

2. Which is true about symptoms of cervical neoplasia?

   a. Postcoital bleeding common symptom of cervical dysplasia

   b. Pelvic pain is presenting symptom of early cervical cancer

   c. Profuse watery discharge consistent with mild dysplasia

   d. Cervical dysplasia usually leaves no visible lesion on examination

3. Diagnostic excisional procedures:

   a. Include LEEP, cold knife conization, and laser conization

   b. Are typically followed by an endocervical curettage at the same time.

   c. Are generally avoided in pregnancy.

   d. All of the above.

4. Which is *not* true about Pap smear and HPV screening?

   a. May be discontinued after age 70 years in women without recent cervical disease

   b. HPV testing recommended for use by college student health services

   c. Normal Pap smear and HPV results do not have to be repeated for 3 years

   d. Women with a hysterectomy for benign disease do not need further Pap smears

See the testbank CD for more self-test questions.

GYNECOLOGIC NEOPLASMS

Michael D. Benson, MD

I. Vulvar Malignancies

A. Epidemiology, presenting symptoms, and diagnosis
1. 3970 new cases in United States and 880 deaths (2004)[1]
2. Peak incidence in women age 70s and 80s
3. 90% are squamous cell carcinoma
4. Symptoms: premalignant and malignant vulvar lesions can give rise to vulvar irritation, pain, dyspareunia, bleeding, or palpable growth
5. Invasive cancer arises typically in two groups of patients 51A
   a. Young smokers with human papillomavirus (HPV); premalignant disease of the vulva; vulvar intraepithelial neoplasia (VIN)
      i. As with cervix, premalignant lesions usually precede invasive cancer; classified as VIN I, II, or III: mild, moderate, or severe
      ii. HPV lesions (condyloma, genital warts) may appear as flat, slightly raised areas flesh-colored or white or as familiar wart—irregular, papillary lesions—typically not premalignant but can sometimes be difficult to distinguish from pre-invasive disease
      iii. Bowenoid papulosis: specific variety of VIN III that appears as multiple red, brown, or purple papules
      iv. Symptoms of VIN: pruritus, irritation, pain with intercourse, raised area (latter less common)
      v. Diagnosis of VIN 41Q, 51B
         (1) Biopsy: shaving or 3–5-mm punch after small subcutaneous injection of local anesthetic; suture may or may not be required
      vi. Treatment of VIN

(1) Local excision with 5-mm margins

(2) Destruction of lesion by laser

    b. Elderly nonsmokers without HPV or VIN: high incidence of lichen sclerosis next to cancer

B. Squamous cell cancers: staging and treatment

    1. Symptoms of vulvar cancer include grossly visible lesion, vulvar mass, vulvar bleeding, pain, and pruritus

    2. Can spread by direct extension or by lymphatic or hematogenous routes

    3. Staging: Tumor, Node, Metastasis (TNM) methodology; vulvar cancer staged surgically

        a. Stage I: tumor <2 cm, confined to vulva

        b. Stage II: tumor >2 cm, confined to vulva

        c. Stage III: tumor spread to adjacent organs by direct extension and/or tumor in groin lymph nodes

        d. Stage IV: tumor invaded rectal or bladder mucosa and/or fixed to bone and/or other distant metastases

    4. Prognosis (5-year survival rate—approximate): stage I, 90%; stage II, 80%; stage III, 50%; stage IV, 20%

    5. Treatment 51C

        a. Stage I: radical vulvectomy with ipsilateral inguinal lymph-node dissection

        b. Stage II and III: radiation treatment or preoperative chemotherapy to shrink tumor before surgery as with stage I

        c. Stage IV: widely metastatic disease

            i. Poor prognosis

            ii. Variety of chemotherapy protocols

C. Paget disease: white, flat lesions with sharp borders

    1. Diagnosis

        a. Erythematous, mottled area with white, raised epithelium interspersed

        b. Large, pale Paget cells on microscopic examination of biopsy

    2. Treatment: wide local excision with frozen section of the margins to ensure they are clear

    3. Associated adenocarcinoma (present in up to 20% of cases) requires same treatment as other invasive vulvar cancers

II. Vaginal Cancer

A. Epidemiology

  1. Rare

  2. Half of cases occur in women older than 70 years

  3. Most cases are squamous cell

B. Symptoms and signs

  1. Painless vaginal bleeding or discharge

  2. Most lesions in upper third of vagina on posterior wall

    a. Easily missed if obscured by blades of speculum

C. Staging: clinical—not based on TNM; uses International Federation of Gynecology and Obstetrics (FIGO) nomenclature

  1. Stage I: limited to vaginal wall

  2. Stage II: invaded beyond vagina but not to pelvic wall

  3. Stage III: extended to pelvic wall

  4. Stage IV: extended beyond true pelvis or has invaded bladder or rectal mucosa

D. Treatment: rareness of disease makes protocol development difficult

  1. Primarily involves external and intracavitary radiation

  2. Surgical excision used in special circumstances (stage I disease in upper vagina)

III. Cervical Cancer

A. When neoplastic epithelium has penetrated below basement membrane, process no longer premalignant but rather invasive cancer

B. Epidemiology, presenting symptoms, and diagnosis

  1. 12,900 new cases in United States in 2001, with estimated 4400 deaths likely to result[2]

  2. Much more prevalent in Third World: roughly 400,000 new cases worldwide annually

  3. Risk factors 52A

    a. Smoking

    b. Antecedent HPV, cervical dysplasia

    c. Immunosuppression

  4. Symptoms (not specific—most with these symptoms do not have cervical cancer): 52C

    a. Abnormal discharge: watery or malodorous

    b. Bleeding after intercourse

    c. Intermenstrual bleeding

5. Diagnosis

    a. Direct biopsy of visible lesion

    b. Follow-up of abnormal cytology with colposcopically directed biopsies

    c. Cone biopsy: removes conical (or hemispherical) central portion of cervix

        i. Cold-knife: typically hospital procedure; preferred in rare cases of suspected early invasion as margin of specimen easier to read pathologically

        ii. Loop electrosurgical excision procedure (LEEP): office procedure under local anesthetic in which central portion of cervix excised by loop electrode

C. Staging 52E

    1. Overview

        a. Established by FIGO (1994)

        b. Does not use TNM classification

        c. Entirely clinical; beyond history, physical examination, and cervical biopsies, can include computed tomography (CT) or x-ray of chest, CT of pelvis and abdomen, or cystoscopy and colonoscopy (often done for stage II or greater)

        d. Postoperative pathology findings do not change staging but can be used to guide treatment

        e. Incidental cervical cancer discovered at time of hysterectomy cannot be staged in this paradigm

        f. Recurrence does not change stage

    2. Specific stages

        a. Stage I: confined to cervix

            i. Stage IA: microinvasion; no lesion visible to unaided eye

                (1) Maximum depth of invasion 5 mm

                (2) Maximum width 7 mm

            ii. Stage 1A1: invasion <3.0 mm

            iii. Stage 1A2: invasion >3.0 mm

            iv. Stage IB: clinically visible or not visible but >1A

                (1) Stage 1B1: ≤4 cm

                (2) Stage 1B2: >4 cm

        b. Stage II: extends beyond uterus but not to pelvic side wall or to lower third of vagina

            i. Stage IIA: no obvious extension into parametrium

      ii. Stage IIB: obvious extension into parametrium

  c. Stage III

     i. Includes any or all of the following

       (1) Extension to pelvic wall: no cancer-free space between tumor and pelvic wall on rectal examination

       (2) Tumor involves lower third of vagina

       (3) Hydronephrosis and/or nonfunctioning kidney (unless known to be due to unrelated cause)

     ii. Stage IIIA: involves lower third of vagina but no extension to side wall

     iii. Stage IIIB: extension to pelvic side wall

  d. Stage IV: extends beyond true pelvis or involves mucosa of bladder or rectum (established by biopsy)

     i. Stage IVA: spread to adjacent organs

     ii. Stage IVB: spread to distant organs

D. Treatment 52E

  1. Stage I

    a. Stage IA1 (microinvasion 3 mm or less)

     i. Cone biopsy required to characterize depth and width of lesion

     ii. Treatment can be limited to cone biopsy or hysterectomy (risk of spread to nodes at this stage <1%) if:

       (1) Margins of biopsy are free of disease *and*

       (2) Endocervical curettage (collection of tissue from remaining cervical canal) result negative

       (3) If (1) and (2) do not apply, patient needs repeat cone biopsy

     iii. Risk of infection on subsequent hysterectomy may be increased so interval of 6 weeks often employed (if patient has positive margins, some proceed with surgery immediately to offset risk of further spread of disease)

    b. Stage IA2 (microinvasion 3–5 mm)

     i. Less information about extent of spread to lymph nodes and less consensus

     ii. For women intent on future childbearing, radical trachelectomy (removal of entire cervix) and pelvic lymphadenectomy may be option (rather than treatments listed below for IB)

   (1) Nonabsorbable cerclage suture place at time of surgery to permit carrying pregnancy to viability; subsequent cesarean required

   (2) Magnetic resonance imaging (MRI) can be used preoperatively to assess spread of disease into corpus of uterus

2. Stages IB1 and IIA: radical hysterectomy or radiation acceptable; both have similar rates of cure and major morbidity

 a. Types of hysterectomy

  i. Type I: extrafacial (simple)

  ii. Type II: (Wertheim): modified radical hysterectomy

   (1) Removal of medial half of cardinal ligaments and proximal uteral sacral ligaments

   (2) Removal of enlarged pelvic nodes

   (3) Performed for stage IB1

  iii. Type III: (Meigs): radical hysterectomy

   (1) Removal of entire cardinal ligament

   (2) Removal of upper half of vagina

   (3) Performed for stage IIA

 b. Complications: bladder dysfunction, sexual dysfunction (related to extent of excision of upper vagina), lymphedema in limbs, urinary tract fistulas (roughly 1%)

 c. Prognosis (and considerations in recommended postoperative radiation)

  i. Tumor size, depth of invasion

  ii. Cell type—small cell less common and poorer prognosis

  iii. Presence of disease in lymph nodes or lymphatic/vascular invasion

  iv. Status of vaginal margins and invasion into parametrial tissue

3. Radiation: treatment of choice for stage IIB or greater and often used for stages IB and IIA

 a. Elements

  i. External beam treatment

  ii. Brachytherapy: short-distance radiation; radiation source directly into cervix (needles) or vagina

b. Chemotherapy in combination with radiation may improve progression-free survival—weekly cisplatin for 6 weeks seems to be best tolerated and most effective regimen

E. Prognosis (5-year survival rate—approximate): stage I, 85%; stage II, 70%; stage III, 35%; stage IV, 10%

F. Adenocarcinoma of the cervix: perhaps 15% of all cervical cancers

  1. Cervical canal has glandular cells that can give rise to adenocarcinoma

  2. More difficult to diagnose in early stages as Pap smears are less sensitive

  3. Generally treated the same stage for stage as squamous cell carcinoma

IV. Uterine Malignancies

A. Can arise in endometrium (adenocarcinoma) or uterine wall (leiomyosarcoma)

B. Adenocarcinoma of endometrium 54A–B

  1. Epidemiology, presenting symptoms, and diagnosis

    a. Most common genital tract malignancy in United States with roughly 40,000 new diagnoses per year and 7300 deaths; almost three-fourths are diagnosed as stage I

    b. Two general pathologic types

      i. Type I

        (1) 90% of cases

        (2) Indolent

        (3) Results from excess estrogen unopposed by progesterone and progresses through endometrial hyperplasia

        (4) Risk factors: nulliparity, infertility, menstrual irregularities, early menarche, late menopause, obesity, hypertension, diabetes, gallbladder disease, thyroid disease, unopposed menopausal estrogens, white race, higher income and educational level

      ii. Type II: more lethal, with high-grade nuclei and serous or clear-cell pathology; associated with atrophic endometrium or polyps

    c. Symptoms

      i. Symptomatic bleeding: postmenopausal bleeding or worsening of menses (frequency, duration, amount)

      ii. 10% of women do not have abnormal bleeding

  d. Family history: genetically linked cancer; Lynch syndrome (hereditary nonpolyposis colorectal cancer [HNPCC])

      i. Carrier risk increased with colorectal cancer or endometrial cancer younger than age 50 years or for those with two or more Lynch syndrome cancers in an individual or family (colorectal, endometrial, ovarian, gastric)

      ii. Commercial test for mutations in three genes (*MLH1, MLH2,* and *MSH6*) that cause most Lynch syndrome cancers

2. Premalignant conditions

  a. Hyperplasia: may not be truly premalignant; usually responds to progestin treatment; may be simple or complex (adenomatous)

  b. Hyperplasia with atypia

      i. Simple

      ii. Complex (adenomatous)

         (1) Occasionally responds to progestin

         (2) Probably a true premalignant condition: 25% may go on to develop invasive cancer

         (3) May be associated with concomitant invasive cancer

  c. Hyperplasia without atypia is probably not a precursor to hyperplasia with atypia

3. Diagnosis 54D

  a. Endometrial biopsy (office procedure) finds 90% of malignancies if present 41G

  b. Fractional dilation and curettage with hysteroscopy 41E, 41J

      i. Endocervical curettage done first and sent separately from endometrial curettings; hysteroscopy allows directed biopsy of suspicious lesions

      ii. If hyperplasia found on an endometrial sampling, fractional dilation and curettage may be desirable to obtain larger tissue sample, particularly in those with abnormal bleeding

      iii. May be done to follow up endometrial biopsy showing adenomatous hyperplasia with atypia to help identify potential concomitant cancer preoperatively

  c. Treatment of adenomatous hyperplasia with atypia

PART

    i. Hysterectomy reasonable treatment in all women with hyperplasia who do not wish to retain their uterus

    ii. For those who wish to avoid hysterectomy

        (1) Provera (medroxyprogesterone acetate) 10 mg 14 days/month in premenopausal women or daily in postmenopausal women

        (2) Alternative treatments include Mirena (progestin intrauterine device [IUD])

        (3) Follow-up biopsy in 3–6 months

        (4) If hyperplasia regresses, long-term progestin treatment or ovulation induction (if appropriate)

        (5) If hyperplasia remains, trial of high-dose progestin: commonly Megace for 3 months followed by repeat biopsy

4. Staging and treatment of endometrial adenocarcinoma `54E-F`

  a. Staging: can be clinical or surgical; surgical takes precedence (defined by FIGO, not TNM)

    i. General concepts

        (1) Clinical stage includes examination, biopsies (including fractional dilation and curettage) as well as ancillary investigations such as cystoscopy, proctoscopy, and imaging procedures

        (2) Surgical staging refers specifically to findings at time of hysterectomy with or without lymph-node biopsies

        (3) Stages modified by histologic grade of 1–3 based on extent of solid growth pattern within tumor; further modified by amount of nuclear atypia

    ii. Specific stages

        (1) Stage I: confined to corpus

          (A) Stage IA: confined to endometrium

          (B) Stage 1B: invades less than half of myometrium

          (C) Stage 1C: invades more than half of myometrium

        (2) Stage II: extension to cervix

          (A) Stage IIA: endocervical glands only

          (B) Stage IIB: extension to cervical stroma

        (3) Stage III

(A) Stage IIIA: extension to uterine serosa, ovaries, or positive peritoneal cytology

(B) Stage IIIB: extension to vagina

(C) Stage IIIC: pelvic or periaortic lymph-node involvement

(4) Stage IV

(A) Stage IVA: invasion of bladder or bowel mucosa

(B) Stage IVB: distant metastases

b. Factors related to increasing risk of lymph-node metastases with resultant poor prognosis (beyond stage, grade, and nuclear atypia)

i. Increasing age

ii. Histology: squamous and papillary components worsen prognosis

iii. Depth of myometrial invasion

iv. Tumor size (>2 cm in diameter worse prognosis)

v. Invasion of lymphatic or vascular vessels

c. Hormone receptor status: presence of estrogen or progestin receptors associated with improved prognosis

d. Surgical treatment and staging

i. Removal of uterus, tubes, and ovaries

ii. Peritoneal washings and fluid for cytology and biopsies of omentum and pelvic and periaortic lymph nodes for selected stage I cases; no universal consensus on indications

iii. Common criteria include

(1) Grade 3 tumor

(2) >50% invasion of myometrium (opened uterus at time of hysterectomy)

(3) Tumor size >2 cm

(4) Presences of enlarged lymph nodes

(5) Poor histologic type

iii. Full perioaortic and pelvic lymphadenectomy

(1) Selected biopsies for staging and assessing utility and type of radiation treatment

(2) Lymphadenectomy for treatment

(A) May be considered for suspicious lymph nodes, spread to tubes or ovaries, and invasion of outer third of myometrium

(B) Lifelong lymphedema with recurrent cellulites is major morbidity

e. Radiation treatment: administered to selected patients after surgical treatment and staging (adjuvant therapy)

i. Generally reserved for patient with grade 3 histology or stage II or higher

ii. Vaginal brachytherapy: helps to reduce disease recurrence at vaginal cuff (most common site of recurrence); can be administered as outpatient; generally low morbidity rate

iii. External pelvic radiation and periaortic radiation

(1) Generally reserved for those with positive pelvic or periaortic lymph-node biopsy results on surgical staging or those at high risk who have not been surgically staged

(2) May not be necessary for those who have had complete lymphadenectomy

(3) Effective for vaginal cuff so brachytherapy not also given

f. Prognosis[3]: individual prognosis highly variable and dependent on specifics of disease (grade, patient age, etc.); 5-year survival rate (approximate): stage I, 90%; stage II, 70%; stage III, 35%–60%; stage IV: 20%

g. Special issues

i. Recurrent disease: commonly treated with radiation for vaginal recurrence

ii. Progestational agents may be palliative for advanced disease

iii. Cytotoxic chemotherapy may also be used for palliation; doxorubicin most effective

iv. Can occur with pregnancy but very rare and typically focal and well differentiated

C. Sarcomas

1. Classification

a. Embryonic origin

i. Pure: derived from mesoderm (such as muscle, vessels)

ii. Mixed: mesoderm and epithelial derivatives (e.g., containing glandular tissue)

b. Derived organ

i. Homologous: arising from tissue normally found in uterus

ii. Heterologous: arising from tissue outside of uterus (cartilage, etc.)

c. Can arise in both endometrium and myometrium

2. Epidemiology and diagnosis of most common sarcoma: leiomyosarcoma

i. Arises in smooth muscle of uterine wall: can arise within fibroid but not common

ii. As tumor grows within uterine wall, diagnosis usually made by pathology examination of hysterectomy or myomectomy specimen; discovered in <1% of hysterectomies for fibroids

iii. Peak incidence age 34–55 years

iv. Symptoms not specific: include abnormal bleeding, pain, or rapid growth of uterus/presumed fibroid

3. Treatment: removal of uterus (and usually both tubes and ovaries); role of radiation and chemotherapy for metastases still evolving

V. Ovarian Neoplasms

A. Types of ovarian neoplasms `55B, 55E`

1. Functional cysts: physiologic occurring, fluid-filled structures in ovary

a. Follicular: site of maturing egg prior to ovulation; multiple cysts typically form with each ovulatory cycle; most mature egg is typically in largest cyst that then ruptures

b. Corpus luteum: follicular cyst that has filled in with blood and progesterone, producing cells immediately after ovulation

c. Theca lutein: associated with pregnancies, particularly molar pregnancies; can grow up to 15 cm

d. Functioning tissue from another organ: endometrioma

i. Endometrial tissue established within ovary by direct extension or hematogenous spread

ii. Can be multiloculated and cause adhesions to adjacent organs (appear and behave similar to a malignancy in some respects)

iii. Can be associated with an elevated CA-125

iv. Treatment usually surgical

e. Polycystic ovaries: name is a misnomer as this condition does not usually result in large ovarian cysts but rather multiple small ones with a thickened ovarian capsule

2. Ovary consists of three distinct tissues that give rise to neoplasia; each tumor type can be benign or malignant

a. Epithelium: 70% of all ovarian neoplasms

  i. Serous cystadenoma/cystadenocarcinoma

   (1) Often (50%) bilateral

   (2) Often unilocular

   (3) Psammoma bodies (round collections of calcifications seen on histology sample)

   (4) Cystic lining with papillary excrescences

  ii. Mucinous cystadenoma/cystadenocarcinoma

   (1) Can grow very large

   (2) Tend to be multilocular

   (3) Mucin within is thick

  iii. Brenner tumors

   (1) Solid tumors

   (2) Also known as transitional cell

   (3) Mimics genitourinary (GU) tract epithelium

  iv. Endometrioid tumor

   (1) Usually malignant

   (2) Associated with endometriosis and concomitant endometrial cancer

  v. Borderline tumor (tumor of low malignant potential)

   (1) On microscopic examination, tumor has greater epithelial proliferation than commonly seen in serous cystadenomas, but no invasion seen

   (2) As implied by its name, borderline tumor falls between purely benign and malignant; occasionally, normal ovaries can be preserved, particularly for those women desiring future pregnancies

b. Sex cord stromal tumors: hormonally active tissue of the ovary

  i. Granulosa cell tumors

   (1) Can produce estrogen

   (2) Can be associated with Meigs syndrome: triad of benign ovarian tumor, ascites, and right-sided pleural effusion

(3) Call-Exner bodies: granulosa cells surrounded by eosinophilic fluid

(4) Coffee bean cells: have nuclei with grooves

ii. Thecomas—sex cord stromal tumors

(1) Can produce estrogen; can be associated with postmenopausal bleeding and Meigs syndrome

(2) Often unilateral

(3) Usually benign

(4) Age usually >35 years

iii. Sertoli-Leydig cell tumors; can produce androgens

c. Germ cells: tumors arising for totipotential cells

i. Benign

(1) Dermoid (mature cystic teratoma): can contain cartilage, hair, and teeth

(2) Struma ovarii: special type of dermoid; consists of thyroid tissue and can rarely produce enough thyroid hormone to cause thyrotoxicosis

ii. Malignant

(1) Dysgerminoma

(A) Uniquely sensitive to radiation therapy and chemotherapy

(B) Solid

(C) Large polygonal cells

(D) Can contain syncytiotrophoblast; 5% produce human chorionic gonadotropin (hCG)

(2) Endodermal sinus tumor (yolk sac tumor)

(A) Very aggressive

(B) Alpha-fetoprotein useful tumor marker

(3) Immature cystic teratoma: malignant behavior related to amount of mitotic activity and differentiation

(4) Gonadoblastoma: typically occurs in congenitally abnormal gonad, such as in patients with gonadal dystenesis; may coexist with other germ cell tumors

iii. Note on treatment

(1) Often found in reproductive-age women

(2) Treatment: removing afflicted ovary and possibly chemotherapy

(3) Removal of uterus and other normal ovary not required

3. Primary peritoneal carcinoma: malignancy that resembles ovarian carcinoma clinically and histologically; arises from peritoneum as a primary site; not truly ovarian cancer but has been confused with it; some refer to it as non-ovarian ovarian cancer

4. Fallopian tube cancer: uncommon
   a. Generally diagnosed and treated in manner similar to ovarian cancer
   b. Linked to mutations in *BRCA-1* and *BRCA-2* genes

B. Epidemiology, screening, and diagnosis
   1. Approximately 25,000 women diagnosed annually in the United States; 16,000 die[1]
   2. No effective screening tests that have appropriate sensitivity and specificity
   3. Epithelial cell malignancies account for 90% of all ovarian malignancies; peak incidence in women in their late 50s
   4. Majority of ovarian cancers are stage III at time of diagnosis; ovary has no peritoneal covering, and malignant cells can spread throughout abdomen relatively early in the process
      a. Stage at diagnosis varies by age (older women tend to have more advanced disease at time of diagnosis) and race (blacks have more advanced disease than whites)
      b. Only 25% of women diagnosed at stage I; remainder have disease that has spread beyond the ovary
   5. 80% of epithelial cell tumors are serous, 10% mucinous, and remainder are Brenner cell, clear cell, or endometrioid cell
   6. Oral contraceptive use for 5 years or more associated with 50% reduction in risk
   7. Risk factors 55D
      a. Low parity (not infertility treatment per se)
      b. Early menarche and late menopause
      c. High body mass index (BMI)
      d. Family history (may be factor in up to 10% of ovarian cancer; most cases sporadic)
         i. *BRCA-1* and *BRCA-2* mutations
            (1) Inherited via autosomal dominance
            (2) Carrier rate for one or more mutations is 2.5% among Ashkenazi Jews

(3) Test those with individual or first-degree relative histories of:
  (A) Breast cancer <50 years
  (B) Ovarian cancer
  (C) Bilateral breast cancer
  (D) Male breast cancer
  (E) Breast cancer in two or more relatives
  ii. Lynch syndrome (hereditary nonpolyposis colorectal cancer syndrome)—see discussion in section on endometrial cancer
  iii. Single, postmenopausal, first-degree relative likely to be sporadic and does not suggest familial pattern

8. Symptoms and signs `55C`
  a. No symptoms specific to ovarian cancer
  b. Nonspecific symptoms
    i. Abdominal bloating/fullness, usually progressive
    ii. Urinary urgency or frequency
    iii. Pelvic or abdominal pain
    iv. Early satiety
  c. Hormonally active tumors (uncommon) can produce virilization or abnormal bleeding
  d. Adnexal mass often (but not always) palpable on examination; ascites can sometimes be suspected

9. Diagnosis: `410, 55A` There is no "standard" protocol or clear consensus on the workup of cystic or solid masses of ovary; elements (other than patient age) found on ultrasound that help guide evaluation and treatment are solid/cystic and absolute size
  a. Premenopausal: functional cysts such as follicular cysts or corpus luteum cysts are common; rarely exceed 6 cm
    i. <8 cm: observation with serial ultrasounds 2–3 months apart; if stable or regress, no intervention necessary
    ii. >8 cm (in absence of ovulation-induction drugs): surgical excision for diagnosis (and treatment)
  b. Postmenopausal: functional cysts stop arising and cancer incidence increases with age, changing threshold of suspicion
    i. Simple cystic masses: in general these can be observed with serial ultrasound

      ii. Solid tumors: index of suspicion much higher; if less than 5 cm, unilateral, without ascites, and no other suspicious findings might be reasonable to watch for 2–3 months with serial ultrasounds

  c. Role of CA-125

      i. For those undergoing surgery for ovarian tumor, generally should be obtained preoperatively so that in the event it is elevated and malignancy discovered, a baseline level has been obtained that can monitor treatment

      ii. Not good screening tool in asymptomatic population due to high false-positive and false-negative rates

      iii. Role in evaluation of patient with adnexal mass controversial; can increase or decrease suspicion but cannot establish or exclude possibility of malignancy

C. Staging surgical

  1. Specifics of staging (actual practice and requirements vary by institution and protocols) typically involve the following:

    a. Free fluid in pelvis submitted for cytology; if none present, saline placed into pelvis to obtain washings, ideally from cul-de-sac, each paracolic gutter, and each hemidiaphragm

    b. Systemic examination of all intra-abdominal surfaces with biopsies of any questionable lesions or adhesions

    c. Diaphragm sampling via biopsy or scraping

    d. Omentum resected

    e. Removal of uterus, tubes, and ovaries

    f. Evaluation of pelvic lymph nodes: microscopic evaluation of enlarged nodes; if nodes not enlarged or frozen section does not confirm metastases, lymphadenectomy performed

    g. Exploration of para-aortic area: remove any enlarged nodes and resect nodes that are not enlarged for histologic evaluation

  2. Stages (FIGO)

    a. Stage I: growth confined to ovaries

      i. Stage IA: one ovary, no ascites, no tumor on external surface

      ii. Stage IB: growth on both ovaries

      iii. Stage IC: growth on surface or malignant ascites/pelvic washings

  b. Stage II: growth on one or both ovaries extends to pelvis
      i. Stage IIA: extension to uterus and/or tubes
      ii. Stage IIB: extension to other pelvic tissues
      iii. Stage IIC: A or B as above but also tumor on surface of ovary and/or positive pelvic washings
  c. Stage III: growth on one or both ovaries within peritoneal cavity outside of pelvis or involvement of retroperitoneal or inguinal nodes
      i. Stage IIIA: grossly limited to true pelvis but with microscopic seeding of peritoneal surfaces
      ii. Stage IIIB: grossly limited to true pelvis with macroscopic peritoneal implants (<2 cm in diameter)
      iii. Stage IIIC: implants >2 cm and/or positive retroperitoneal or inguinal nodes
  d. Stage IV: distant metastases: parenchyma of liver or malignant pleural effusion
D. Treatment surgical
  1. Seeks to excise all tumor or minimize volume of malignant cells that remain ("tumor debulking"); optimal staging may be associated with higher survival rate, perhaps because there is a more formal effort in identification (and eradication) of small tumor foci
  2. Chemotherapy indications continuously evolving; intended to eradicate microscopic foci of tumor
      a. Stage III and IV epithelial cell tumors require chemotherapy; some use it for lower stages that have not been optimally staged (biopsied)
      b. Two most active agents are carboplatin and paclitaxel; different protocols are being tested
E. Approximate 5-year survival rates: 55F stage I, 80%; stage II, 60%; stage III, 45%; stage IV: 10%

VI. Gestational Trophoblastic Neoplasia (GTN) (Benign and Malignant Tumors of Placenta)

A. Classification of disease (see section on diagnosis)
  1. Benign: hydatidiform mole
      a. Complete mole
          i. Embryo commonly absent
          ii. Karyotype: 46 XX or XY

> **b.** Partial mole
>> i. Gestational sac, embryo, or fetus commonly present
>> ii. Usually 69 XXX or XXY

2. Malignant types
  a. Invasive mole: invasion of chorionic villi into myometrium
  b. Placental site trophoblastic tumor: absence of villi; proliferation of intermediate trophoblast cells
  c. Gestational choriocarcinoma: malignancy involves syncytiotrophoblast and cytotrophoblast (no chorionic villi): metastases outside of uterus commonly to vagina, lung, liver, brain

3. Classification of malignant types: divided into good and poor prognosis; good prognosis if:
  a. <4 months since pregnancy
  b. hCG <40,000 mIU/mL
  c. No brain or liver metastases
  d. No antecedent term pregnancy
  e. No prior chemotherapy

B. Epidemiology
  1. 1 in 1500 pregnancies for hydatidaform mole
  2. 20% of those with molar pregnancies have subsequent malignant disease
  3. Gestational choriocarcinoma occurs in 1 in 20,000–40,000 pregnancies

C. Diagnosis `50A-B`
  1. Symptoms
    a. Uterine size greater than expected for gestational age
    b. Abnormal bleeding
    c. Metastases can cause symptoms depending on affected organ (lung: hemoptysis; brain: neurologic symptoms)
    d. Pregnancy-induced hypertension
    e. Hyperemesis gravidarum
    f. Hyperthyroidism
    g. Anemia
    h. Large theca lutein cysts
  2. Imaging and laboratory tests
    a. Commonly made by ultrasound
      i. Classic appearance is uterus filled with grape-like structure

      ii. In early pregnancy absence of gestational sac or fetal heart tones can raise possibility

  b. hCG: typically much higher than expected for given gestational age

  c. Histology

      i. Commonly diagnostic

      ii. Malignancy can develop after pregnancy (20% after complete mole; <5% after partial mole)

      iii. Histology not required for diagnosis of malignant disease

        (1) hCG titers typically used

        (2) Biopsy of malignant lesions such as invasive mole or lesions outside of uterus can lead to considerable bleeding and are generally avoided

3. Diagnosis of malignant disease after evacuation of molar pregnancy

  a. Serial weekly hCG levels that plateau over 3 weeks (stay within 10%) or rise over 2 weeks

  b. Persistence of elevated hCG levels 6 months or more after evacuation

  c. New pregnancy has to be excluded

D. Treatment 50C

  1. Molar pregnancy: surgical evacuation of uterus (dilation and curettage); medical abortion generally not recommended

    a. Preoperative evaluation

      i. Complete blood count (CBC) with platelets

      ii. Clotting studies

      iii. Renal and liver functions

      iv. Chest x-ray (spiral CT much more sensitive)

      v. Blood type and antibody screen

      vi. hCG level

    b. Intra-operative considerations

      i. Bleeding and uterine perforation risks higher

      ii. Some physicians routinely crossmatch patients

      iii. Intra-operative ultrasound may be helpful to confirm complete evacuation of products of conception

      iv. Respiratory distress has been reported after evacuation for a variety of reasons; treated with central venous monitoring and respiratory support as needed

c. Hysterectomy is alternative for women who have completed childbearing; associated with lower (not zero) risk of subsequent malignant disease

2. Molar pregnancy and co-existent fetus: relatively uncommon; for those continuing the pregnancy:
   a. Karyotype recommended
   b. Ultrasound to look for anomalies and placenta abnormalities
   c. Serial hCG levels monitored
   d. Increased risk for complications of pregnancy such as bleeding, preterm labor, pregnancy-induced hypertension

3. Malignant disease (choriocarcinoma): GTNs very sensitive to chemotherapy
   a. Additional workup (beyond that recommended pre-evacuation of mole)
      i. MRI or CT of brain
      ii. Pelvic ultrasound
      iii. CT of lungs
      iv. CT or MRI of abdomen (with special attention to liver for metastases)
   b. Nonmetastatic disease
      i. Weekly intramuscular (IM) methotrexate ($30–50$ mg/m^2)
      ii. Continue 1 week past first normal hCG level
      iii. Laboratory monitoring
         (1) CBC with platelets before each dose
         (2) Renal and liver functions (excreted by kidney; can be hepatotoxic)
      iv. Produces complete remission in 80% of population
   c. Low-risk metastatic disease
      i. Single-agent 5-day methotrexate treatment or IV dactinomycin every 14 days
      ii. Successful 60% of time
      iii. Hysterectomy reduces amount of chemotherapy needed
   d. High-risk disease
      i. Multiple chemotherapy agents
      ii. Two common protocols
         (1) Methotrexate, dactinomycin, cyclophosphamide
         (2) Etoposide sometimes added
      iii. Radiation therapy sometimes used for brain metastases

MENTOR TIPS

- Vulvar cancer is rare.
- Cervical cancer is typically treated with radiation. Surgery (radical hysterectomy) is typically reserved for Stage I or early Stage II in younger patients in otherwise good health.
- Cervical cancer adenocarcinoma is a small minority of cervical cancers and not reliably screened for by cervical cytology.
- Adenocarcinoma of uterus is surgically staged to determine the need for subsequent radiation therapy.
- For ovarian cancer, there is no particularly effective screening tool, even including CA-125 and ultrasound.
- Ovarian cancer is surgically staged, and treatment requires maximum effort to surgically remove as much tumor as possible.
- Gestational trophoblastic neoplasia is a rare placental tumor; of these, 80% are benign (although not necessarily benign clinically).

References

1. Jemel A, Tiwari RC, Murray T, et al: Cancer statistics 2004. CA: A Cancer Journal for Clinicians 54:8–29, 2004.
2. Greenlee RT, Hill-Harmon MB, Murray T, et al: Cancer statistics 2001. CA: A Cancer Journal for Clinicians 51:15–36, 2001.
3. Creasman W, Odicino F, Masionneuve P, et al: Carcinoma of the corpus uteri: Annual report of the results of treatment in gynecological cancer. Journal of Epidemiology and Biostatistics 6:45–86, 2001.

Resources

Textbook

Berek JS, Hacker NF (eds): Practical gynecologic oncology, 4th ed. Sydney, Australia: Lippincott Williams & Wilkins, 2005.

ACOG Practice Bulletins

ACOG Practice Bulletin 35. Diagnosis and treatment of cervical carcinomas. Washington, DC, American College of Obstetricians and Gynecologists, May 2002.

ACOG Practice Bulletin 53. Diagnosis and treatment of gestational trophoblastic disease. Washington, DC, American College of Obstetricians and Gynecologists, June 2004.

ACOG Practice Bulletin 65. Management of endometrial cancer. Washington, DC, American College of Obstetricians and Gynecologists, August 2005.

Chapter Self-Test Questions

Circle the correct answer. After you have responded to the questions, check your answers in Appendix A.

1. Malignancies of which organ are only clinically staged?

   a. Vulva

   b. Cervix

   c. Uterus

   d. Ovary

2. Which is an ovarian stromal tumor?

   a. Thecoma

   b. Endodermal sinus tumor

   c. Brenner tumor

   d. Endometrioid tumor

3. An ultrasound shows a 5-cm unilocular cyst in the right ovary in a 40-year-old woman with vague abdominal pain. The next step is to:

   a. Repeat the ultrasound in 4 weeks.

   b. Do a CA-125.

   c. Schedule for laparoscopy.

   d. Obtain *BRCA-1* and *BRCA-2* markers.

4. Which cancer causes the most deaths annually in the United States?

   a. Vulvar

   b. Cervical

   c. Endometrial

   d. Ovarian

See the testbank CD for more self-test questions.

17

SPECIFIC GYNECOLOGIC PROCEDURES, TECHNIQUES, AND INSTRUMENTS

Michael D. Benson, MD

I. Indications and Complications of Gynecologic Surgery

A. Indications discussed throughout the text for specific problems

B. Complications of obstetric and gynecologic surgery can include (not exhaustive): 33D

   1. Blood loss requiring blood transfusion

   2. Deep venous thrombosis and pulmonary embolus

   3. Infection that can lead to a wide variety of other complications including pneumonia, abscesses and septic shock

   4. Damage to other organs requiring additional surgery to repair either that day or in subsequent operation(s); ureter, bladder, blood vessels, and bowel are at particular risk from gynecologic procedures

   5. Anesthetic complications (risk of death from anesthesia generally at least 10 times less that of gynecologic surgery)

   6. Failure to benefit

   7. Failure to complete procedure

C. Procedure costs often difficult to establish because third-party payers often have contractual (legislated, in the case of Medicare) discounting; out-of-pocket cost to patients highly variable and specific to region and health insurance available

II. Dilation and Curettage With Hysteroscopy 33E

A. Pelvic examination under anesthesia to determine size and orientation of uterus and check for adnexal masses (commonly done before most gynecologic procedures)

B. Dilation

1. Paracervical block given (if patient not under general anesthesia)
   a. 4 mL 1% lidocaine into side of cervix where it meets vagina at 3:00 and 9:00
   b. Aspirate first to avoid intravascular injection
2. Place single-tooth tenaculum on cervix for traction
3. Endocervical curettage (if appropriate); gently curette endocervical canal with Kevorkian curette; send sample separately to pathology laboratory
4. Sound uterus
   a. Advance sound through cervical canal into uterus until resistance encountered, then stop
   b. Note cavity length (sound has cm markings)
5. Dilate cervix by passing steel rods of increasing diameter through cervix
   a. Extent of dilation varies with needs of procedure
   b. Sound diameters
      i. mm
      ii. French: diameter of sound in mm X 3 (roughly corresponds to circumference; 3 French is 1 mm in diameter

C. Hysteroscopy
   1. Hysteroscope with sheath inserted gently into uterus
   2. Distention media infused through sheath for better visualization
      a. Typically, normal saline or glycine
      b. Usually introduced under pressure
D. Curettage
   1. Polyp forceps introduced to remove bulky tissue
   2. Sharp curette used to gently scrape all four surfaces of uterus; tissue collected and sent to pathology laboratory
E. Instruments in uterus and cervix removed; cervix inspected for hemostasis (tenaculum and paracervical block puncture sites)

III. Suction Curettage (for Evacuation of First-Trimester Pregnancy With Miscarriage)

A. Paracervical block and dilation as above
B. Endocervical curettage and sounding of uterus not done
C. Suction curette passed through cervix, advanced to fundus, and withdrawn 1 cm; suction applied, and curette slowly withdrawn

1. Diameter of curette (mm) generally corresponds to gestational age in weeks
2. Straight suction can be rotated about its longitudinal access as it is withdrawn; curved curette can be tilted slightly to right and left to help evacuate uterine cornua
3. Vacuum pressure should generally read over 60 mm Hg; gauge should be visible
4. After suction curette performed, polyp forceps followed by sharp curettage

D. Cycle of suction, polyp forceps, and sharp curettage repeated until uterus empty; sharp curette has gritty rough feeling as it moves over each uterine surface when pregnancy tissue no longer present

IV. Diagnostic Laparoscopy (Fig. 17.1) 33E, 41K

A. Preparation
  1. Pelvic examination under anesthesia performed; patient prepared and draped in dorsal lithotomy position

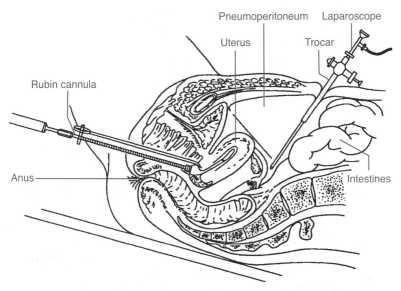

FIGURE 17.1 Gynecologic laparoscopy. (Redrawn and adapted from Cavanaugh BM: Nurse's Manual of Laboratory and Diagnostic Tests, ed 3. Philadelphia, FA Davis, 1999, p 571, with permission.)

2. Bladder catheterized
3. Uterine manipulator placed (different options)
   a. Ring forceps with 4 × 4-in sponge at end
   b. Rubin cannula: tenaculum placed on cervix; cannula placed into cervix and attached to tenaculum
   c. HUMI cannula: tenaculum placed; HUMI placed through cervix into uterus; balloon gently inflated; tenaculum removed
4. Insufflation of abdomen
   a. Veress needle placed through small incision made immediately below umbilicus
      i. Needle directed downward toward uterus at angle (not perpendicular to floor)
      ii. Needle kept in midline
      iii. Syringe half filled with normal saline used to aspirate to ensure needle not in a gas- or blood-filled place
      iv. Saline placed into end of Veress needle; abdomen tented, creating negative pressure that should suction drop into the needle if needle tip properly in peritoneal cavity
   b. CO_2 gas under pressure placed through Veress needle
      i. Abdominal pressure monitored and should be under 15 mm Hg; if not, obstruction to flow is suggested, which might mean needle tip not free in abdomen
      ii. Flow of 14–20 L/min generally used
      iii. 3–4 L CO_2 gas typically insufflated, gas turned off, and needle removed
5. Placement of laparoscope
   a. Umbilical incision enlarged to size of scope
   b. Appropriate-size laparoscopy sleeve with trocar placed through skin incision and pushed through abdominal wall along same path as Veress needle
   c. Trocar removed and laparoscope inserted promptly to ensure correctly located within peritoneal cavity and no obvious bleeding or injury
   d. Gas tubing attached to sleeve and CO_2 placed on low flow (3 L/min)
6. Placement of second port

    a. Transverse incision made in midline at pubic hairline

    b. Laparoscopy sleeve with trocar placed through incision while watching tip emerge through parietal peritoneum with laparoscope

    c. Trocar removed and probe or other instrument placed through sleeve

  7. Closure

    a. Instrument removed through second port while watching through laparoscope

    b. Laparoscope removed

    c. Gas allowed to escape through both sleeves

    d. Both sleeves removed

    e. Incisions greater or equal to 10 mm; absorbable suture placed in fascia

    f. Skin incisions closed with dissolving suture

    g. Instruments in vagina removed (if any)

V. Abdominal Hysterectomy and Bilateral Salpingo-oophorectomy (Fig. 17.2) `33E, 41H`

A. Abdominal incision

  1. Transverse (Pfannenstiel, Mallard)

  2. Vertical midline

B. Preparation of pelvis

  1. Pelvis and abdomen examined

    a. Self-retaining retractor placed with care to keep blades off psoas muscles

    b. Bowel packed away with moist laparotomy pads

  2. Grasp uterus across either cornua with 8-inch Kocher clamp

  3. Round ligament

    a. Place clamp across a few centimeters lateral to uterus

    b. Divide

    c. Suture ligate; hold suture long for traction and identification

  4. Visceral peritoneum

    a. Dissect uterus anteriorly above bladder by undermining with closed scissors

    b. Open scissors as withdrawing to create plane

    c. Divide in semicircular fashion down to midline of lower uterine segment

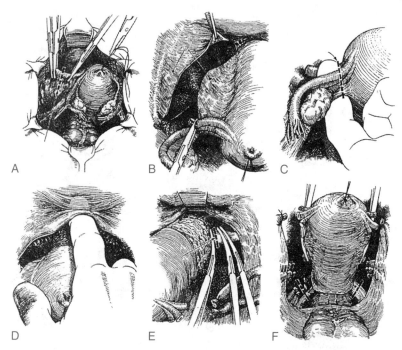

FIGURE 17.2 Abdominal hysterectomy. *A,* Clamping and dividing the round ligament. *B,* Dividing the vesico-uterine peritoneum. *C,* Site of division of the fallopian tube and ovarian suspensory ligament (with ovarian preservation). *D,* Dissection of the bladder off the lower uterine segment. *E,* Clamping and dividing uterine blood vessels. *F,* Uterine vessels and cardinal ligament cut and ligated; location of uterosacral ligaments (from posterior aspect of uterus). (Redrawn and adapted from Wheeless, CR Jr: Atlas of Pelvic Surgery. Copyright Lea & Febiger, Philadelphia, 1981, pp 213, 215, with permission. Illustrations by John Parker.)

5. Secure infundibulopelvic ligament (name given to ovarian vessels and their enveloping peritoneum)
  a. Identify location of ureter in retroperitoneal space on medial leaf of the broad of the infundibulopelvic ligament (generally well beneath this)
  b. Skeletonize by gently dissecting peritoneum off vessels
  c. Doubly clamp
  d. Cut between clamps

    e. Suture ligate (O-vicryl or O-chromic commonly used throughout)

    f. Place free tie around pedicle proximal to suture ligation

6. Repeat process for contralateral side

7. Dissect bladder off uterus and cervix

    a. Typically done by gentle blunt dissection using finger or moist sponge

    b. Can be done with sharp dissection if scarring and adhesions present

8. Uterine arteries (first one side, then the other)

    a. Skeletonize by dissecting peritoneum off vessels

    b. Doubly clamp

    c. Divide between two clamps

    d. Suture ligate

9. Cardinal ligaments

    a. Place single clamp close to uterus

        i. Stay inside uterine artery pedicle

        ii. Back-bleeding (bleeding from tissue being removed) less of a problem once uterine arteries secured; many surgeons place clamp on contralateral cardinal ligament before dividing either one

    b. Divide

    c. Suture ligate

10. Uterosacral ligaments: same steps as for cardinal ligament

11. Lateral vaginal apex

    a. Be sure bladder away from field

    b. Place curved clamp across both lateral vaginal apices (immediately beneath cervix)

    c. Divide pedicle, and remove cervix and uterus from patient

    d. Suture-ligate both pedicles; sutures often held long for identification and traction

12. Closure of vaginal cuff

    a. Running locking suture

    b. Cuff can be left open by placing running baseball-type suture along rough edges of vaginal mucosa (leaving cuff open allows pelvis to drain vaginally)

13. Closure

    a. Pedicles inspected for hemostasis

    b. Irrigation often used

    c. Self-retaining retractor removed

    d. Remainder of closure similar to that of cesarean section

C. Vaginal hysterectomy (Fig. 17.3)

    1. Preparation and start

        a. Patient prepared and draped in dorsal lithotomy position (usually not catheterized)

        b. Pelvic examination under anesthesia

        c. Weighted speculum placed into vagina to hold posterior vaginal wall out of the way while assistant positions

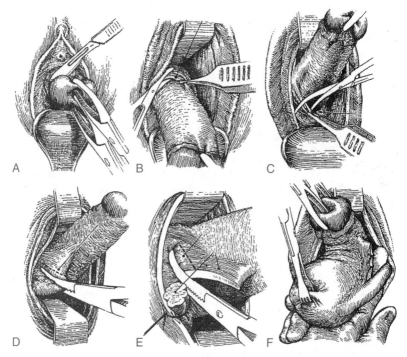

FIGURE 17.3 Vaginal hysterectomy. *A,* Incising the cervix. *B,* Incising the anterior cul-de-sac (vesico-uterine peritoneum). *C,* Incising the posterior cul-de-sac. *D,* Clamping and dividing the uterosacral ligament. *E,* Clamping and dividing the cardinal ligament. *F,* Inverting the uterus for better exposure of the round ligaments and fallopian tubes. (Redrawn and adapted from Wheeless, CR Jr: Atlas of Pelvic Surgery. Copyright Lea & Febiger, Philadelphia, 1981, pp 203, 205, with permission. Illustrations by John Parker.)

right-angle retractor to keep anterior vaginal wall out of surgical field

d. Tenaculum placed on cervix

e. Circumferential incision made around cervix close to level of internal os, just distal to beginning of vaginal mucosa

f. With a combination of blunt dissection with moist sponge and sharp dissection with Metzenbaum scissors, anterior cul-de-sac and then posterior cul-de-sac entered

2. Ureteral sacral ligaments

a. Clamp, divide, suture-ligate

b. Repeat on contralateral side

3. Cardinal ligaments: same steps for uterosacral ligaments

4. Uterine arteries: same steps as above

5. Uterine fundus

a. Delivered through vaginal opening

b. Remaining pedicle of ovarian suspensory ligament, round ligament, and proximal fallopian tube clamped, divided, suture-ligated, and free-tied

c. Repeated on contralateral side; separates uterus from patient

6. Closure of visceral peritoneum (optional)

7. Closure of vaginal cuff

a. "Figure 8" sutures placed in either lateral corner

b. Remainder of cuff closed with running suture

VI. Other Types of Hysterectomies

A. The same pedicles have to be secured, so the procedures are similar; the specific surgical instruments and techniques to secure these specimens and separate the uterus from the patient vary

B. Laparoscopic-assisted vaginal hysterectomy: upper portion of uterus secured via laparoscopy down to uterine arteries; remainder of procedure completed vaginally with specimen removed vaginally

C. Supracervical hysterectomy: uterine fundus removed, leaving cervix

1. Abdominal: laparotomy used to gain access

2. Laparoscopic: uterus usually cut into small pieces ("morcellated") to facilitate removal through small laparoscopy ports

D. Laparoscopic total hysterectomy: removes fundus and cores out central portion of cervix

E. Bilateral salpingo-oophorectomy: not integral part of hysterectomy (vaginal or abdominal); decision to remove ovaries separate from decision to remove uterus

VII. Burch Procedure

A. Indicated for urinary stress incontinence

B. Also known as retropubic urethral suspension; similar to Marshall-Marchetti-Krantz operation

C. Begins with Pfannenstiel abdominal incision that stops short of entering peritoneal cavity

1. Enter space of Retzius, between back of symphysis pubis and bladder; fat overlying vesicovaginal fascia (typically has gray, smooth appearance) and then fat overlying Cooper ligament bluntly dissected away (tendinous tissue inserting into top lateral aspect of symphysis pubis)

2. Distend bladder slightly with 100–200 mL of indigo carmine dye while clamping off Foley drainage to facilitate bladder identification

3. Place nondominant hand into vagina to facilitate placing traction on Foley as well as to push up on periurethral tissue; bladder neck identified by virtue of the Foley bulb, which can be palpated by abdominal hand while gently tugging downward with the vaginal hand

4. With assistant providing exposure with sponge sticks (4 × 4-in gauze folded in a ring forceps) and retractors, surgeon places suture into vesicovaginal fascia 1 cm lateral to proximal point of urethra: where urethra enters bladder (demarcated by palpating Foley bulb); many surgeons place suture through this tissue twice, so-called "double throw"; absorbable and nonabsorbable sutures used, each type having its advocates

5. Second suture placed 1 cm lateral to urethra, 1 cm distal to first suture; needle left attached to each of these sutures for further use

6. Repeat on contralateral side of urethra so it is supported by two sutures on either side of it in vesicovaginal fascia

7. Sutures in vesicovaginal fascia brought through Cooper ligament; distal urethral suture placed through medial aspect of Cooper ligament while proximal suture placed 1 cm lateral to this (sutures do not cross or rub against each other); sutures tied down in sequence by assistant

8. Tensioning sutures: no rigorously tested, reproducible answers; if too little tension maintained, patient's stress incontinence may not be helped; excessive tightening can result in prolonged urinary retention; some physicians place cotton swab in urethra and pull up on sutures until swab parallel to floor; others leave small amount of space between urethra and back of symphysis

9. Closing: fascia and skin closed in usual fashion

10. Placement of suprapubic catheter (if desired): facilitates "bladder training" postoperatively

   a. Fill bladder with 400 mL of indigo carmine

   b. Make stab wound a few centimeters away from the incision

   c. Place catheter with trocar in place directly through skin, fascia, and into bladder while watching tip enter bladder

   d. Remove trocar; some catheters have a balloon to inflate, others stay in bladder because they curl into a pigtail when trocar removed

   e. Secure catheter with suture (such as 3-0 silk) in skin

VIII. Anterior Colporrhaphy

A. Can be done with uterus in place at time of hysterectomy or after

B. Make transverse vaginal incision at apex of cystocele (proximal aspect of vagina)

C. Dissect vaginal mucosa off underlying fascial tissue with combination of sharp and blunt dissection with scissors; proceed to limit of repair: typically bladder neck or start of proximal urethra

D. Peel vaginal mucosa off underlying tissue laterally by sharp dissection with knife or scissors and blunt dissection with forefinger or moist sponge

E. Trim excess vaginal mucosa (typically held up and lateral with several Allis clamps on each side)

F. Place horizontal mattress sutures laterally in vesicovaginal fascia to plicate material in midline

G. Close vaginal mucosa with running or interrupted absorbable suture

H. Posterior colporrhaphy is similar in approach on back wall of vagina

IX. Tension-Free Vaginal Tape (TVT) Urethral Sling: Retropubic Approach (Fig. 17.4)

A. Drain bladder

B. Make small (5-mm) skin incisions immediately above pubic bone 2–3 cm to either side of midline

C. Make 1–2-cm midline incision in vaginal mucosa underneath mid-urethra

D. Dissect vaginal mucosa off underlying tissue for 1–2 cm bilaterally

E. Place rigid guide in Foley catheter, place into bladder, affix distal end of Foley to drapes overlying patient's left side (this moves bladder to patient's right)

F. Attach needle guide to sling material; direct needle through vaginal incision, beneath vaginal mucosa, behind (and in close proximity to) symphysis pubis in direction of patient's left shoulder, and out through skin incision

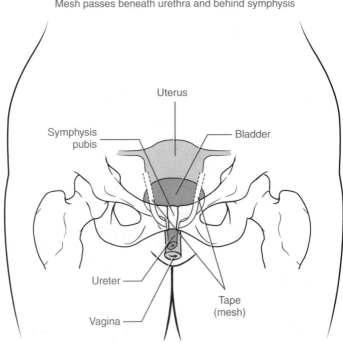

FIGURE 17.4 Retropubic urethral sling, tension-free vaginal tape (TVT) type. (Redrawn and adapted from an image by Gynecare.)

G. Hold needle in place while cystoscopy done
H. Remove Foley and do cystoscopy with 70-degree cystoscope and fully distended bladder to check for bleeding, bladder perforation, or foreign body
I. If needle in proper position (no perforation), may detach guide and pull needle through so that sling emerges 1–2 cm through skin incision
J. Drain bladder; repeat on other side (repeat cystoscopy)
K. Fine positioning of sling material: adjust each limb of sling so that material close to underside of mid-urethra but not displacing it; most surgeons also place small scissors or hemostat between urethra and sling to ensure proper positioning and leave instrument in place when plastic sheath removed
L. Assistant removes both arms of plastic sheath by pulling evenly and steadily upward while surgeon provides slight countertraction with hemostat so that sling not made tighter than intended
M. Steri-Strip or glue skin incisions
N. Place running absorbable suture in vaginal incision

X. Sutures
A. Suture gauge
  1. Small gauge
    a. Designated by a number followed by a dash and a zero
      i. Zero often called the letter O
    b. *In*creasing numbers indicate *de*creasing suture diameter (e.g., 3-0 suture smaller than 2-0 suture)
  2. Large gauge
    a. Larger-suture diameters not commonly used in obstetrics-gynecology (occasional exception is fascial closure in heavy patients or those with malignancy or diabetes)
    b. Designated by the word "number" before numeral; become larger in size with increasing number (e.g., #2 suture *bigger* than #1 suture)
B. Nonabsorbable sutures
  1. Not commonly used in obstetrics-gynecology
  2. Examples: silk, nylon, Gore-Tex, Tevdek (braided polyester), and Prolene (polypropylene)
C. Absorbable sutures
  1. Plain suture (untreated mammalian intestine) most rapidly absorbed and weakens significantly after a few days

2. Chromic suture consists of mammalian intestine strips specially treated with chromic salts; maintains strength somewhat longer: 7–10 days
3. Vicryl and Dexon are polyglycolic acid suture (made by different companies); maintain 50% of their strength at 3 weeks and take 2–3 months to resorb totally
4. Polydioxanone (PDS) maintains 60% of strength at 6 weeks (3-0 and larger); takes longer than polyglycolic acid to disappear completely

XI. Needles (Fig. 17.5 and Fig. 17.6)

A. Straight: not commonly used except occasionally on skin (e.g., Keith needle)
B. Curved
　1. Degree of curve
　　a. 3/8 circle and 1/2 circle are used frequently

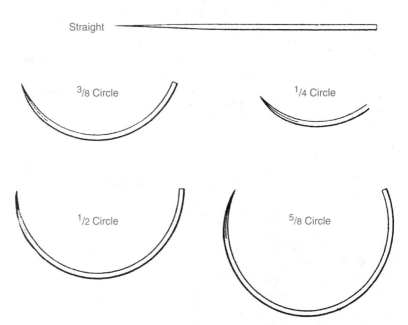

Straight

3/8 Circle　　　　1/4 Circle

1/2 Circle　　　　5/8 Circle

FIGURE 17.5 Suture needles. (Redrawn and adapted from Anderson, RM and Romfh, RF: Technique in the Use of Surgical Tools. Appleton-Century-Crofts, New York, 1980, p 198, with permission of the McGraw-Hill Companies.)

Hand-honed cutting

Lancet

Inverted lancet

Reverse cutting

Conventional cutting

Spatula

Blunt

Taper

FIGURE 17.6 Needle cross sections. (Redrawn and adapted from Anderson, RM and Romfh, RF: Technique in the Use of Surgical Tools. Appleton-Century-Crofts, New York, 1980, p 199, with permission of the McGraw-Hill Companies.)

b. 1/4 circle and 5/8 circle are used only in special circumstances

2. Shape of shaft cross section

a. Circular is called taper-point needle; used for sewing easily penetrated tissue such as peritoneum or bowel

b. Cutting needles are triangular or polygonal

  i. Typically have one of the angles sharpened to facilitate tissue penetration

  ii. Conventional needles have sharpened inside edge and used for sewing fascia and skin

3. Atraumatic needle: suture wedged into shaft of needle rather than being threaded through an eye at the end (as it is in sewing needles for clothes)

4. Pop-off needles have suture affixed in such a way that sudden, moderate force applied to needle will remove it from the suture

XII. Instruments

A. Instruments used in laparotomy and cesarean section (Table 17.1; Fig. 17.7 and Fig. 17.8)

B. Laparoscopy instruments

TABLE 17.1

Surgical Instruments

Instrument	Description	Figure Number and Letter
Cutting Instruments: Knives		
#10 blade	Large, curved; most commonly used	Figure 17.8E
#11 blade	Pointed, triangular; for small, precise incisions	
#15 blade	Small, curved	
Cutting Instruments: Scissors		
Mayo	Curved, thick blades; cuts heavy tissue	Figure 17.8A
Metzenbaum	Curved, thin blades; dissection; cuts thin tissue	Figure 17.8B
Suture	Thick, straight blades; suture cutting dulls blades	Figure 17.8D
Bandage	Angled, thick jaws	Figure 17.8E
Retractors		
Haney	Long, right-angle retractor; useful in vaginal hysterectomy	
Deaver	Straight handle, curved blade; for abdominal wall	
Malleable	Can be bent to conform to situation	
Army-Navy	Right-angle blades on both ends	
Richardson	Similar to Army-Navy retractor except that tips are slightly curved; used in opening and closing abdomen	Figure 17.7F
Jackson	Wide, right-angle retractor; commonly used in cesarean sections	Figure 17.7E
Grasping Instruments		
Forceps	With and without teeth	Figure 17.7F
Adson forceps	Small, delicate; with and without teeth	Figure 17.7B

Surgical Instruments (continued)

Instrument	Description	Figure Number and Letter
Russian forceps	Bear-paw end for grasping thick tissue	Figure 17.7D
Hemostats	Straight and curved; for clamping blood vessels	Figure 17.7H
Curved 6	6-inch curved clamp	
Curved 8	8-inch curved clamp	
Kocher clamp	Straight clamp with teeth at end	Figure 17.7J
Heaney clamp	Heavy clamp with teeth near but not at tip; straight and curved; clamps large tissue bundles	
Ring forceps	Long, straight; often used to hold sponges	Figure 17.7K
Babcock clamp	Ends are half circles; grasps fallopian tubes	
Allis clamp	Flared end with teeth; provides firm grasp	Figure 17.7I

1. Veress needle:
   a. Long steel tube with a sharp tip covered by a spring-loaded sheath; in theory, sharp tip exposed only when it encounters significant resistance such as offered by abdominal fascia
   b. Two common lengths: 120 mm, 150 mm
2. Trocars:
   a. Bladed (sharp) and atraumatic (no conclusive evidence regarding superior safety of either)
   b. Available in variety of sizes: 5-mm to 15-mm common range in gynecology
3. Insufflators
   a. Rate of flow gauge—rate of CO_2 introduction through Veress needle; low flow typically 3 L/min; high flow 20 L/min; at higher pressures vena cava compression and inhibition of diaphragmatic descent possible
   b. Abdominal pressure gauge

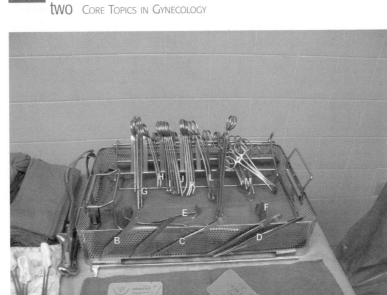

FIGURE 17.7 Surgical instruments. *A*, Sponge stick (4 × 4" sponge loaded onto ring forceps). *B*, Adson forceps. *C*, Forceps with teeth. *D*, Russian forceps. *E*, Jackson retractor. *F*, Richardson retractor. *G*, Needle holders. *H*, Curved hemostats. *I*, Allis clamps. *J*, Kocher clamps. *K*, Curved 6-inch clamps. *L*, Ring forceps. *M*, Towel clips.

      i. Usually desirable to keep this pressure below 20 mm Hg

      ii. Higher pressures may mean that the sheath introducing CO_2 is not free in the abdomen but rather is in an enclosed space such as a hollow viscus or a mass of scar tissue

      iii. Typically has a setting that prevents gas flow if the pressure exceeds this value

  c. Volume gauge: records absolute volume of gas introduced—typically 2.5–4 L for placement of trocars

4. Laparoscopes: vary in size 5–10 mm

5. Light source: can be off, stand-by, or on; if light on and laparoscope tip is resting on paper drapes, fires can be (and have been) started

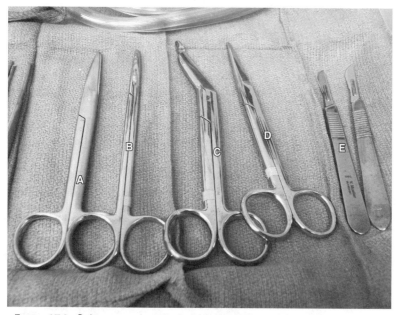

FIGURE 17.8 Scissors and scalpel. *A*, Curved Mayo scissors. *B*, Metzenbaum scissors. *C*, Bandage scissors. *D*, Straight Mayo scissors ("suture scissors"). *E*, Scalpel with #10 blade.

6. Variety of other instruments may be placed through the various-size sheaths: Babcock clamps, staple applicators, scissors, and cautery devices; most rapidly expanding part of the market is disposable instruments

C. Devices using power to cut and coagulate

    1. Lasers 33E

        a. General concepts

            i. Not many specific uses in gynecology; lasers tend to be expensive and technically cumbersome

            ii. Biggest advantage is ability to precisely control depth of destruction

            iii. Safety: it is important to know which type of laser is in use in the operating room: laser light easily reflected and different wavelengths require different types of eye protection; laser energy can set operating drapes on fire; in many cases, drapes are first wetted with water

   b. CO_2 laser

      i. Invisible and thus requires a second, low-power helium-neon laser to provide visible, red aiming point

      ii. Usefulness limited because laser cannot penetrate blood

      iii. Most commonly used for destroying transformation zone of the cervix and large condylomata of lower genital tract

   c. Yttrium-aluminum-garnet (YAG) laser

      i. Capable of tissue destruction down to 4 mm, much deeper than CO_2 laser

      ii. Depth of destruction actually a disadvantage and has been circumvented through use of sapphire tips that limit depth of energy penetration; unfortunately, laser tips get hot and require constant cooling with high-flow gas stream, typically nitrogen

      iii. Laser sometimes used to destroy endometriosis because laser absorbed by darkly pigmented tissue and, with sapphire tips, has a precisely controlled effect

   d. Potassium-titanyl-phosphate (KTP) laser similar to YAG laser with respect to its precision

2. Electrocautery

   a. General concepts

      i. Electrosurgical devices much less expensive than lasers and easier to maintain

      ii. For laparoscopic surgery, have largely replaced lasers for both cutting and cautery

      iii. Chief drawbacks of electrosurgery are limited control over the depth of tissue destruction and ever-present possibility that current will not flow in expected path but will damage tissue adjacent to field of surgery; generators are now so well engineered that uncontrolled flow of current (a highly undesirable event) is extremely uncommon

   b. Unipolar cutting and cautery

      i. Require a ground; can be a grounding pad attached to patient or surgical table

      ii. Current travels from the tip of cautery device to the ground

      iii. Most commonly used

iv. Type of current varies
  (1) When cutting chiefly desired, continuous current generated so that water in cells adjacent to tip heats very quickly, causing these cells to burst; prevents conduction of heat into deeper tissue
  (2) For cautery, current generated in pulses, allowing time for heat to be conducted away from site
  c. Bipolar cautery: current passes between two tips of cautery instrument; occasionally used in tubal ligations and for controlling bleeding from small vessels
  d. When using electrosurgery, important to ground patient properly so that current leaves patient in controlled manner
3. Harmonic scalpel
  a. Almost exclusively a laparoscopic instrument
  b. Used to cut and coagulate
  c. Uses rapid vibration of blade (55,500 Hz) to create ultrasound energy
  d. Heats tissue to 50°–100°C; denatures protein to form coagulum (laser and electrocautery heat tissue to 150°–400°C; desiccate tissue and cause eschar to form)

XIII. Techniques

A. Most important objective in learning surgery is to understand goal of operation and steps used to reach goal
B. Anticipating next step is absolutely necessary for surgical proficiency
C. Scalpel
  1. Should be held with thumb opposing other four fingers so that steady downward pressure can be maintained, particularly when incising abdominal wall
  2. Stabilize tissue to be incised with nondominant hand; try to stay in same vertical plane as the incision is made deeper into the tissue
D. Clamps with locking teeth should be fully closed
E. Cutting suture: stabilize dominant hand with the other (if possible) and simply use tips of the scissors; never cut what you cannot see
F. Suture material being tied determines specific type of knot to be used; for instance, sutures that hold knots well, such as plain and

chromic catgut, can be secured with three half-hitches; suture material prone to slippage, such as Vicryl, Dexon, and polydioxanone (PDS), often better secured with a surgeon's knot (two initial throws) followed by three or four additional half-hitches; leave substantial suture material beyond the knot when cutting excess suture, particularly in deeper layers, where the excess will not protrude through skin

G. Suturing around clamps—fixation sutures

1. The most common way to suture a pedicle is to place the needle just beneath the tip of the clamp and tie behind the clamp.

2. Haney suture: needle passes beneath tip of clamp, suture brought around clamp, and needle brought through again through middle of pedicle; many surgeons keep needle passage above loop of suture so that, if second passage pierces a blood vessel, this perforation will be distal to the suture when it is tied

3. Pulley suture: needle passes through middle of pedicle and then brought around front of clamp clockwise while back of suture brought around front of clamp counterclockwise; suture tied behind clamp so entire pedicle within tied ligature

XIV. Safety in the Operating Room (OR)

A. After 150 years of surgery performed under effective anesthesia, only now is safety in the OR getting a real push.

1. Anything with an energy source can cause a fire, including focal light sources and cautery; alcohol in some antibacterial solutions is volatile and can flash over if not completely dry

2. In practically every hospital in the country, the wrong surgery has been done on the wrong part of the wrong patient; patients now mark their bodies with a marker over the site to be operated on before going into the OR; once there, the patient name and procedure to be performed read aloud and confirmed by all present before incision made

3. Sponges, needles, and instruments are counted before patient enters OR and then, for open abdominal cases, three times during surgery: immediately before closing peritoneum (if it is closed), before fascia, and before skin closure; if count not correct, patient x-rayed for material left behind before leaving OR; needles easy to misplace so they should be handed back to scrub nurse very deliberately

MENTOR TIPS

- There is no one right way to perform any specific procedure. Over time, each surgeon develops preferences. Flexibility and open-mindedness about surgical approaches are very desirable, particularly as one is learning, and throughout a surgical career.
- Beware of tradition. Much about surgery is taught by specific mentors in a physician's life, and not every step is the result of double-blinded placebo-controlled trials.
- When tying the knot at the end of a running suture, most surgeons add at least one extra half-hitch because the end with three strands is the one more likely to become undone.
- Every new innovation is not necessarily a good innovation. Consider the case of endometrial ablation, which was initially performed with a YAG laser with a 0.6-mm width of destruction. In view of the current "low-tech" methods that are fast, easy to perform, and more effective, the use of the laser for this procedure seems almost bizarre, in retrospect.
- Apprentices should pay careful attention to every step. Even for those not planning to go into a surgical- or procedure-oriented specialty, being attentive will help the physician in training get the most value out of the time spent. Consider (1) How is the patient positioned? (2) Is the bladder catheterized? (3) Are prophylactic antibiotics used? (4) What are the specific steps of the procedure? (5) What sutures are used?
- Pay attention to safety in the OR (e.g., laser light, fire risks, areas to be operated on, and counts of sponges, needles, and instruments).

Resources

Anderson RM, Romfh RF: Technique in the use of surgical tools. New York, Appleton-Century-Crofts, 1980.

Rock JA, Jones HW: TeLinde's operative gynecology, 9th ed. Philadelphia, Lippincott Williams & Wilkins, 2003.

Wheeless CR Jr, Parker J: Atlas of pelvic surgery. Philadelphia, Lippincott Williams & Wilkins, 1997.

Chapter Self-Test Questions

Circle the correct answer. After you have responded to the questions, check your answers in Appendix A.

1. Order of structures encountered during an abdominal hysterectomy:

    a. Uterine artery, cardinal ligament, uterosacral ligament

    b. Cardinal ligament, uterine artery, uterosacral ligament

    c. Uterosacral ligament, cardinal ligament, uterine artery

    d. Uterine artery, uterosacral ligament, cardinal ligament

2. Which is the largest suture?

    a. 3-0

    b. 2-0

    c. 0

    d. 1

3. Which is absorbable?

    a. Tevdek

    b. Prolene

    c. Polydioxanone

    d. Nylon

4. Which cuts and coagulates at the lowest temperature?

    a. Unipolar cautery

    b. CO_2 laser

    c. Bipolar cautery

    d. Harmonic scalpel

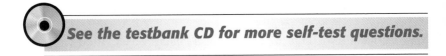

See the testbank CD for more self-test questions.

18

EMOTIONAL AND SEXUAL HEALTH IN WOMEN

Michael D. Benson, MD

I. Premenstrual Dysphoric Disorder [49A]

A. Definition[1]

1. Symptoms confined to last week of luteal phase

2. Symptoms present for most of preceding 12 months

3. Five or more of the following

a. Sadness, hopelessness (may have transient suicidal ideation)

b. Tense

c. Marked lability of mood with frequent tearfulness

d. Irritability, anger

e. Decreased interest in social activities

f. Difficulty concentrating

g. Fatigue

h. Marked change in appetite

i. Sleep disorder (too much, too little)

j. Feeling out of control

k. Physical symptoms (breast tenderness, headache, bloating, weight gain, muscle pain)

4. May co-exist with other psychiatric conditions

B. Incidence

1. 75% of women report some premenstrual symptoms/ discomfort

2. Estimated 3%–5% meet formal criteria

3. Majority of women in research protocols are in their mid-30s, but no systematic population-based estimates available

4. Symptoms do not occur during pregnancy or menopause

C. Etiology [49B]

1. Unknown

2. Measurements of a variety of hormones including estrogen and progesterone not linked to occurrence of symptoms, whether comparing different women or levels within same woman
3. Response to selective serotonin reuptake inhibitors (SSRIs) different from that classically seen with depression
   a. Response for premenstrual dysphoric disorder (PMDD) seen in 24–48 hours in prospective placebo-controlled double-blinded trials
   b. For depression, response typically not seen for 14–21 days
   c. SSRIs improve bloating and breast tenderness though mechanism not known

D. Diagnosis 40C
1. Daily symptom log
   a. Classic recommendation for diagnosis: prospective daily log of all symptoms for 3 months
   b. Not practical in everyday practice
      i. Delays treatment for 3 months
      ii. Patients seeking treatment usually want immediate relief
      iii. Compliance poor even in motivated patients
2. History usually sufficient; patient usually presents with self-diagnosis (e.g., PMS) and is more often than not correct
3. Differential diagnosis: diagnosis usually fairly straightforward and emphasis is on symptoms being confined to week before menses; differential possibilities include depression, bipolar disease, substance abuse, thyroid disease, and irritable bowel syndrome

E. Treatment 40D
1. Symptom relief: diuretics, pain relievers
2. Ovulation suppression
   a. Cyclic oral contraceptives do not reliably provide benefit
   b. Noncyclic combination contraceptives might (Seasonale, Lybrelle)
   c. Gonadotropin-releasing hormone (GnRH) agonists rarely appropriate
3. SSRIs
   a. Proven efficacy
   b. Two approaches: continuously or last 14 days of cycle
4. Anxiolytics for those with only 1 or 2 days of anxiety or irritability; benzodiazepines are reasonable alternative

II. Psychiatric Disorders in Pregnancy

A. Normal, commonplace feelings of pregnancy `29A`
  1. Stress
  2. Anxiety (many sources, including fetal health, maternal health, finances, employment, lifestyle, relationship, childbirth pain, parenting)
B. Baby blues
  1. Self-limited, transient condition
  2. Occurs in over half of postpartum women
  3. Onset by day 3
  4. Resolution by day 14
  5. Symptoms: tearfulness/crying, mood shifts, anxiety, irritability
  6. Not consistently disabling
  7. Not considered psychiatric disorder
C. Postpartum depression `29B–C`
  1. Same diagnostic criteria as depression, simply occurring post partum
  2. Differing views of onset in postpartum state
    a. DSM-IV TR defines onset as occurring within 4 weeks
    b. Most physicians consider the diagnosis for an onset within 12 weeks of birth
  3. Definition of major depressive disorder
    a. Five or more of the following:
      i. Depressed sad mood for most of the day nearly every day
      ii. Markedly diminished interest or pleasure in all or almost all of activities
      iii. Significant weight loss (>5% in 1 month)
      iv. Sleep disturbance (too much, too little)
      v. Psychomotor agitation or retardation
      vi. Fatigue
      vii. Feelings of worthlessness or excessive guilt
      viii. Impaired thinking, concentration
      ix. Thoughts of death
        (1) Recurrent
        (2) Recurrent suicidal ideation without plan
        (3) Recurrent suicidal ideation with a plan
        (4) Suicide attempt
    b. Symptoms do not meet criteria for bipolar disease

  c. Symptoms cause significant distress or impairment in social functioning

  d. Not direct effect of medication, substance abuse, or medical condition

  e. Symptoms not result of bereavement

 4. Diagnosis

  a. Definition often sufficient

  b. Edinburgh Postnatal Depression Scale[2] (Box 18.1)

   i. Good screening tool: easy to administer and effective

   ii. Developed for postnatal use, but also useful during pregnancy; typically given at 28 weeks

 5. Epidemiology and risk factors

  a. 8%–15% of population (most common postpartum complication[3])

  b. Risk factors: prior depression history (risk 30%), adolescence (risk 30%), or prior postpartum depression (risk up to 70% with subsequent pregnancy)

 6. Treatment

  a. SSRIs safe during pregnancy and nursing

  b. Exception: Paxil (paroxetene); concern over increased risk of heart defects (not seen with other SSRIs)

  c. Other antidepressants safe during pregnancy

   i. Wellbutrin (bupropion): not anxiolytic; may inhibit smoking desire

   ii. Effexor (venlafaxine)

  d. Early recognition and treatment lead to better results

   i. Depression disruptive for patient

   ii. Depression disrupts maternal and infant bonding and can affect child development

   iii. Depression not benign: suicide can result

  e. Suicidal ideation with a plan requires immediate steps to ensure patient safety to self and others (these patients must not drive)

D. Postpartum psychosis 29B–C

 1. Occurs 1 in 1000 deliveries

 2. Symptoms

  a. Confusion, disorientation

  b. Difficulty separating reality from fantasy (including visual and auditory hallucinations)

BOX 18.1   Edinburgh Postnatal Depression Scale (EPDS)

Instructions for users

Administering:

1. The mother is asked to underline the response which comes closest to how she has been feeling in the previous 7 days.
2. All ten items must be completed.
3. Care should be taken to avoid the possibility of the mother discussing her answers with others.
4. The mother should complete the scale herself, unless she has limited English or has difficulty with reading.

Scoring:

Questions 1, 2, and 4 (without an asterisk [*]) are scored 0, 1, 2, or 3, with the top answer scored as 0 and the bottom answer scored as 3.

Questions 3 and 5–10 (marked with an asterisk [*]) are reverse-scored, with the top answer scored as 3 and the bottom answer scored as 0.

The total score is the sum of all the scores for each of the ten items.

Maximum score: 30

Possible depression: 10 or greater

Always look at item 10 (suicidal thoughts).

Reproducing:

Users may reproduce the scale without further permission providing they respect copyright (which remains with the British Journal of Psychiatry) by quoting the names of the authors, the title, and the source of the paper in all reproduced copies.

Administered/Reviewed by: _____

Date: _____

Name: _____

Address: _____

Phone: _____

Your date of birth: _____

Baby's due date (if not yet born): _____

Baby's date of birth (if already born): _____

As you are pregnant or have recently had a baby, we would like to know how you are feeling. Please UNDERLINE the answer which comes closest to how you have felt IN THE PAST 7 DAYS, not just how you feel today.

Here is an example, already completed.

I have felt happy:

Yes, all the time

Yes, most of the time

(continued on page 310)

Edinburgh Postnatal Depression Scale (EPDS) (continued)

No, not very often
No, not at all

This would mean: "I have felt happy most of the time" during the past week. Please complete the other questions in the same way.

In the past 7 days:
1. I have been able to laugh and see the funny side of things
As much as I always could
Not quite so much now
Definitely not so much now
Not at all

2. I have looked forward with enjoyment to things
As much as I ever did
Rather less than I used to
Definitely less than I used to
Hardly at all

*3. I have blamed myself unnecessarily when things went wrong
Yes, most of the time
Yes, some of the time
Not very often
No, never

4. I have been anxious or worried for no good reason
No, not at all
Hardly ever
Yes, sometimes
Yes, very often

*5. I have felt scared or panicky for no very good reason
Yes, quite a lot
Yes, sometimes
No, not much
No, not at all

*6. Things have been getting on top of me
Yes, most of the time I haven't been able to cope at all
Yes, sometimes I haven't been coping as well as usual
No, most of the time I have coped quite well
No, I have been coping as well as ever

*7. I have been so unhappy that I have had difficulty sleeping
Yes, most of the time
Yes, sometimes
Not very often
No, not at all

Edinburgh Postnatal Depression Scale (EPDS) (continued)

*8. I have felt sad or miserable
  Yes, most of the time
  Yes, quite often
  Not very often
  No, not at all
*9. I have been so unhappy that I have been crying
  Yes, most of the time
  Yes, quite often
  Only occasionally
  No, never
*10. The thought of harming myself has occurred to me
  Yes, quite often
  Sometimes
  Hardly ever
  Never

    c. Paranoid ideation
    d. Difficulty caring for infant
  3. Risk factors: other psychiatric illness; family history
  4. Treatment: generally requires specific psychiatric consultation

III. Sexual Health
  A. Physiology (based on Masters and Johnson[4]) 56A
    1. Female sexual response
      a. Excitement
        i. Vaginal lubrication
        ii. Inner vagina expands
        iii. Vaginal walls thicken
        iv. Cervix and uterus move up
        v. Nipple erection
        vi. Sexual flush

  b. Plateau
   i. Further expansion of inner vagina
   ii. Withdrawal of clitoris
   iii. Carpopedal spasm
   iv. Increase in vital signs
  c. Orgasm: contractions of uterus, rectal sphincter
  d. Resolution
 2. Male sexual response
  a. Excitement
   i. Erection
   ii. Elevation of testes
  b. Plateau: further enlargement of penis, testes
  c. Orgasm: penile contractions with ejaculation of seminal fluid
  d. Resolution
 3. Effect of aging
  a. Libido diminishes
  b. Sexual response for both genders takes longer and becomes somewhat less intense

B. Sexual expression `56B`
 1. Homosexuality (women: 1%–3%; men: 3%–6%)
 2. Heterosexual behavior (90% participate in oral sex; 10% participate in anal sex)
 3. Influences
  a. Presence of Y chromosome
  b. Endocrine factors at puberty
  c. Social taboos and attitudes play large role
  d. Many behaviors learned during childhood
  e. Many aspects unknown, particularly role of genetics versus environment in sexual preference

C. Sexual dysfunction in women `56C`
 1. Dyspareunia (painful intercourse)
  a. Most common cause: loss of libido (due to ambivalence about partner or to depression or anxiety)
  b. Other causes include pelvic disorder (such as ovarian masses, uterine masses, or endometriosis) or childbirth injuries
 2. Vaginismus: involuntary contraction of vaginal musculature preventing intercourse; usually psychological in origin

3. Decreased libido

    a. Primary: never had interest

    b. Secondary: initial interest lost (cause usually relationship difficulties or depression/anxiety)

IV. Sexual Assault 57A-C

A. Definitions

    1. Sexual assault: unwanted (nonconsensual) sexual contact or touching

    2. Specific types (depending on legal and social relations of the perpetrator and victim): marital rape, acquaintance rape, incest, rape by a stranger, and statutory rape (although sexual contact may be consensual, issue is whether individual old enough to give consent)

B. Incidence 58A

    1. 20%–25% of adult women in the United States report unwanted sexual contact at some time

    2. Majority of rapes (~70%?) go unreported

    3. Acquaintance sexual assault much more common than assault by strangers

        a. Major issue in adolescence and college age

        b. Alcohol consumption by perpetrator and/or victim very often a common denominator

    4. Estimated 500,000 cases of child abuse in United States annually

    5. Elder abuse: data lacking

C. Victim presentation 58B

    1. Symptoms

        a. Presenting complaint often not "rape"

        b. Patient presents with:

            i. Complaints of "mugging"

            ii. Concern about acquiring a sexually transmitted disease

            iii. Psychiatric issues such as suicide attempt

    2. Emotional response to sexual assault

        a. Short term:

            i. Loss of emotional control

            ii. Detached calm

        b. Medium term: (2 weeks to months)

            i. Initial reactions abate

        ii. Emotional distress returns; often causes victim to seek care

    c. Long term: post-traumatic stress disorder

        i. Intense distress

        ii. Reliving trauma

        iii. Avoidance of situations that remind patient of the event

  3. Injuries

    a. 40% sustain some sort of injury

    b. 1% require hospitalization or surgery

    c. 1 in 1000 killed

D. Medical evaluation (establishes a legal record)

  1. Careful (and intrusive) history: cannot have any party other than medical personnel with specific need to attend

    a. Specifics of assault

        i. Date, time, place

        ii. What exactly occurred

        iii. Ejaculation?

        iv. Condom use

        v. Weapons/threats

    b. Victim past history

        i. Last consensual intercourse

        ii. Last bath/shower

        iii. Sexual patterns (number of partners, type of partners)

  2. Physical examination

    a. Thorough body evaluation, including general appearance, emotional status, vital signs, and body surface (with particular attention to signs of trauma)

    b. Genital examination: attention to signs of trauma

  3. Forensic evidence collection

    a. Photographs of any signs of trauma

    b. Toxicology screen

    c. Collection of tissues (sperm/semen, nail clippings, pubic hair combings, blood samples)

    d. Cultures (or DNA probes) for gonorrhea and chlamydia

    e. Wet preparation for motile sperm, trichomonads

    f. Collect clothing

    g. Serology (rapid plasma reagin [RPR], human immunodeficiency virus [HIV], hepatitis B and C)

E. Treatment

1. All trauma and injuries as appropriate
2. Tetanus toxoid
3. Hepatitis B vaccine (two follow-up doses needed)
4. Antibiotic prophylaxis:
   a. Ceftriaxone 125 mg IM *and*
   b. Metronidazole 2 g orally *and*
   c. One of the following:
      i. Erythromycin 1 g orally *or*
      ii. Doxycycline 100 mg orally twice daily for 7 days
5. Emotional care: counseling
6. Follow-up
   a. Counseling
   b. Repeat sexually transmitted infection (STI) testing at 2–3 weeks and repeat serologies at 3–6 months
   c. Hepatitis B repeat vaccine at 1–2 months and 4–6 months
F. Special case: children
   1. 90% victimized by someone known to them
   2. Parents and relatives cannot be present during interview
   3. Mandatory legal reporting (specifics vary by state)

V. Domestic Violence 58A-B

A. Types of abuse: spouse, children, parents
B. Among women
   1. 40% beaten by mates
   2. 10% raped
   3. Violence may increase during pregnancy
   4. 10% reported (estimated) and 1%–2% result in arrest
   5. Alcohol and/or substance abuse very commonly involved
   6. Domestic violence calls have one of the highest rates of injury for police officers
C. Screening
   1. "Do you feel safe at home?"
   2. Can ask specifically about types of abuse (emotional, physical, unwanted sexual contact, fear of partner or others)
D. Treatment 58C-E
   1. Domestic violence provides real health threat
      a. Huge source of emotional and psychiatric distress
      b. Real risk of permanent injury or death
   2. Chief effort is patient safety

a. Very difficult; no universal answer
b. Most localities have shelter for women, only short-term solution
c. Police involvement may (or may not) be helpful
d. Victims often feel powerless and paradoxically unwilling to take obvious and even easy steps to leave situation
   3. Legal reporting: varies by state
a. Spouse/ partner abuse: reporting often not required
b. Child abuse: reporting almost always required
c. Elder abuse: reporting commonly required
   4. Help patient to seek resources (local agencies, Family Violence Prevention Fund, National Resource Center, shelters)

MENTOR TIPS

- For premenstrual dysphoric disorder, you can usually rely on self-diagnosis of patient. SSRIs (either continuously or cyclically) are very effective.
- Most women have some premenstrual change in mood. Extent of change and distress varies.
- Symptoms of baby blues and postpartum depression overlap; key distinguishing feature is duration of symptoms.
- Screening for depression in pregnancy is becoming mandatory in many states.
- Physician must be looking for signs and symptoms of assault and domestic violence, as victims only rarely directly complain of these events.
- Emotional distress or symptoms without clear physical causes can be tip-offs to abuse.
- Marriage is no guarantee against sexual assault.
- Good counseling for young women: (1) avoid being around intoxicated men; (2) know where you are and where you are going at all times; (3) make sure someone else knows your plans.

References

1. Diagnostic and statistical manual of mental disorders, 4th ed, text revision (DSM-IV-TR). Arlington, Va., American Psychiatric Association, 2000.
2. Cox JL, Holden JM, Sagovsky R: Detection of postnatal depression. Development of the 10-item Edinburgh Postnatal Depression Scale. British Journal of Psychiatry 150:782–786, 1987.
3. Wisner KL, Parry BL, Piontek CM: Postpartum depression. New England Journal of Medicine 347:194–199, 2002.
4. Masters WH, Johnson VE: Human sexual response. Toronto and New York, Bantam Books, 1966.

Resources

Flitcraft A: Violence, abuse, and assault over the life phases. In Wallis LA, et al (eds): Textbook of women's health. Philadelphia, Lippincott-Raven, 1998, pp 249–258.

Chapter Self-Test Questions

Circle the correct answer. After you have responded to the questions, check your answers in Appendix A.

1. Which is true about premenstrual dysphoric disorder?

   a. Specific hormone levels have been linked to symptoms.

   b. Response to selective serotonin reuptake inhibitors similar to that of depression.

   c. The most clinically useful diagnostic tool is patient history.

   d. Symptoms can persist into pregnancy and menopause.

2. Which treatment is *not* effective for premenstrual dysphoric disorder?

   a. Cyclic oral contraceptives

   b. Diuretics

   c. Selective serotonin reuptake inhibitors

   d. Benzodiazepines

3. Which is *not* true about sexual expression?

   a. Majority of people have oral sex.

   b. Same-sex expression more common among men than women.

   c. Mechanism of sexual preference is well understood.

   d. Social taboo plays a large role.

4. Evaluation of the rape victim typically includes all of the following *except:*

   a. Sexual history.

   b. Explicit details of assault.

   c. X-ray of limbs to check for fractures.

   d. Collection of pubic hair combings.

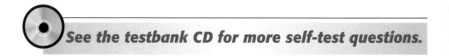

See the testbank CD for more self-test questions.

PART three

CORE TOPICS IN OBSTETRICS

19

PRENATAL CARE

Michael D. Benson, MD

I. Preconception Counseling [10J]

A. A naïve ideal?

1. Many pregnancies are not planned
2. For those that are, most women do not seek preconception counseling
3. Most pregnancies do well with no planning

B. For minority who do seek counseling

1. Social, demographic issues: physician advice not typically sought for these issues yet they may be most important for health and welfare of mother and child

a. Completion of education

b. Marriage?

i. Conceptions that occur without this formal, legal, and social sanction more likely to end in failed relationship

     ii. Single parenthood much more difficult in terms of financial and social support

  c. Financial resources: employment and savings are considerations

  d. Advanced age `9D`

     i. Does not greatly increase maternal risk of morbidity or mortality

     ii. Gradually increases risk of chromosome abnormalities

     iii. Not associated with increased neonatal morbidity/mortality beyond possible link to intrauterine fetal demise (in absence of other maternal illness)

     iv. Can significantly reduce chance of conception

2. Nutrition `10F`

  a. Body mass index (BMI) should be between 19 and 25; excess BMI at start of pregnancy more important in determining macrosomia than development of gestational diabetes

  b. Advice needs to be realistic; no effective medical interventions for weight loss (other than bariatric surgery)

  c. Folic acid

     i. Only supplement that can reduce incidence of a rare birth defect

     ii. Neural tube defects are decreased with folic acid supplementation at least 3 months in advance of conception

       (1) General population: 400 mcg/day (almost all multi-vitamins in United States have at least this amount)

       (2) For those with a personal history of a child with a neural tube defect: 4 mg daily

3. Exercise: improves long-term health but does not specifically improve ease or outcome of pregnancy or labor

4. Genetic screening: carrier status for single-gene defects contingent on ethnicity/ancestry (see Chapter 20: Obstetrical Genetics) `10C`

5. Rubella titer: live vaccine may be offered to those not immune `10H`

6. Substance abuse: tobacco, alcohol, and illicit drugs ideally stopped 3 months before conception `9E, 10E, 10G`

a. Tobacco: associated with increased risk of miscarriage, low birth weight, abruption, and perinatal mortality

b. Alcohol

   i. Leading preventable cause of mental retardation in United States

   ii. No known safe level

   iii. Fetal alcohol syndrome (FAS)

      (1) Threshold not conclusive: probably near four drinks daily (binge drinking may be more or less damaging)

      (2) Brain damage and facial abnormalities common

      (3) Associated with heart defects, spina bifida, limb defects, and urinary tract anomalies

   iv. Fetal alcohol effects

      (1) Lower threshold than FAS (but not clear what that is)

      (2) Milder impact on fetus than FAS, such as behavior problems

c. Illicit drug use (including improper prescription-drug use): depends on drug; not well characterized; risks include neonatal withdrawal, neurologic injury, and possibly subsequent behavior/learning problems in child

7. Prescription medication: many medications can (and should) be continued, particularly those for asthma, depression, and anxiety (see Chapter 20: Obstetrical Genetics) `10G`

8. Chronic medical conditions `9A-B`

a. Asthma: not predictably affected by pregnancy; continue medications

b. Heart disease: significant cardiac impairment associated with substantial increased risk of maternal mortality

c. Hypertension: associated with increased risk of pre-eclampsia and intrauterine growth restriction

d. Diabetes: insulin needs will increase

e. Epilepsy: minority have increased seizure frequency (~20%?)

   i. Increased risk of low birth weight, congenital anomalies, perinatal mortality, neurologic damage: treatment or disease etiology unclear

   ii. Many anticonvulsants have some risk of teratogenicity; use fewest drugs at lowest dose

II. Prenatal Visits

A. Timing: frequency chiefly related to screening for pre-eclampsia

    1. Every 4 weeks from initial presentation through 28 weeks

    2. Every 2 weeks from 28 weeks through 36 weeks

    3. Weekly at 36 weeks and thereafter

B. Initial visit `1A, 10A`

    1. History

        a. History of present illness: should focus on prior types of contraception, menstrual history, first positive pregnancy test, symptoms of pregnancy

        b. Gravidity (total number of pregnancies)

            i. Includes present one

            ii. Multiple gestations counted as only one pregnancy

        c. Parity (pregnancy outcomes): TPAL system:

            i. T: term deliveries; fetuses delivered at 37 completed weeks or beyond

            ii. P: preterm deliveries (after 20 weeks and before term)

            iii. A: abortions: intended or unintended delivery of pregnancy before fetus completed 20 weeks or achieved 500 g

            iv. L: number of offspring currently living

        d. Past medical history: prior abdominal surgery, major medical conditions, and previous pregnancy outcomes are of special interest

        e. Family history

            i. Predispositions for illness in mother

            ii. Genetic history: birth defects in families of either parent-to-be, as well as families' ethnic backgrounds

        f. Social history

            i. Substance abuse (tobacco, alcohol, illicit drugs, or use of prescription medication)

            ii. Marital status

                 (1) Number of sexual partners in last year, if single

                 (2) Name of baby's father if single: may be helpful in paternity issues postpartum

        g. Review of systems: inquire about symptoms characteristic of pregnancy: fatigue, heartburn, gas, constipation, nausea, breast tenderness, and so on

    2. Initial physical examination `10H`

a. General: all major body systems
b. Special emphasis: abdomen and pelvis
    i. Scars
    ii. Presence of heart tones
    iii. Uterine size
    iv. Cervical dilation and effacement
c. Historical signs of pregnancy
    i. Chadwick sign: blue discoloration of cervix
    ii. Goodell sign: softening of cervix
    iii. Hegar sign: softening of lower uterus
d. Pelvimetry (estimation of size of bony pelvis) difficult for beginners, but effort can be made to note some of the most obvious landmarks, which are indicated as follows and in Figure 19.1
    i. Measurements
        (1) Conjugate diameter (CD): distance from lower aspect of pubic symphysis to sacral promontory

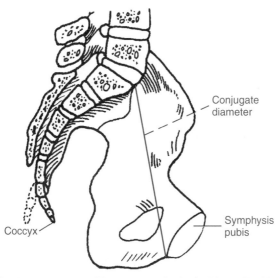

FIGURE 19.1 Maternal pelvis. (Redrawn and adapted from Bonica JJ: Principles and Practice of Obstetric Analgesia and Anesthesia. FA Davis, Philadelphia, 1967, p 851, with permission.)

       (A) Palpate as far upward and backward as possible

       (B) Often not able to feel sacral promontory: note that CD is greater than measured length of your outstretched fingers (in cm)

    (2) Sacrum: hollow or flat (subjective assessment)

    (3) Coccyx: anterior or posterior (subjective judgment)

    (4) Ischial spines: bony protuberances at 4 and 8 o'clock, 2 inches or so into vaginal canal along vaginal sidewalls; are they prominent?

    (5) Transverse diameter: distance between ischial tuberosities; best examined with patient flat with legs adducted and dorsiflexed (position for routine pelvic examination); broad bony prominences palpable on medial aspect of buttocks, inferior to anus

    (6) Pubic arch angle: can be estimated by sweeping two fingers under pubic arch; women commonly have arch angle of 110° or greater

  ii. Four pelvic types

    (1) Gynecoid: ideal: round/oval inlet

    (2) Android: triangular inlet, prominent ischial spines, narrow pubic arch angle

    (3) Anthropoid: transverse diameter of inlet greater than outlet

    (4) Platypelloid: flat inlet with shortened conjugate diameter

  iii. Limitations of pelvimetry

    (1) Available evidence does not support prognostic significance of pelvimetry for predicting vaginal birth or course of labor

    (2) Not reliably reproducible among different observers

    (3) Maternal pelvis dimensions change (up to 25%) depending on position

    (4) Still taught and occasionally charted, but probably not clinically relevant

C. Assignment of estimated date of confinement: single most important task of prenatal care [10B]

1. Last menstrual period (LMP)
   a. 40% of women do not accurately recall LMP
   b. First day of LMP and whether it was normal
   c. Length and variability of patient's menstrual cycles (when not on oral contraceptives)
   d. Presence or absence of pill use or breastfeeding within 6 months prior to conception; these factors can result in delayed ovulation for several subsequent cycles
   e. Naegle rule: subtract 3 months and add 7 days to first day of LMP for estimated date of confinement (EDC)
2. First fetal movement (quickening)
   a. Primigravidas generally feel first fetal movement at 18–20 weeks
   b. Multigravidas generally feel first fetal movement at 16–18 weeks
3. Fetal heartbeat: usually heard with Doppler by 12 weeks (*Note:* In first 2 trimesters, fetal heartbeat most commonly heard close to midline.)
4. Fundal height: measure from top of symphysis pubis
   a. 12 weeks: palpable abdominally just at symphysis pubis
   b. 16 weeks: palpable midway between symphysis and umbilicus
   c. 20 weeks: palpable at umbilicus
   d. 20–32 weeks: height in centimeters above symphysis parallels gestational age in weeks
   e. Although these guidelines can serve as a rule of thumb, interobserver and intraobserver variability very high; assuming that one ultrasound has been done to confirm due date, additional scans based on discrepancies in physical examination warranted only in more extreme cases
5. Ultrasound
   a. First trimester: crown-rump length predicts EDC to within 7–10 days
   b. Second trimester: biparietal diameter (BPD) or femur length predicts EDC to within 7–10 days
   c. Third trimester: scans postponed to this time not very helpful in predicting EDC and are accurate only to within 3 weeks either way

      d. Ultrasound conflicts with LMP: when early ultrasound prediction disagrees with an EDC assigned by LMP by more than 1 week, ultrasound dates assigned; if scan and LMP agree to within 1 week, EDC based on LMP used

D. Nutrition: excessive starting weight and/or excessive gain associated with increased fetal weight and possibly lifelong risk for chronic disease such as obesity and diabetes 9F, 10F

  1. BMI <19: 15 lb

  2. Normal BMI: 20–30 lb

     a. 3 lb first trimester

     b. 12 lb second trimester

     c. 11 lb third trimester

     d. Alternatively, half pound per week for first 28 weeks and 1 pound weekly thereafter

  3. BMI >25: 15 lb

  4. BMI >30: <15 lb

  5. BMI >40: no weight gain; occasionally a few pounds net loss observed as patients become more focused on eating balanced diet

  6. Pregnant women usually aware of their weight and weight gain; gain unpredictable and can be difficult to control

  7. Women with BMI or weight gain issues should be referred to dietitian

  8. 300 kcal/day increase over maintenance

  9. Increased needs

     a. Iron: 1 g over course of pregnancy: supplement for low hemoglobin

     b. Calcium: fetus requires 30 g; suggest 1200 mg/day supplementation depending on diet

     c. Vitamin D: 200 IU daily recommended supplement

E. Blood pressure (see Chapter 26, Medical Complications of Pregnancy, regarding pre-eclampsia)

F. Urinalysis: trace and 1+ proteinuria relatively common in absence of disease; 2+ or more requires timely investigation as it may suggest pre-eclampsia, particularly after 20 weeks (see Chapter 26, Medical Complications of Pregnancy)

G. Fetal heart tones: present or absent (if absent after 12 weeks, ultrasound required for follow-up); for any concern about fetal well-being, other evaluation required (ultrasound, monitoring)

H. Cervical examination

    1. Often begun weekly at 36 weeks

    2. Weak correlation among effacement, dilation, and onset of labor

    3. Bishop score (see Chapter 27, Table 27.1)

        a. Score <5: induction less likely to be initiated successfully

        b. Score of ≥9 suggests labor will occur spontaneously; alternatively induction likely to be successful

I. Maternal-fetal medicine consultation may be advisable for: `10C`

    1. History of preterm delivery (<36 weeks or weight <5 lb, 8 oz)

    2. Prior intrauterine fetal demise

    3. Pregnancy loss between 14 and 20 weeks (suggestive of incompetent cervix)

    4. Multiple gestation

    5. Third-trimester bleeding or discovery of placenta previa after 26–28 weeks' gestation

    6. Isoimmunization

    7. Presence of serious systemic disease, such as diabetes, hypertension, asthma, renal or cardiac disease, and so on

    8. History of deep venous thrombosis (not varicose veins) or pulmonary embolus

III. Common Concerns of Pregnancy `10I`

A. Fetal movement

    1. Stillbirth rate has generally not been shown to decrease significantly among mothers who monitor their baby's movements daily

    2. Variety of different protocols for instructing patients checking to be sure there are at least 10 movements in 8 hours is one such protocol

    3. A key principle is that any large change in fetal daily activity requires medical evaluation

    4. Poor specificity: generally hundreds of fetal assessments will be conducted for every fetus in jeopardy

    5. Instructions commonly given at 24 weeks

        a. Maternal perception of fetal movement more difficult before

    b. Viability before 24 weeks problematic so that intervention less beneficial

    c. Norms for fetal monitoring before 24 weeks less well established

  6. Medical assessment of maternal concern over fetal movement

    a. Most common evaluation nonstress test (NST)

    b. For nonreassuring NST or where suspicion remains high, biophysical profile or contraction stress test may obtain additional information

B. Sex

  1. No restrictions placed on sex for pregnant woman without specific medical or obstetrical problems

  2. Air emboli resulting in maternal death have been reported in medical literature from blowing air under pressure into vagina during oral sex

C. Abdominal pain

  1. Most pregnant women eventually complain of lower abdominal discomfort or pain. Sometimes pain may actually be a uterine contraction.

  2. Patients at 24 weeks and beyond should be advised to call if they have frequent contractions (more than four per hour) for 2 consecutive hours because this may be an early sign of preterm labor. This discomfort may be Braxton Hicks contractions (isolated, generally mild tightening sensations of uterus), but it is often difficult to find a specific cause.

  3. Round ligament pain

    a. Occasionally patients will complain of cramping or aching pain along lateral aspects of uterus, commonly worse with activity/movement

    b. Examination generally reveals tenderness in portion of round ligament (runs from symphysis pubis along lateral border of pelvis to top of uterus)

    c. Treatment: moist heat and acetaminophen

  4. Mild abdominal aches and pains are common and can be treated with a heating pad and acetaminophen.

D. Leg cramps

  1. Common, particularly in calves at night

  2. Cause unknown

  3. No remedy

    4. Pain that is severe, unilateral, persistent, or associated with redness, swelling, or fever should prompt further investigation for deep vein thrombosis (DVT)

        a. Physical examination not sensitive or specific

        b. Doppler flow study of circulation between groin and knee may be indicated

E. Exercise

    1. Supine position: after 20 weeks, growing uterus can reduce venous return by compressing vena cava; generally, exercises on back discouraged after this point.

    2. Third-trimester aerobic exercise

        a. Some studies show dose-response relationship between sustained aerobic exercise and decreased newborn birth weight: exercising muscles divert blood flow from uterus

        b. Individual instruction

            i. Normal or low BMI: generally restrict aerobics in third trimester

                (1) Can advise pulse restriction (somewhat arbitrary)

                (2) Commitment to exercise among fit women can be very strong: exercise restriction may not be well received

            ii. Elevated BMI: generally do not restrict aerobics

                (1) Continued weight gain poses significant maternal and fetal health threat

                (2) Available evidence suggests that those with elevated BMI do not elevate pulse as high or for as long

F. Meaning of EDC (due date)

    1. Roughly 90% of patients will deliver within a 4-week period centered on a due date

    2. In statistical terms, due date is midpoint of a Gaussian probability distribution with two standard deviations being roughly 2 weeks

    3. 5% will deliver prematurely and perhaps 5% will go into labor post term

    4. Probability of delivering on due date roughly 4%

G. Common myths

    1. "NutraSweet is not safe during pregnancy."

        a. Sweetener is safe for all except women known to be homozygous for phenylketonuria.

   b. NutraSweet is a combination of two amino acids, phenylalanine and aspartic acid.
2. "The fetal heart rate is linked to gender." Heart rate varies from instant to instant, so this idea falls apart under briefest scrutiny.
3. "Women are more likely to go into labor during a full moon." Scientifically, this is simply not true.
4. "Pregnant women are more likely to rupture membranes before storms." Although it is true that atmospheric pressure drops with rain, so does pressure within the body, which is equal at all times with external pressure. If it were not, more than amniotic membranes would burst.
5. "Pregnant women should not sleep on their back." Its origins can probably be traced to the observation that labor in supine position can compromise uterine blood flow. This is not relevant to non-laboring patients (and not important for those in labor). Although many women are uncomfortable flat on their back and can even develop symptomatic hypotension, those who can tolerate this position will not cause fetal injury. Those who cannot will avoid the position naturally.
6. "Hot baths can injure fetus."
   a. Some data link increases in maternal core temperatures with birth defects
   b. Nearly impossible to raise core temperature from a hot bath
      i. Total body immersion in warm water may raise body temperature.
      ii. Studies have found that people become very uncomfortable with a rise of a single degree in their core temperature.
   c. Because significant increases in core heat can result in unconsciousness, general precautions regarding body immersion in whirlpools also apply to pregnant women; limit total time, and get out if dizziness or discomfort occurs

IV. Prenatal Laboratory Test Results 10E
A. First visit
1. Urine culture
2. Gonorrhea and chlamydia screening (some omit for married women)

3. HIV antibodies, rapid plasma regain (RPR) for syphilis, and hepatitis B surface antigen
4. Blood type and antibody screen
5. Rubella titer
6. Other
   a. Toxoplasmosis titer for animal-care workers and patients who own cats
B. Subsequent visits
   1. 24–28 weeks
      a. Hemoglobin
      b. 1-hour glucose screen post 50-g glucose load
      c. Antibody screen; for Rh-negative mothers, screen done before administration of Rho(D) antibody to ensure isoimmunization has not already occurred
   2. 36 weeks: vaginal/rectal culture for group B streptococcus
C. Genetic testing (see Chapter 20: Obstetrical Genetics)
   1. Single-gene defect screening
      a. Cystic fibrosis: universally offered
      b. Hemoglobin electrophoresis: African American (and for those with anemias and poor response to iron)
      c. Ashkenazi Jews: screening for Tay-Sachs disease, Canavan disease, familial dysautonomia, Niemann-Pick (type A) disease, Fanconi anemia (group C), Bloom syndrome, Gaucher disease (non-neuronopathic type), mucolipidosis type IV, and glycogen storage disease type 1
      d. Other: as indicated by family genetic history
   2. Chromosome abnormality screening: generally one or other (using both raises false-positive rate substantially)
      a. Nuchal translucency at 11–13 weeks
      b. Alpha-fetoprotein (AFP) (multiple markers) at 15–20 weeks
   3. Fetal karyotyping: for abnormal screens or specific risk factors such as advanced maternal age
      a. Chorionic villus sampling: at 11–13 weeks
      b. Amniocentesis: at 15–18 weeks
   4. Neural tube defects: AFP blood test at 15–20 weeks
   5. Anatomical abnormalities: targeted genetic ultrasound (typically at 18–20 weeks), most often referred to as a level II ultrasound

V. Postpartum Care 13A-C

A. Inpatient care after vaginal birth

1. Recovery period: patients typically given 2 calendar days following birth to recover in hospital

   a. Postpartum examination in hospital

   i. Breasts: erythema, localized tenderness, or nipple cracking should be noted

   ii. Uterus: top of fundus commonly palpable at level of umbilicus or 1–2 cm below

   iii. Lochia (vaginal discharge) is generally bright red blood for first few days and usually does not soak more than one to two pads per hour; clots greater than 50 mL are abnormal; most common cause of excessive postpartum bleeding is uterine atony

   iv. Generally, perineum does not need to be examined unless patient has a fever or complains of severe pain in region; most easily examined by viewing it posteriorly, having patient lie on her side and lift superior leg

B. Inpatient care after cesarean section

1. Progress notes: guidelines here are one approach to documentation on a postoperative patient; usual postpartum hospital stay following a cesarean section is 3–4 days

   a. For first 2 days or so following cesarean birth, progress notes should include:

   i. Vital signs and urine output

   ii. Breasts (lactation progress)

   iii. Lungs

   iv. Abdomen: bowel sounds/distention/tenderness/uterine firmness

   v. Incision

   vi. Quantity of lochia

   vii. Lower extremities: tenderness, palpable cords, edema

   b. Following first 1–2 days, notes can be less extensive as long as patient is doing well; abdominal examination and reference to incision remain important

2. Follow-up laboratory tests: complete blood count (CBC) on first day following surgery; occasionally, urinalysis and/or culture obtained on removal of Foley catheter

3. Special problems following cesarean section

a. Return of bowel function

    i. Ileus uncommon after cesarean (postpartum endometritis is risk factor)

        (1) Bowel sounds are usually reasonably active by 24 hours following surgery. Passage of flatus is variable but usually occurs between days 2 and 4.

        (2) Generally, a clear liquid diet is offered shortly after surgery and advanced as tolerated.

    ii. Removal of Foley catheter

        (1) The Foley catheter is necessary only during surgery to keep the bladder deflated.

        (2) Many patients will have urinary retention during emergence from anesthesia.

        (3) The longer the catheter is kept in, the greater the risk of infection. Generally, it is retained for the first night.

    iii. Staple removal

        (1) Commonly day 3 for a transverse incision and day 4 (or later) for a vertical incision

        (2) Steri-Strips should be removed after 7 days

    iv. Activity

        (1) Thrombosis is a concern, and early ambulation should be encouraged.

        (2) Sequential compression boots are being increasingly utilized and should be worn at least for the first night (studies showing benefit in nonpregnant patients show a benefit only after several days of continuous use in immobilized patients).

        (3) Incentive spirometer is not typically utilized in those with regional anesthesia, although advisable in those with general anesthesia.

4. Discharge checklist

  a. If temperature has been over 100.4°F (some use 99.4°F) in last 24 hours, consider further observation. Examine patient thoroughly for a source. The most likely possibilities are endometritis and mastitis.

  b. If the patient is Rh-negative and the baby is Rh-positive, confirm Rho(D) antibody administration.

  c. CBC

i. Patients who have a hemoglobin level >7 are rarely transfused if they are not symptomatic.

ii. Oral iron is usually sufficient to reverse a postpartum anemia. It is typically given for 4–8 weeks postpartum.

iii. Ferrous sulfate (325 mg) is often poorly tolerated.

iv. Depending on extent of anemia, nature and timing of follow-up, and patient's preferences, smaller, branded iron tablets may result in better compliance.

v. Continue prenatal vitamins.

vi. Constipation is a common complaint with iron supplementation.

C. Instructions and miscellaneous considerations

1. Sex

a. It is reasonable to advise abstinence for 4–6 weeks. This is an arbitrary period, but it usually allows vaginal lacerations and episiotomy to heal enough to permit intercourse without great discomfort.

b. Most women will have at least some discomfort with resumption of sexual activity.

2. Some patients may notice inadequate vaginal lubrication

a. Should be reassured that this is a temporary condition that resolves within a few months

b. K-Y jelly or other water-soluble lubricants may be suggested

3. Contraception

a. Initiation

i. Some centers start some patients on oral contraception on postpartum day 14. A delay of 2 weeks is recommended to avoid peak of hypercoagulability from pregnancy.

ii. An alternative is to wait to prescribe pill until postpartum check-up.

b. Avoid interference with lactation

i. Estrogen tends to reduce milk supply: typically not prescribed for this reason

ii. Progestin-only pill or injection often preferred

c. Intrauterine device (IUD)

i. Often ideal for postpartum patients

    ii. Typically not placed before 4–8 weeks (to reduce risk of perforation)

    iii. May be inserted without waiting for menses

        (1) Confirm no contraceptive failures in prior 3 weeks

        (2) Do urine pregnancy test

4. Driving

    a. Driving poses no inherent dangers to new mother.

    b. Postpartum pain may result in slight braking hesitation.

    c. Mothers who are anemic or very fatigued may not be as attentive as they should be while driving.

    d. Prohibiting driving for the first few weeks may be prudent, although advice should be individualized.

5. Bathing

    a. Vaginal birth: tub baths can be very soothing for lacerations and episiotomy repairs

    b. Cesarean section: many physicians prefer to avoid soaking incision for 1–2 weeks after surgery, although there is no harm in getting an incision wet during a shower

6. Activity

    a. A commonsense rule: "If it hurts, don't do it."

    b. Resume exercise on an individual basis, typically by 4 weeks postpartum.

7. Vaginal bleeding

    a. Can persist for 3–4 weeks, although it should not be heavier than a period; passage of blood clots alone does not signify abnormally heavy bleeding

    b. Women who change more than one or two pads an hour for several hours should call; reasonable to restrict tampon use for first 2–4 weeks to allow lacerations to heal and cervix to constrict

8. Bowel care

    a. Most mothers somewhat fearful of first postpartum bowel movement because of constipation or stitches close to anus

    b. Call if no bowel movement by postpartum day 4

    c. Laxatives: recommend to facilitate first bowel movement and as needed thereafter for constipation

        i. Milk of magnesia

        ii. Bisacodyl (Dulcolax; two tablets per day)

    iii. Add fiber and fluid to diet to reduce constipation; simply increasing vegetables usually not enough, and specific diet additives such as Metamucil or Fiberall may be more helpful

  9. Hemorrhoids: invariably improve at least somewhat with birth

    a. Avoid traumatizing the area. This can be accomplished by minimizing wiping after defecation or by using soft medicated pads such as Tucks.

    b. Ease pain and swelling by using rectal suppositories after each bowel movement (over-the-counter Preparation H). An alternative prescription medication is Anusol-HC (topical anesthetic and hydrocortisone) on awakening and at bedtime (and after each bowel movement).

  10. Pain medication: encourage 24-hour use of nonsteroidal anti-inflammatory drugs (NSAIDs) for first several days (synergistic with narcotics)

    a. Acetaminophen with codeine (Tylenol No. 3), two tablets every 4 hours (high doses have been associated with neonatal respiratory depression and death in nursing mothers)

    b. 100 mg propoxyphene with 650 mg acetaminophen (Darvocet-N 100), one tablet every 4 hours as needed

  11. Swelling

    a. Often increases paradoxically 4–7 days after birth

    b. Resolves spontaneously

D. Fever in postpartum patient

  1. Risk factors `28A`

    a. Cesarean section

    b. Premature rupture of membranes or membranes ruptured longer than 18 hours

    c. Fever during labor

    d. Prolonged labor

  2. Differential diagnosis (vaginal birth) `28B`

    a. Postpartum endometritis

      i. Suggested by fever, uterine tenderness, and purulent vaginal discharge (very uncommon finding)

      ii. Diagnosis of exclusion to some extent

      iii. Organisms

        (1) Aerobes

(A) Gram-positive: streptococci, enterococcus, *Staphylococcus aureus* and *Staphylococcus epidermidis*, *Gardnerella vaginalis*

(B) Gram-negative: *Escherichia coli*, *Klebsiella*, *Proteus*

(2) Anaerobes: *Peptococcus*, *Peptostreptococcus*, *Bacteroides*, *Clostridium*, *Prevetella*

(3) Others: *Neisseria gonorrhoeae*, *Chlamydia trachomatis*, *Mycoplasma*

iv. Prophylaxis: generally, first-generation cephalosporin administered 28D

b. Mastitis

c. Pyelonephritis

d. Septic pelvic vein thrombophlebitis

   i. Diagnosis: often empirical; suggested by fever that does not respond to multiple antibiotics

   ii. Computed tomography (CT) scan may or may not be diagnostic

   iii. Treatment: 7–10 days of full anticoagulation with heparin (diagnosis further validated by defervescence within 3 days)

   iv. Need for prolonged anticoagulation uncertain

3. Differential diagnosis (cesarean section): same as for vaginal birth plus

a. Endometritis more common

b. Respiratory causes (atelectasis, pneumonia)

c. Wound infection

4. Diagnosis 28C

a. History and physical examination in effort to localize infection to specific organ (often few signs and symptoms, which leaves endometritis as most likely)

b. Radiology studies as suggested by clinical findings

c. Blood cultures and urine culture (not typically very helpful but advisable before start of antibiotic prescription)

5. Treatment of endometritis

a. Gentamicin 1.5 mg/kg and clindamycin 900 mg intravenous piggy-back (IVPB) every 8 hours: >90% efficacy

b. Third-generation cephalosporins

c. Extended-spectrum penicillins

    E. DVT/pulmonary embolism

        1. Both uncommon, but suspicion must remain high in those with unusual leg complaints, chest discomfort, or increased respiratory rate

        2. Doppler flows of legs, pulse oximetry, and spiral CT of chest remain mainstays of diagnosis: history and physical examination not sensitive or specific

    F. Outpatient postpartum visit

        1. Timing

            a. 6 weeks following vaginal birth

            b. 4 weeks following cesarean section

            c. Sooner as needed for specific follow-up

        2. History: nursing, sleep, mood, bladder/bowel function, pain, bleeding, contraception plans

        3. Examination

            a. Breasts: typically engorged if nursing

            b. Abdomen: uterus should no longer be palpable abdominally

            c. Vulva: lacerations? episiotomy healing well? (sutures should largely have disappeared)

            d. Vagina: lacerations generally resolved; should not be tender

            e. Cervix: may appear patulous and irregular

            f. Uterus: typically under 12-week size at 4 weeks and less than 8-week size at 6 weeks postpartum

            g. Adnexa

            h. Rectal examination (for vaginal birth): assess tone

            i. Lower extremities: edema resolved?

        4. Assessment/plan

            a. Contraception

            b. Address specific concerns or examination findings

            c. Establish follow-up time for return examination (individualize: may just need annual follow-up)

VI. Lactation

    A. Changes of breast during pregnancy `14A`

        1. Breast tenderness often first symptom of pregnancy

        2. In third trimester

            a. Breasts have marked swelling

    b. Areola darken

    c. Colustrum: clear watery fluid often secreted

B. Benefits of breastfeeding `14C`

  1. Newborn

    a. Transfers passive antibodies and enhances passive immunity

    b. Babies may be less prone to excessive weight gain

    c. Formula contamination and expense are avoided

    d. Bonding enhanced

  2. Maternal

    a. Partial contraceptive effects

    b. Faster uterine involution, reduced blood loss

    c. Decreased risks of breast and ovarian cancer

    d. Reduced risk of osteoporosis and obesity

C. Contraindications to breastfeeding

  1. Infections: HIV, cytomegalovirus, areolar herpes infection, acute hepatitis B (and C)

  2. Maternal need for contraindicated medication

  3. Infant with galactosemia

D. Breastfeeding technique and advice `14E`

  1. 500 kcal/day increased calorie needs over maintenance

  2. Sooner initiated after birth, faster milk will come in

  3. Frequent feedings (every 2–3 hours) advantageous

  4. Baby should be held so that it does not have to strain for nipple

  5. Neonates are obligate nose-breathers: keep breast tissue from blocking nares

  6. To remove baby from breast, mouth suction on nipple can be gently broken by inserting finger into side of baby's mouth

  7. Baby may need a few days to get used to breastfeeding; mothers so inclined should be encouraged to persist

  8. Babies normally lose up to 10% of body weight postpartum, although they rapidly regain

  9. Many drugs can be excreted in breast milk, but few of them pose a threat to the baby; see following section on drug safety

E. Lactation suppression

  1. Tight bra and cold packs

  2. Analgesics frequently necessary because resulting breast engorgement can be painful

3. Pharmacologic suppression (beyond combination oral contraceptives, which have limited effect) not recommended

    a. High-dose estrogens in immediate postpartum period seemed to make process less painful but has been linked to increased risk of thromboembolism

    b. Bromocriptine (Parlodel) promised some benefit but has been linked to an increased risk of seizures, stroke, and myocardial infarction

F. Breast engorgement and mastitis `14B`

  1. Debate whether severe breast engorgement can cause low-grade fever; rarely a cause of spiking fevers of temperatures above 101°F

  2. Mastitis suggested by localized warmth, tenderness, and erythema in one breast

    a. Can happen throughout lactation period and shortly thereafter

    b. Continue breastfeeding

    c. Pain relief: warm packs, acetaminophen, prescription narcotics

    d. Pathogens: *S. aureus,* beta-hemolytic streptococci, *E. coli,* and *Haemophilus influenzae* (bacteria often enter breast through a cracked nipple)

    e. Treatment

      i. Initial antibiotic of choice for mastitis is dicloxacillin 500 mg orally four times a day for 1 week. Cephalosporins are an alternative.

      ii. For those allergic to penicillin, 250 mg of erythromycin four times a day may be used.

      iii. Those who are not significantly better within 48 hours should be examined for a breast abscess. These lesions frequently require incision and drainage. Early administration of antibiotics is usually effective in preventing this complication.

G. Drug safety during lactation `14D`

  1. Most drugs are secreted in breast milk in small amounts; many do not pose a threat to the baby

  2. Drugs acceptable for nursing mothers

    a. Most antibiotics

    b. Asthma medications

   c. Most pain relievers including NSAIDs and narcotics (newborn respiratory depression possible with high-enough doses)

   d. Thyroid medication

   e. Insulin

   f. Most antihypertensives

3. Drugs with safety concerns for nursing mothers

   a. Illicit drugs

   b. Radiopharmaceuticals

   c. Some psychotropic medications, such as lithium

   d. Chemotherapy agents

MENTOR TIPS

- Even though preconception counseling and planning is ideal, most pregnancies proceed without such benefit. Most important aspects of planning pregnancy in terms of good outcome and health and happiness of all concerned (marriage, completion of education, and financial security) are not typically sought (or heeded) bits of medical advice.

- Pelvimetry (assessment of maternal bony pelvis) is mentioned here for historical interest, although it is still taught occasionally.

- Although BMI and maternal weight gain are important and relevant concerns, medical humility is in order here. Weight gain during pregnancy is unpredictable and often difficult to control. Other than bariatric surgery, there are not very effective treatments for elevated BMI.

- First-trimester ultrasound remains the best method for confirming EDC and correlating it with the last menstrual period. Clinical signs suggestive of a specific gestational age are mentioned for historical interest.

- The emphasis on lactation by medical schools and government has become extensive. There is a modicum of scientific evidence for modest benefits from nursing. (In Third World countries where contaminated water is used for preparing formula, infant mortality is much higher than for nursing mothers, but this is a specific problem.) Mothers who decline to nurse should not be made to feel guilty.

Resources

Briggs GG, Freeman RK, Yaffe SJ: Drugs in pregnancy and lactation, 7th ed. Philadelphia, Lippincott Williams & Wilkins, 2005.

Cunningham G, Leveno KJ, Bloom SL, et al: Williams obstetrics, 22nd ed. New York, McGraw-Hill, 2005.

Chapter Self-Test Questions

Circle the correct answer. After you have responded to the questions, check your answers in Appendix A.

1. Which disease is *not* significantly affected by pregnancy and does not affect pregnancy?

   a. Asthma

   b. Heart disease

   c. Diabetes

   d. Hypertension

2. A patient's uterus is midway between symphysis and umbilicus. The patient is how many weeks along?

   a. 12

   b. 14

   c. 16

   d. 18

3. Which is *not* true about pregnancy?

   a. Sex is generally not restricted without a specific pregnancy complication.

   b. NutraSweet is safe throughout pregnancy.

   c. Pregnant women should feel free to take hot tub baths.

   d. Monitoring fetal movement has been clearly shown to reduce stillbirth rate.

4. Which is *not* true about postpartum recovery following a vaginal birth?

   a. Driving may resume after 1 week.

   b. Exercise may resume after 4 weeks.

   c. Combination birth control pills can be started before the patient leaves the hospital.

   d. Coitus may resume after 4 weeks.

See the testbank CD for more self-test questions.

20 CHAPTER

OBSTETRICAL GENETICS

Michael D. Benson, MD

I. General Concepts: What Is a "Birth Defect"?

A. Background risk of birth defects: 2%–3% of newborns have a structural defect at birth (extent of severity highly variable—extra digit at birth is different from three heart chambers)

B. Relationship of genes to function

    1. Number of genes in human genome still subject to dispute—estimates vary 30,000–100,000

    2. Paradox: common estimate of number of different antibodies in people approximately one billion—results from combination of limited numbers of heavy chain (with variations in "constant" and variable chain) with light chain

C. How knowledge is gained about teratogens

    1. Human experience—typically empirical (retrospective) observations during times of population stress

        a. Medication exposure

        b. Infection

        c. Radiation (atomic bomb effects on population at Hiroshima and Nagasaki)

        d. Famine

    2. Animal studies

        a. Typically chemical and medication exposure at higher doses than would be encountered in normal human usage

        b. Must use caution in extrapolating—adverse effects in other species do not precisely predict human responses

    3. Databases

        a. At least 600 medical journals that cover genetic subjects

        b. Service available that provides new, searchable updated world literature on DVD quarterly

II. Causes of Congenital Anomalies 9C-D

A. Chromosome errors (missing or extra chromosomal material)

1. Etiology

a. Extra or missing entire chromosomes (aneuploidy) typically result from problems during meiotic non-disjunction: chromosomes fail to pair or fail to separate

b. Translocation: portion of chromosome rearranged

i. Balanced translocation: no genetic material gained or lost

ii. Not balanced: can have effect of deleting or duplicating portion of chromosome (and multiple genes)

c. Deletions: occasionally portion of chromosome missing

d. Autosome abnormality: duplication or absence of large portions of the 22 autosome pairs generally result in serious or lethal damage

e. Sex chromosome errors tend to be less deleterious

f. Recurrence: recurrence risk in subsequent pregnancy rises to 1% until background risk of maternal age predominates

g. Mosaicism

i. Two different cell lines present (typically one with normal chromosome complement and one abnormal)

ii. Error in mitosis (in contrast to most chromosome abnormalities, which result from defective meiosis)

iii. Phenotype depends on relative proportion of normal versus mosaic cell lines

2. Incidence

a. Rises with maternal age

b. Down syndrome frequency is commonly cited to patients because it is most common trisomy observed at birth (can be lethal in that it is associated with increased risk of miscarriage, stillbirth, and shortened life expectancy)

c. Risk of all chromosome errors is summarized in Table 20.1

3. Common abnormalities

a. Trisomy 21 (Down syndrome)

i. Appearance: small head, loose skin at nape of neck, single palmar crease

ii. Heart defects common

iii. Gastrointestinal malformation

iv. Childhood leukemia, thyroid disease

TABLE 20.1	
	Chromosome Errors as a Function of Age
Maternal Age	**Risk of Any Chromosome Error**
20	0.2%
25	0.2%
30	0.2%
35	0.5%
40	1.6%
45	5%

Adapted from Hook EB: Rates of chromosome abnormalities at different maternal ages. Obstet Gynecol 1981; 58:282.

     v. Significant mental retardation

b. Trisomy 18 (Edwards syndrome)

     i. Three to four times more common in females

     ii. Profoundly retarded

     iii. Less than 10% survive to age 1 year; hospice is option for those born alive

c. Trisomy 13 (Patau syndrome)

     i. Cardiac defects in majority

     ii. Most also missing portions of brain

     iii. Less than 10% survive to age 1 year

d. 45X (Turner syndrome)

     i. Estimated 98% abort in first trimester

       (1) Most common aneuploidy in miscarriages

       (2) 20% of all chromosome abnormalities in first-trimester losses

     ii. Most of the few fetuses that survive first trimester have anatomical abnormalities seen on ultrasound (cystic hygroma, hydrops)

     iii. Small minority live-born (1 in 5000 live births)—typically have only minor problems

       (1) Appearance

         (A) Short stature

         (B) Low hairline, webbed neck

         (C) Congenital lymphedema

       (2) Usually normal intelligence although subtle impairments commonly present (problems with social keys, nonverbal problem solving)

          (3) Up to half have cardiac anomalies usually involving root of aorta (bicuspid valve or coarctation)

          (4) Ovarian dysgenesis (90% incidence) requires hormone replacement therapy at start of adolescence

  e. Extra Y chromosomes

     i. XYY

       (1) Normal intelligence

       (2) Tall

       (3) Emotional difficulties, learning disability (not criminal behavior)

     ii. With more than two Y chromosomes, mental retardation and physical abnormalities occur

  f. Extra X chromosome (Klinefelter syndrome)

     i. XXY: phenotypic male

     ii. Small testes, reduced fertility

     iii. Increased risk for germ-cell tumors and breast cancer

     iv. Normal intelligence

     v. Minority have breast development sufficient to warrant surgery

B. Single-gene mutations

  1. Mutations for thousands of diseases have been identified, with more on the way; continuously growing category; mutations classified by location of gene (Table 20.2).

    a. Autosome

    b. Sex chromosome

      i. X-linked dominant: males and females can have abnormal phenotype

        (1) Sons of male with disorder not affected

        (2) Offspring of females with disorder have 50% chance of inheriting it

      ii. X-linked recessive: females typically unaffected; males display abnormal phenotype

      iii. Y-linked (always dominant): associated with male infertility

    c. Mitochondrial: egg (not sperm) contributes mitochondria; exclusive maternal inheritance (can affect both genders)

  2. Classical mendelian genetics

    a. Alteration in DNA occurs in a single gene

    b. Gene is one of pair residing in identical places on chromosome pairs (homologous chromosomes)

TABLE 20.2 Inheritance Patterns of Single-Gene Mutations	
Pattern	**Examples**
Autosomal-dominant	Achondroplasia
	Adult polycystic disease
	Amyotrophic lateral sclerosis (Lou Gehrig disease)
	BRCA mutations
	Factor V Leiden mutation
	Familial hypercholesterolemia
	Hereditary nonpolyposis colorectal cancer
	Huntington chorea
	Marfan syndrome
	Neurofibromatosis
	Tuberous sclerosis
Autosomal-recessive	Most inborn errors of metabolism, e.g.:
	Tay Sachs
	Phenylketonuria
	Gaucher disease
	Albinism
	Cystic fibrosis
	Deafness
	Sickle-cell anemia
	Thalassemias
X-linked: dominant (females can display abnormal phenotype)	Aicardi syndrome
	Hypophosphatemia
X-linked: recessive (females typically unaffected phenotype; all males affected)	Color blindness
	Duchenne muscular dystrophy
	Fragile X syndrome
	Hemophilia
	Ocular albinism
Y-linked	Male infertility
Mitochondrial	Leber hereditary optic neuropathy

    c. A specific gene is known as an allele

    d. One (heterozygous) or both (homozygous) members of pair may be affected

    e. Hemizygous: defective gene on sex chromosome in males

  3. Effect on organism (phenotype) dependent on specific nature or defect

    a. Recessive: requires both genes (maternal and paternal) in pair to be defective for significant effect to be observed

    b. Dominant: single gene in pair can produce adverse result

    c. Genes themselves are not recessive or dominant

    d. Gene products can be absent or defective

    e. Specific phenotype can result from different mutations in same gene

      i. Cystic fibrosis example

        (1) Dozens of gene mutations identified in cystic fibrosis

        (2) Some mutations much more common in specific ethnic groups: Ashkenazi Jews, Cajuns, and Northern Europeans have increased incidence but have different mutations within each population

      ii. *BRCA-1* and *BRCA-2*

        (1) One of a very few clinical tests that involves direct sequencing of portion of genome (approximately 30,000 base pairs)

        (2) More than 2000 mutations identified

        (3) Significance (if any) uncertain; many appear benign

        (4) Example of autosomal-dominant inheritance: gene products repair DNA

          (A) Defect in one gene permits survival

          (B) Environmental damage can often knock out function of other gene, leaving cell with no intact repair mechanism and greatly increasing malignant potential

C. Polygenic (multifactorial) disorders

  1. Result of interaction of several genes inherited as a group

    a. Examples: height, skin color, hair color

    b. See Table 20.2 for examples of inherited disease

  2. Risk of disorder in general population 1 in 1000

  3. Disorder typically affects one organ system

4. Once disorder identified in offspring, risk of subsequent offspring with disorder increases substantially
   a. Often 5- to 10-fold (1 in 1000 risk rises to 1 in 100)
   b. Risk of recurrence not typically 25%–50% as seen with risk of mendelian inheritance of single-gene defects
   c. Risk related to severity: more severe the defect, higher the risk of recurrence in subsequent offspring
D. Environmental damage to genome 9G-H
   1. General concepts
      a. Effect of teratogen highly dependent on time of exposure
         i. First 14 days after conception
            (1) Empirical observation
               (A) Radiation exposure and other teratogens less likely to result in damaged offspring than later in pregnancy
               (B) Speculative explanation is that any damage to early embryo more likely to be catastrophic and result in pregnancy loss (not clinically recognized) than subcritical damage (resulting in birth defect)
         ii. First trimester usually most vulnerable (not always)
      b. Embryo most vulnerable; very few agents damage gametes (as they are not dividing)
   2. Radiation
      a. Medical and nonmedical radiation
         i. Background radiation: roughly 2.4 millisieverts (mSv) per year
         ii. Nuclear weapon radiation most dangerous at 8–15 weeks' exposure
      b. Diagnostic x-rays
         i. Fetal risk related to total dose of radiation and direction of and proximity to rays
         ii. With commonly used x-rays, no known or suspected risk of teratogenicity, particularly if radiation is less than 50 mSv (minimum theoretical threshold for fetal injury)
         iii. Risk of neurologic injury thought to begin at 200 mSv if exposure 8–15 weeks (derived atomic weapon data)

    iv. Table 20.3 lists typical radiation exposures from common diagnostic imaging

    v. Long-term carcinogenesis is a different issue

       (1) Risk not as clear

       (2) Risk debated in adults

       (3) Fetus may be more vulnerable

         (A) More cells dividing

         (B) Radiation carcinogenesis risk may be cumulative exposure; fetus getting early start

  c. Ultrasound: no known or suspected risk; numerous studies

  d. Magnetic resonance imaging: no known or suspected risk; risk, if present, must be low

3. Pharmacologic

  a. FDA classification of drug safety in pregnancy (Table 20.4)

    i. Classification generally poor (practically worthless) for clinical use; however, patients (and pharmacists) will raise questions regarding it

    ii. Problems include:

       (1) Often out of date

       (2) Specific type of injury and probability of injury not specified

       (3) Data often derived from animal data (which may not be applicable) or anecdotal human evidence (such as case reports)

  b. Genetics database (Reprotox) or large, frequently revised books on the topic are often much better sources of information (see Resources at end of chapter)

TABLE 20.3	Radiation Doses of Common Diagnostic Imaging
Test	**mSv**
Dental x-ray	0.06
Chest x-ray	0.1
Abdominal CT	5.3
Chest CT	5.8
Head CT	1.5

TABLE 20.4	FDA Drug Safety Classifications for Pregnancy
Category	**Interpretation**
A	Adequate, well-controlled studies in pregnant women have not shown increased risk of abnormalities to fetus in any trimester of pregnancy
B	Animal studies have revealed no evidence of harm to fetus; no adequate, well-controlled studies in pregnant women **OR** Animal studies have shown adverse effect; adequate, well-controlled studies in pregnant women have failed to demonstrate risk to fetus in any trimester
C	Animal studies have shown adverse effect; no adequate, well-controlled studies in pregnant women **OR** No animal studies have been conducted; no adequate, well-controlled studies in pregnant women
D	Adequate, well-controlled or observational studies in pregnant women have demonstrated risk to fetus; however, benefits of therapy may outweigh potential risk (e.g., drug may be acceptable if needed in a life-threatening situation or serious disease for which safer drugs cannot be used or are ineffective)
X	Adequate, well-controlled or observational studies in animals or pregnant women have demonstrated positive evidence of fetal abnormalities or risks; use of product contraindicated in women who are or may become pregnant

    c. Table 20.5 lists some important safe and unsafe drugs in pregnancy. (Again, consult appropriate sources for the latest and most detailed information.)

    d. Safety in pregnancy is not the same as safety during lactation

4. Infections (see also Chapters 9 and 26): syphilis, rubella, cytomegalovirus, toxoplasmosis, parvovirus (this list does not include injuries from newborn infection—confined to congenital anomalies from infection prior to birth)

TABLE 20.5

Safe and Unsafe Drugs in Pregnancy*

Generally Safe	Known Teratogens
Narcotics	Alcohol (most clinically important teratogen on list—no known safe threshold)
Non-steroidal anti-inflammatory drugs (concern about interference with closure of ductus if given close to labor)	Angiotensin-converting enzyme inhibitors (Enalapril, Captopril)
Glucocorticoids	Aminopterin (folate antagonist)
Fluoxetine	Lithium
Albuterol	Isotretinoin (Accutane)
Terbutaline	Diethylsilbestrol (DES)
Heparin	Cyclophosphamides
Penicillin	Methotrexate
Cephalosporins	Warfarin (Coumadin)
Gentamicin	Lithium
Clindamycin	Tetracycline
Sulfonamides	Thalidomide
Metronidazole	Valproic acid
Nitrofurantoin	Phenytoin (Dilantin)
Terazol	Carbamazepine (Tegretol)
Doxylamine	Live vaccines (generally not known to be teratogenic but concern remains): rubella
Pyridoxine	
Vaccines (influenza, hepatitis B)	

*This list is a general overview and is not all-inclusive. Good sources for more exhaustive information are Reprotox (http://www.reprotox.org/) (subscription Web service) and Briggs GG, Freeman RK, Yaffe SJ: Drugs in pregnancy and lactation, 7th ed. Philadelphia, Lippincott Williams & Wilkins, 2005.

5. Chemical
   a. Heavy metals: mercury and lead are both associated with mental retardation
   b. Pesticides: data inconclusive (clinical issue when treating lice)
   c. Organic solvents: occupational exposure may be associated with increased risk of pregnancy loss and major malformations

III. Genetic Testing

A. Evaluation for chromosome errors

  1. Screening procedures: typically 5%–8% of population has abnormal screen; only 5% of those with abnormal screen has affected fetus

    a. Alpha-fetoprotein (AFP) test: depressed value suggests chromosome errors

      i. Most common version of test consists of four markers: AFP, human chorionic gonadotropin (hCG) (as entire molecule and as free beta subunit), inhibin, and estriol

      ii. Four markers are combined with maternal demographics algorithm that combines maternal age, gestational age, diabetes, race, singleton

      iii. Abnormally low screen typically followed up by amniocentesis for direct determination of karyotype

      iv. Gestational age window: 15–20 weeks

    b. Nuchal translucency testing

      i. Two components

        (1) Ultrasound: determination of nuchal translucency (echolucent area in back of fetal neck)

        (2) Serum markers: free beta-hCG and pregnancy-associated plasma protein A (PAPP-a)

      ii. Done between 11 and 13 weeks

      iii. Algorithm including maternal demographics and gestational age produces risk estimate

      iv. Abnormal screen typically followed up by amniocentesis for direct determination of karyotype

    c. Sensitivity and specificity of tests very dependent on where cut-off values are set

    d. Combination of first-trimester and second-trimester screening tests: work in progress

      i. Amniocentesis follow-up if either test is abnormal might subject 20% of population to invasive testing

      ii. Alternative: computation of risk only after all data available (combined testing)

        (1) Requires withholding test result from patient for weeks *or*

        (2) Advising patient of potentially abnormal result and suggesting follow-up screening test several weeks later

(3) Both approaches clinically unpalatable to the patient

   iii. Common current practice is to offer both tests, have patient pick one, and act on that basis

2. Who should be screened?

  a. Historical background

    i. Procedure-related pregnancy loss rate was initially thought to be 1 in 200 from mid-trimester amniocentesis until definitive study published in 2006 (FASTER trial)[1] showing minimal to no excess risk

    ii. For live births, risk of any chromosome error did not exceed 1 in 200 threshold until maternal age-at-delivery of 35 years

    iii. Coincidence of unrelated statistics resulted in a recommendation that all women 35 years and older receive amniocentesis (and resulted in a completely mistaken lay impression that pregnancies over age 35 are therefore "high risk")

  b. Ever-accelerating expansion of knowledge and availability of new screening procedures allow for more specific risk assessment for the index pregnancy and suggest maternal age–based paradigm should be changed but common practice taking time to catch up (and protocols are changing with new information)

  c. Genetic screening/testing should be optional but should be offered to everyone

    i. Key limitation for most genetic defects and anomalies: no treatment in most cases beyond pregnancy termination (fetal surgery fraught with problems for neural tube defects and remains largely experimental)

    ii. "Time to prepare" is an argument, but in many cases would only start parental distress earlier (and possibly make it worse as human imagination can exceed reality)

    iii. Minority of couples would not terminate pregnancy in any circumstance: these couples would not benefit from advance knowledge and would still be subject to the disadvantages of false-positive screens and small risk of loss of a normal pregnancy from invasive procedures

3. Diagnostic procedures

   a. Amniocentesis `32C`

      i. At 15–18 weeks, minimal excess risk of miscarriage over those who do not have test: 1 in 1600 or fewer

      ii. Amniocentesis prior to 15 weeks associated with increased risk of 1 in 100

      iii. Obtaining karyotype requires tissue culture and typically takes 2–3 weeks before results are available

      iv. 20 mL of amniotic fluid removed under ultrasound guidance (out of total of 300 mL: promptly regenerated)

   b. Chorionic villus sampling (CVS): small amount of placental tissue aspirated under ultrasound guidance `32B`

      i. Typically between 11 and 13 weeks

      ii. Placental cells divide rapidly, permitting karyotyping within 1 week

      iii. Miscarriage risk: studies vary from "no excess risk" to possibly "1 in 100 risk of miscarriage"

   c. Pre-implantation genetics—for in vitro fertilization

      i. Can be done via assessment of polar body or biopsy of 10-cell embryo

      ii. Assessed by fluorescent in situ hybridization (FISH); see following

      iii. Can evaluate most common chromosome abnormalities or a few single-gene mutations

      iv. Technique and capabilities rapidly developing

      v. Done after fertilization has taken place in vitro before embryo transfer into uterus

   d. Percutaneous umbilical cord blood sampling (also known as cordocentesis) `32C`

      i. Can get karyotype more quickly: 1–2 days

      ii. More often used for other fetal tests (alloimmunization, fetal infection) and in utero transfusions

      iii. Under ultrasound guidance, 22-gauge needle used to sample umbilical vein near placental site of insertion

4. Diagnostic laboratory tests

   a. Karyotype: direct determination of chromosome integrity

      i. Chromosomes counted

      ii. Chromosomes banded so that significant additions and deletions can be determined

b. FISH

  i. Probes for specific DNA sequences

  ii. Can be used for common chromosome abnormalities and single-gene mutations

B. Single-gene mutations

  1. Screening: carrier status can be determined for several thousand mutations

  a. Ethnicity

  b. Specific family history: specific mutation usually needs to be known

  2. Diagnosis: fetal status can be determined through amniocentesis or CVS

  a. Specific mutation needs to be known

  b. Parental gene status important: testing not usually done for recessive traits unless both parents are known gene carriers

  3. Available screening tests for carrier status

  a. Cystic fibrosis

    i. Progressive disease of pulmonary, pancreatic, gastrointestinal, and reproductive system

    ii. Autosomal-recessive

    iii. Mutation in "cystic fibrosis transmembrane conductance regulator" gene

    iv. Median age of survival 30 years

    v. Carrier prevalence (approximate): Ashkenazi Jews and Northern Europeans, 1/25; Hispanic Americans, 1/46; African Americans, 1/65; Asian Americans, 1/94

    vi. Test sensitivity drops as prevalence drops

    vii. More than 1000 mutations identified—only approximately two dozen used in general population screening (generally identifies more than 95% of carriers: population group–dependent)

  b. Fragile X syndrome

    i. Occurs in 1/4000 males and 1/8000 females

    ii. Can lead to developmental delay, autism, mental retardation

    iii. X-linked recessive

    iv. Specific trinucleotide segment repeated variably and leads to abnormal transcription of "fragile X mental retardation 1" gene

v. Four clinical classes recognized: unaffected, intermediate, permutation, full mutation

vi. May be suggested in women under age 40 years with elevated follicle-stimulating hormone

c. Ashkenazi Jews genetic screening

   i. Screens for many syndromes and diseases, including Tay-Sachs disease, Bloom syndrome, Canavan disease, familial dysautonomia, Fanconi anemia group, Gaucher disease, mucolipidosis IV, and Niemann-Pick disease type A.

C. Polygenic mutations

1. Ultrasound for anomalies

   a. Even in tertiary care centers, directed cardiac ultrasound misses 50% of anomalies

   b. Detection rate improves as pregnancy progresses

   c. Many renal, gastrointestinal, cardiac, extremity, and neurologic anomalies detectable

2. AFP: only serum marker currently recommended for universal screening for polygenic anomalies

   a. If elevated, suggests increased risk for neural tube defect

   b. Precise risk determined by algorithm using gestational age, actual value, and maternal demographic variables (age, diabetes, ethnic group, singleton, etc.)

   c. Follow up

      i. 90% of open neural tube defects detectable by ultrasound

      ii. Amniocentesis confirmation: amniotic fluid AFP (elevated) and acetylcholinesterase (presence)

MENTOR TIPS

- Most babies with chromosome errors are born to women younger than age 35 years.
- Risk presented by amniocentesis now thought to be minimal (if any), but chromosome error screening tests have multiplied and improved. The question "Should women older than age X automatically be offered amniocentesis?" remains open, and the answer probably lies with the patient's individual preferences after genetic counseling.
- Of the thousands of prescription and over-the-counter medications, only a few dozen are known teratogens.
- X-ray studies during pregnancy pose two risks to fetus: teratogenicity (almost always quite low) and carcinogenicity (low, but probably not zero, and not as well characterized)
- Four general causes of birth defects, each with its own risk profile: chromosome errors, single-gene defects, polygenic defects, and environmental hazards.
- The only birth defects related to parental age are chromosome errors.
- Nucleated fetal cells known to be circulating in maternal blood are the future source of prenatal genetic testing.
- Gene sequencing knowledge is exploding in terms of number of genetic markers identified and basic laboratory rates of sequencing DNA.
- Prenatal genetics will probably pose a paradigm-changing moral dilemma; namely, a consensus as to what a "birth defect" is.

References

1. Eddleman KA, Malone FD, Sullivan L, et al (FASTER Trial Research Consortium): Pregnancy loss rates after midtrimester amniocentesis. Obstetrics and Gynecology 108:1067–1072, 2006.

Resources

ACOG Practice Bulletin 44. Neural tube defects. Obstetrics and Gynecology 102:203–213, 2003.

Briggs GG, Freeman RK, Yaffe SJ: Drugs in pregnancy and lactation, 7th ed. Philadelphia, Lippincott Williams & Wilkins, 2005.

Jenkins TM, Wapner RJ: Prenatal diagnosis of congenital disorders. In Creasy RK, Resnik R, Iams JD (eds): Maternal-fetal medicine: Principles and practice, 5th ed. Philadelphia, WB Saunders, 2004.

Simpson JL, Elias S: Genetics in obstetrics and gynecology, 3rd ed. Philadelphia, WB Saunders, 2003.

ACOG Committee Opinions

ACOG Committee Opinion 296. First-trimester screening for fetal aneuploidy. Obstetrics and Gynecology 104:215–217, 2004.

ACOG Committee Opinion 298. Prenatal and preconceptional carrier screening for genetic diseases in individuals of Eastern European Jewish descent. Obstetrics and Gynecology 104:425–428, 2004.

ACOG Committee Opinion 318. Screening for Tay-Sachs disease. Obstetrics and Gynecology 106:893–894, 2005.

ACOG Committee Opinion 325. Update on carrier screening for cystic fibrosis. Obstetrics and Gynecology 106:1465–1468, 2005.

ACOG Committee Opinion 338. Screening for fragile X syndrome. Obstetrics and Gynecology 107:1483–1485, 2006.

Chapter Self-Test Questions

Circle the correct answer. After you have responded to the questions, check your answers in Appendix A.

1. Which of the following is *not* a birth defect as traditionally understood?

a. Extra digit

b. Clubfoot

c. Patent ductus arteriosus

d. Coarctation of the aorta

2. Which is *not* inherited as a single-gene defect?

   a. Cleft palate

   b. Marfan syndrome

   c. Deafness

   d. Familial hypercholesterolemia

3. Which drug is *not* considered generally safe in pregnancy?

   a. Dilantin

   b. Ibuprofen

   c. Bactrim

   d. Prozac

4. Which is *not* part of the Ashkenazi Jewish genetic screen?

   a. Fragile X syndrome

   b. Gaucher disease

   c. Canavan disease

   d. Fanconi anemia

See the testbank CD for more self-test questions.

21

LABOR

Michael D. Benson, MD

I. Definitions
A. Labor: progressive cervical dilation in the presence of regular contractions ⅡA
   1. Necessarily retrospective diagnosis
   2. Difficult to establish precise start
   3. Pragmatic alternative is to assign start of labor as time of admission to hospital (also arbitrary as criteria for admissions differ)
B. First stage: begins with cervical effacement and dilation and ends with complete dilation
   1. Latent phase begins with cervical change in presence of regular contractions
   2. Active phase begins with increasing rate of cervical dilation
   3. Divisions are retrospective diagnoses; in most women, latent phase ends and active phase begins at 4 cm dilation
C. Second stage: begins with complete dilation and ends with birth of baby; mothers push during this stage
D. Third stage: begins with delivery and ends with delivery of placenta

II. Assessment of Fetal Orientation and Progress During Labor ⅡB
A. Effacement: normal cervix 2–3 cm long by palpation and shortens during labor; expressed two ways:
   1. Absolute length (cm)
   2. More commonly as a percentage; a cervix that has no length left is 100% effaced
B. Dilation: determine by placement of one or two fingers into cervix and assessing diameter of opening

1. External os may be distinguished from internal os if cervix not fully effaced; internal os dilation generally more important
2. Varies from closed to 10 cm dilated (synonym for completely dilated)

C. Station: distance in centimeters between the lowest bony portion of the fetus and the maternal ischial spines
   1. Ischial spines midway between pelvic inlet and outlet
   2. Distance expressed as a number between -5 (above the spines) and +5 (below the spines)
   3. Station given as numerator divided by 5, to distinguish this from the former nomenclature in which the station was described in thirds
   4. Can be source of confusion because many maternity personnel do not know that there are (were) two different systems of describing station
   5. Engagement
      a. Synonymous with zero station
      b. Lowest portion of scalp is at level of ischial spines: usually implies that biparietal diameter of fetal head (its greatest dimension) is below pelvic inlet

D. Presenting part: the part of the fetus that is coming first; almost invariably the head but can be hand, arm, buttocks, feet, chin (mentum), or brow

E. Position: orientation of presenting part with respect to maternal pelvis
   1. For vertex presentation, orientation of occipital sutures are fetal reference; for breech, fetal sacrum used
   2. Maternal references are left, mid-position, and right; and anterior, transverse, and posterior
      a. For example, head-down fetus with occipital bone on maternal left and closer to the symphis than the sacrum is designated left occiput anterior (LOA)
   3. Position not always able to be determined, particularly if patient less than 5 cm or so dilated; swelling of fetal scalp and molding of fetal bones that occur naturally during labor can make position determinations difficult

F. Asynclitism
   1. Tilt anterior or posterior of saggital suture in transverse plane of pelvic inlet

2. Not usually noted in most examinations
3. If extreme, can prevent fetus from delivering
G. Status of membranes: either intact or ruptured
   1. Three common methods of determining that membranes are ruptured; diagnosis usually requires collecting fluid sample from vagina via sterile speculum examination.
     a. Fluid, often with white flecks of vernix, gushing from vagina (no speculum examination required)
     b. Nitrazine-positive sample; amniotic fluid has pH 7.1–7.4, whereas 90% of women have acidic urine, thus allowing nitrazine paper to help distinguish between them
     c. Presence of "ferning" in sample: small sample of fluid allowed to dry on a glass slide and viewed with microscope; crystalline ferning (crystal-like structure resembling branches of a Christmas tree) results from salt content of amniotic fluid and is virtually diagnostic of membrane rupture; occasionally cervical mucus can fern, so it is important to collect fluid from posterior vault rather than from cervix
   2. Can be difficult to determine: occasionally patient asked to walk around the unit wearing a sanitary napkin lined with nitrazine paper for subsequent evaluation
   3. Indicate presence or absence (clear) of meconium
     a. Fetal colon contents; sterile
     b. Seen in 20% of term deliveries; can be a sign of fetal stress although does not require specific management during labor as long as fetal heart rate is reassuring
     c. Generally described as thin (consistency of water) or thick (pea-soup–like).

III. Progress of Labor [IIB]

A. Most of the information about the length of normal labors and labor curve itself comes from investigations conducted by Emanuel Friedman. The data were collected from roughly 12,000 laboring patients in the 1950s and 1960s and published in *Labor: Clinical Evaluation and Management* (two editions, 1967 and 1978).[1] Obstetrical practice of the era was considerably different, with no computerized infusion pumps controlling oxytocin drips, no electronic monitoring of fetus or contractions, and no epidural anesthesia. Subsequent studies have been published, but usually not with more than 1000 patients or so. Thus, the frequent references to the *Friedman curve* in the labor suite.

B. The following limits are prescribed by Friedman. (It is critical to realize that these numbers are not averages but limits of normal. A given portion of labor is accomplished by 95% of laboring women within the time interval in the following list.)

1. First labors

    a. First stage

        i. Latent phase 20.1 hours (mean 6.4 hours)

        ii. Active phase 11.7 hours (mean 4.6 hours)

          (1) Minimum dilation >1.2 cm/hr (mean 3 cm/hr)

          (2) Minimum descent >1 cm/hr (mean 3.3 cm/hr)

    b. Second stage: 2.9 hours

2. Second labors

    a. First stage

        i. Latent phase 13.6 hours (mean 4.8 hours)

        ii. Active phase 5.2 hours (mean 2.4 hours)

        iii. Minimum dilation >1.5 cm/hr (mean 5.7 cm/hr)

        iv. Minimum descent >2.1 cm/hr (mean 6.6 cm/hr)

    b. Second stage: 1.1 hour

C. American College of Obstetricians and Gynecologists definitions

1. Prolonged second stage—first labor

    a. >2 hours

    b. With epidural >3 hours

2. Prolonged second stage—second labor: >1 hour

IV. Movement of Vertex Fetus Down Birth Canal (Six Movements)

A. Descent: after head engaged, moves below level of ischial spines

B. Flexion: as head moves down, chin tucks toward chest to present smallest aspect of head to birth canal

C. Internal rotation: occiput of head moves from transverse position toward symphysis (or, less commonly, sacrum)

D. Extension: as top of head reaches perineum, occiput extends so that it follows curve of pelvis

E. External rotation: head rotates back to its original orientation to the left or right (and to line up with spine)

F. Expulsion: delivery of shoulders and body

V. Admission of Laboring Patient to Maternity Unit

A. Patients present to maternity unit at all gestational ages and for a wide variety of problems. The workup here refers to healthy patient at term. `11B`

B. History

    1. Chief complaint: contractions and/or spontaneous rupture of membranes (SROM).

    2. History of present illness

        a. Patient is an _____ (age) G_____ P _____ (term-preterm-abortion-living), LMP _____, EDC_____ [by dates, examination, ultrasound (include those that are appropriate)] who presents to labor and delivery at_____ weeks complaining of_____. Contractions are _____ out of 10.

    3. Past medical history: hospitalizations, surgeries, illnesses, chronic medical conditions, medications, drug allergies

    4. Past obstetrical history: brief summary of prior pregnancy outcomes and relevant facts

    5. Social history

        a. Substances: drugs, alcohol, tobacco

        b. Other aspects of social history such as employment or marital status

    6. Family history: relevant positives

    7. Review of system: relevant positives

C. Physical examination: portions unique to labor

    1. Abdomen

        a. Fundal height

        b. Leopold maneuvers

        c. Estimate of fetal weight

        d. Reference to contraction strength and frequency (by palpation and/or monitor)

        e. Reference to fetal heart rate (by auscultation and/or monitor)

    2. Vaginal examination

        a. Effacement

        b. Dilation

        c. Presenting part (and position able to be determined)

        d. Station

        e. Status of membranes

    3. Lower extremities

    a. Deep tendon reflexes (DTRs): patients in labor normally
       have slightly increased DTRs (see section on "Edema")
    b. Clonus: up to two beats of clonus considered normal
    c. Edema: up to 75% of pregnant women develop ankle
       edema at some point
    d. Calf tenderness
 D. Prenatal laboratory tests
    1. Record noteworthy test results
    2. Prenatal record usually available as it is transferred from
       office or clinic to the maternity ward several weeks in
       advance of EDC
    3. Group B streptococcus vaginal colonization status (positive,
       negative, unknown)
 E. Impression: Patient is a ___-year-old, G ___ P ___ female at ___
    weeks who presents to labor and delivery....
 F. Plan: admit; monitor; anticipate spontaneous vaginal birth

VI. Progress Notes
 A. When to write
    1. When
       a. Patient examined
       b. Patient given pain medicine
       c. Significant intervention or change in status occurs
    2. Policy on medical student documentation in the labor record
       varies among institutions
    3. Not written for "incident reports," which are internal hospital
       communications regarding errors or quality issues and are
       considered communications protected from legal proceedings
       in most states
 B. Content
    1. Subjective: patient perception of contractions
    2. Objective
       a. Frequency of contractions (by palpation, tocodynamometer,
          oxytocin use and dose, or intrauterine pressure catheter)
       b. Dilation/effacement/presenting part/station
       c. Statement about fetal heart rate and variability
    3. Assessment: i.e., progress in labor
    4. Plan: pain medicine, continued observation, etc.
 C. Where to write
    1. Formal progress note section of chart

2. Graph area where dilation and station are plotted
3. Directly on fetal heart rate tracing (however, paper copy often destroyed after electronic archiving, so handwritten notations lost)
4. In the electronic medical record

VII. Prescribing Pain Relief

A. Narcotic pain relief
   1. "Not too early, not too late"
      a. Narcotics administered during normal latent phase may prolong labor; therapeutic "sleep" with narcotics may truncate protracted latent phase
      b. If narcotics given too close to time of birth, newborn may have respiratory depression in immediate neonatal period (reversible by naloxone)
      c. In practice:
         i. Narcotics are not often given before the patient is dilated 4 cm unless sequential cervical change (indicating true labor) has been demonstrated.
         ii. Sequential cervical change (indicated true labor) has been demonstrated.
         iii. If birth is anticipated within 1–2 hours, only an IV dose is given (if anything).
         iv. If birth is expected within the next 60 minutes, most physicians do not administer narcotics.
   2. What and how much to prescribe (Table 21.1)

TABLE 21.1	Equivalent Narcotic Doses (for IM Injection)
Drug	**Dose**
Morphine	10 mg
Hydromorphone (Dilaudid)	1.5 mg
Meperidine (Demerol)	100 mg
Butorphanol (Stadol)	2 mg
Fentanyl (Sublimaze)	0.1 mg
Alphaprodine (Nisentil)	45 mg

    a. Common dose: butorphanol (Stadol) 1 mg IV push and 1 mg intramuscular (IM)

    b. IV dose provides relief in minutes but wears off rapidly

    c. IM dose provides longer relief, usually for 1–2 hours

    d. Sometimes higher dose given more frequently than every 2 hours required

    e. Each subsequent dose of narcotic provides less relief than preceding dose

    f. Other drugs given with narcotics

        i. Hydroxyzine pamoate (Vistaril) can be used with narcotics to provide additional pain relief. This drug potentiates the analgesic effects of narcotics and also has antiemetic, antipruritic, and antianxiety effects. Common doses are 25–75 mg IM or 12.5 mg IV every 4 hours.

  3. Precautions and side effects

    a. Newborn respiratory depression if narcotic given too close to birth

        i. Naloxone hydrochloride (Narcan) can be given IM, and the baby can be assisted for a few minutes with a bag and mask.

        ii. The usual dose of Narcan is 0.01 mg/kg. Because Neonatal Narcan is supplied in 0.02-mg/mL solutions for neonatal use, 1–2 mL IM usually suffices.

        iii. The half-life of Narcan is substantially less than that of many narcotics so that the newborn can experience respiratory depression again; newborns receiving Narcan need to be monitored for several hours post dose.

    b. Narcotics commonly cause decrease in variability on a monitor tracing; may cause some health-care professionals to withhold medication from women in whom there is some question about an indeterminate fetal heart rate tracing

    c. Maternal side effects

        i. Largely the same type of side effects within the class, although response of individual patients may vary

        ii. All narcotics can cause sedation and nausea

B. Epidural pain relief

  1. Delivers intermittent or continuous flow of local anesthetic and/or narcotics through small catheter placed into lumbar epidural space and maintained in position for hours or days; most often referred to as continuous lumbar epidural (CLE)

2. Advantages
    a. Local anesthetic provides significant pain relief
    b. Addition of narcotic potentiates pain relief; because placed close to spinal nerves, much less is needed, thereby reducing systemic side effects of sedation and nausea
    c. Analgesic effect dramatically better than narcotic and longer lasting; benefit continues as long as infusion does
    d. Unlike narcotic, which is labor analgesic only, epidural can also provide labor analgesia and significant analgesia/ anesthesia for delivery

3. Disadvantages/risks
    a. Hypotension: can cause hypotension due to venodilation (sympathetic block) in the veins of pelvis and legs
        i. Rarely, hypotension can lead to uterine hypoperfusion manifesting as abnormalities in fetal heart rate tracing
        ii. Prevented by giving fluid bolus of 500–1000 mL in advance
        iii. Treated with 5–10 mg of ephedrine IV
    b. Pruritus: from narcotic in epidural (histamine release); treated with diphenhydramine hydrochloride (Benadryl) 25–50 mg IV or IM
    c. "Wet tap" recognized: epidural needle advanced beyond epidural space, through dura and arachnoid membrane; spinal fluid leaks out
        i. Incidence perhaps 1%
        ii. Risk of spinal headache up to 50% (needle bigger than that normally used for deliberate spinal anesthesia)
        iii. Characterized by postpartum headache than can last for several days, most commonly postural; worse with sitting or standing
        iv. Treated by epidural blood patch: blood removed from arm, placed into epidural space to help plug hole in dura; very effective
    d. Wet tap unrecognized: dose intended for epidural administration introduced directly into spinal fluid
        i. Much higher dose of medication than usually administered for spinal

      ii. Rare occurrence but can occur

      iii. Paralysis of diaphragm with significant respiratory impairment possible (note: patient initially conscious and aware; feels suffocation)

      iv. Treated with sedation and respiratory support (and commonly prompt delivery by cesarean)

   e. Epidural space hematoma, infection: rare but measurable— 1 per 10,000–100,000 administrations

   f. Prolonged labor

      i. Longer first stage of labor—typically a result of decreased contraction frequency; treated with oxytocin augmentation of labor

      ii. Longer second stage of labor—maternal expulsive efforts may be less effective due to loss of rectal pressure/urge to push leading to misdirected or less forceful pushing; treated with allowing a longer second stage

 4. Administration (Table 21.2)

   a. Test dose (small local anesthetic dose given after catheter placement to prove subarachnoid space not entered; response would be as with spinal anesthesia)

   b. Bolus

   c. Continuous infusion

   d. Patient-controlled analgesia: patient occasionally given device to self-administer small boluses in addition to continuous infusion

 5. Timing: varies among obstetricians

   a. Beginning: some require an absolute amount of cervical dilation, and others administer as soon as progressive dilation occurs

   b. Cessation: some stop or reduce in second stage of labor; others maintain through third stage and repair of any lacerations

C. Walking epidural: administration of spinal narcotic in early labor followed by placement of epidural

 1. Advantage: spinal narcotic provides pain relief without blocking motor or sensory nerves; permits patient to walk during labor

 2. Disadvantage: two anesthetic procedures

D. Other techniques

TABLE 21.2	Common Dosages of Regional Anesthesia*		
Type of Regional Anesthesia	Type of Dose	Common Dosage	Notes
Epidural anesthesia	Test dose	3 mL 1% lidocaine with 1:200,00 epi	As patient weight increases, dosage trends downward due to greater compression of epidural space
	Bolus	5–7 mL 1/8% bupivacaine (narcotic 10 mcg fentanyl)	
	Continuous dose	0.1%–0.25% bupivacaine at 5–12 mL/hr (as concentration increases, rate decreases)	
	Patient-controlled bolus	80% of hourly rate	
Spinal anes-thesia		Bupivicaine 0.75% 1–1.5 mL	For postoperative analgesia, 0.15–0.2 mg preservative-free morphine often added

*Highly variable among institutions and individual practitioners

1. **Paracervical block** (for labor): local anesthetic injected at 3 and 9 o'clock into cervix after aspirating to avoid intravascular injection

2. **Pudendal block** (for delivery): local anesthetic injected just beneath ischial spine through sacrospinous ligament; blocks innervation of perineal skin for delivery (after aspirating to avoid intravascular injection)

3. **Local infiltration in perineum**: commonly used as anesthesia in absence of regional to facilitate repair of lacerations

MENTOR TIPS

- Contractions that result in cervical dilation may be indistinguishable from those that do not—the only way to differentiate true labor from false labor is often observation to assess cervical change over a period of hours.
- Tips on performing a history and physical examination on a laboring patient:

Brevity and speed are important. These patients are typically in pain and are anxious. A focused history and physical are appropriate.

Most of the history is already available in the prenatal record; brief history-taking should focus on (1) contraction information and membrane status, (2) current medication and allergies, and (3) review of systems (brief, positives only).

Epidural anesthetics are very safe and effective for labor pain relief; in hospitals where they are readily available, up to 90% of first-time mothers chose to avail themselves.

Review your findings with a more experienced health professional before committing them to the medical record. Seemingly innocuous statements such as "estimated fetal weight of 11 pounds" or "fetal presentation unable to be determined" can have important clinical implications (if true).

References

1. Friedman EA: Labor: Clinical evaluation and management, 2nd ed. New York, Appleton-Century-Crofts, 1978.

Resources

Cunningham FG, Leveno KJ, Bloom SL, et al: Williams obstetrics, 22nd ed. New York, McGraw-Hill, 2005.

Chapter Self-Test Questions

Circle the correct answer. After you have responded to the questions, check your answers in Appendix A.

1. A 29-year-old G1 P0 at term presents complaining of regular, frequent contractions that she rates as a 5 on a pain scale of 10. She does not believe she needs pain medication at this time. She is 1 cm/20% effaced, 0 station, and vertex on vaginal examination. After monitoring for 20 minutes to obtain a normal fetal heart rate pattern, the appropriate clinical management of this patient is to:

  a. Admit to maternity unit as she is clearly in labor.

  b. Discharge from maternity unit with instructions to return when contractions are stronger.

  c. Observe for several hours and recheck cervix as needed. Permit ambulation, clear liquids, and intermittent monitoring.

  d. Observe for several hours, and recheck cervix as needed. Start IV and continuous monitoring.

2. A laboring patient with a baseline blood pressure of 90/60 experiences dizziness and a blood pressure of 60/30 a few minutes after epidural administration. Actions include which of the following?

  a. Ephedrine 5–10 mg IV push

  b. IV fluid bolus

  c. Confirm patient is in lateral decubitis tilt

  d. All of the above

3. Which of the following is true about the diagnosis of labor?

  a. Classically defined as regular contractions that lead to progressive cervical dilation

  b. Is a retrospective diagnosis

  c. For practical reasons, often said to start with admission to hospital

  d. All of the above

4. True statements about Friedman's labor curve include each of the following *except:*

    a. It represents the largest number of observations of laboring patients to date.

    b. Friedman identified a latent and active phase of labor.

    c. The first and second stages of first-time labors are longer than for subsequent labors.

    d. The data included corrections for the use of oxytocin labor augmentation and epidural administration.

See the testbank CD for more self-test questions.

FETAL MONITORING

Michael D. Benson, MD

I. Procedures to Facilitate Maternal or Fetal Monitoring

A. Artificial rupture of membranes (AROM)

  1. Indications

    a. Induction or augmentation of labor

    b. Placement of internal monitoring devices

  2. Precautions

    a. Incidence of spontaneous cord prolapse (obstetrical emergency requiring urgent cesarean section) roughly 3 in 1000 among women laboring with vertex (head presenting) fetuses at term

    b. Small but real risk from AROM

    c. Risk of prolapse reduced if fetal vertex well applied to cervix

      i. Fetal vertex can be at relatively high station but still be in good approximation with cervix

      ii. Sometimes AROM is only way to obtain critical information about fetal well-being

    d. Requires that cervix be dilated sufficiently for access to membranes (typically at least 1 cm)

  3. Methods

    a. AmniHook (Fig. 22.1)

      i. Identify and stabilize cervix with one hand and snag membranes with AmniHook in other hand

      ii. Leave examining hand in place for a few moments to detect any change in fetal presentation or station as fluid leaks out

      iii. Assess amniotic fluid: clear, meconium, blood

    b. Placement of internal fetal electrode (IFE) (see following section)

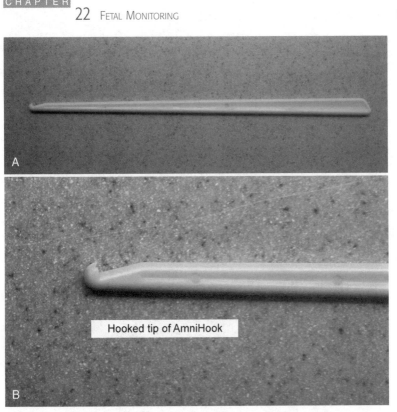

Hooked tip of AmniHook

FIGURE 22.1 *A*, AmniHook amniotome. *B*, Close-up of AmniHook tip.

    i. As uterus contracts, membranes sawed through by wire
    ii. May take several contractions to assess adequately
       amount and color of fluid

B. Placement of IFE (Fig. 22.2)
   1. Identify cervical opening and fetal scalp with forefinger of
     nondominant hand
   2. Guide spiral electrode in its sleeve over forefinger onto fetal
     scalp
   3. Press scalp electrode onto fetal scalp while rotating device
     clockwise
   4. Withdraw guide and hand; connect to fetal monitor leads

C. Placement of intrauterine pressure catheter (IUPC) (membranes
   must be ruptured prior to placement) (Fig. 22.3 and Fig. 22.4)

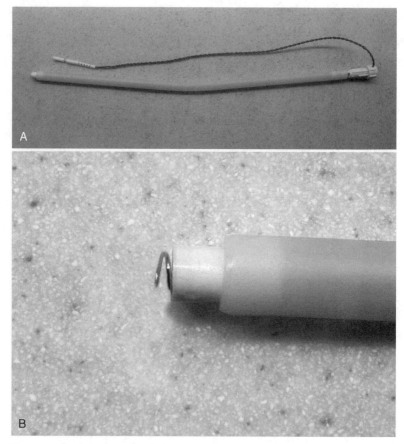

FIGURE 22.2 *A,* Internal fetal electrode (IFE). *B,* This close-up shows the spiral electrode at the end.

1. Zero sensor (instructions vary by manufacturer)
2. With nondominant hand, identify cervical opening
3. Slide catheter with external guide tube through cervix
4. Feed catheter through guide tube to pass it into uterus and alongside fetus
5. Remove guide tube (typically, tube separates along score that runs down its length)
6. Check placement and sensitivity by having patient cough once: pressure should rise at least 10 mm Hg

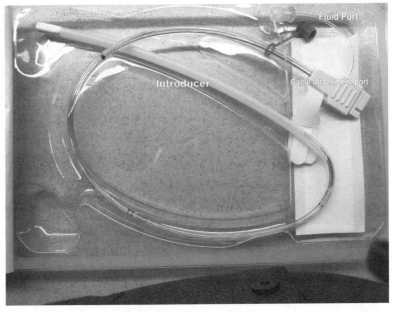

FIGURE 22.3 Intrauterine pressure catheter (IUPC).

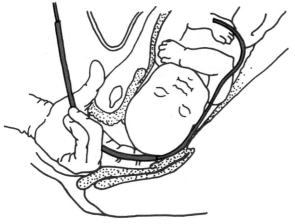

FIGURE 22.4 IUPC placement. (Redrawn and adapted from Freeman, RK and Garite, TJ: Fetal heart rate monitoring. Williams & Wilkins, Baltimore, 1981, p 45.)

7. Amnioinfusions can be administered through side port of IUPC

D. Scalp pH (Fig. 22.5): rarely done in current practice; many maternity units do not have the equipment available

1. Indication: uncertain or difficult to interpret fetal heart rate (FHR) tracings

2. Preparation: ensure there are at least two scalp pH cartridges at room temperature and that machine is on for 30 minutes before starting

3. When machine indicates "stand by," slip a fresh cartridge in close door and wait until machine indicates "ready"; requires about 2–3 minutes after inserting cartridge

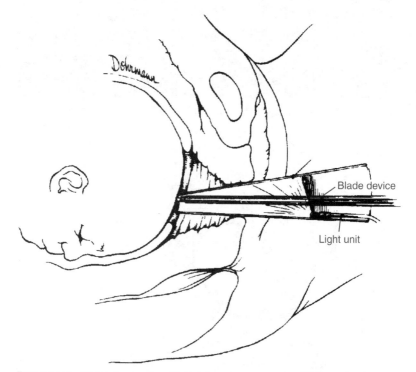

FIGURE 22.5 Obtaining scalp pH. Fetal scalp exposed to hollow plastic cone; nick made in fetal scalp. (Redrawn and adapted from Creasy, RK and Parer, JT: Prenatal care and diagnosis. In Rudolph, AM [ed]: Pediatrics, ed 16. Appleton-Century-Crofts, New York, 1977.)

4. Patient may be in supine or lateral decubitus position, with buttocks flush with edge of bed

  a. Open kit and put on sterile gloves

  b. Slide white plastic truncated cone into vagina

  c. Have nurse affix light source to cone

  d. Slide cone in far enough to visualize fetal scalp; press to form a seal between cone and fetal scalp so that amniotic fluid and cervical mucus do not enter field

  e. With dry swabs, clean scalp

  f. Apply silicone preparation with additional swabs; helps blood form droplets on scalp rather than disperse

  g. Study razor orientation on long handle; make an X in fetal scalp with very firm pressure (may need repeat effort if scalp soft and edematous)

  h. With long capillary tube, dab at blood as it wells up; while holding the tube transversely, dip distal end into the clay and give tube to an assistant, who should slide the capillary tube into the upright receptacle within cartridge; machine will provide pH printout within about 15 seconds; new cartridge should be inserted immediately to prepare for second sample

  i. Fill a second capillary tube for a second sample and then observe the site to be sure bleeding stops; if necessary, apply pressure with a swab

  E. Amnioinfusion

   1. Indications

     a. Mitigation of variable decelerations

     b. Prophylaxis for labor with oligohydramnios (evidence mixed)

     c. Dilution of meconium-stained fluid (evidence mixed)

   2. Saline administered through IUPC infusion port

     a. Bolus: 500–800 mL

     b. Constant infusion: 180 mL/hr

   3. Complications (uncommon): cord prolapse, amnionitis, cardiorespiratory compromise

II. Congenital Fetal Neurologic Injury and Stillbirth

  A. Adverse fetal outcomes identified at or presumed to be present at birth

1. Stillbirth (developed countries)
   a. Antepartum: 5.2/1000 births; rate has not substantially dropped over past several decades
   b. Intrapartum: 0.9/1000 births; rate has declined over several decades but still accounts for 20% of all stillbirths
2. Mental retardation (rate has not changed over past several decades)
   a. Severe: 3.5/1000 population
   b. Mild: 23–31/1000 population[1]
3. Cerebral palsy (rate has not changed over past several decades)
   a. 5/1000 births
   b. Prevalence among school-age children: 1–2/1000
   c. 90% or more of cases believed to originate in events occurring prior to labor
      i. Single strongest demographic or clinical association with prematurity
      ii. Inflammation (not necessarily linked to infection) believed to play a role
      iii. Inflammation also thought to be a factor in preterm birth and initiation of spontaneous labor at term
B. Physiology of fetal oxygen transfer
   1. Resting pressure of myometrium and amniotic fluid 10 mm Hg
   2. Mean arterial blood pressure of uterine spiral arteries typically 85 mm Hg
   3. Fetal oxygenation
      a. Concentration higher than in adults
      b. Fetal cardiac output higher than adult per weight
      c. Fetal hemoglobin binds oxygen at low P_{O_2} more strongly than adult hemoglobin
   4. Spiral arteries deliver maternal blood to intervillous space and to fetal capillaries contained within the chorionic villi that project into this space
   5. 85% of maternal uterine blood flow estimated to go to intervillous space and remainder goes to myometrium
   6. Oxygen available to fetus closely related to maternal blood flow to placenta
      a. No known method of increasing flow
      b. Many things will decrease flow

     i. Exercise

     ii. Supine position after 20 weeks

     iii. Uterine contractions

     iv. Hypotension (sufficient to cause maternal symptoms)

     v. Hypertension

C. Physiology of FHR control

    1. Parasympathetic

       a. Originates in brainstem; carried over vagus nerve

       b. Slows heart rate

    2. Sympathetic

       a. Originates in brainstem; carried over cervical sympathetic fibers

       b. Speeds heart rate

    3. Instantaneous heart rate (inverse of time interval between individual heartbeats) changes constantly and reflects balance between sympathetic and parasympathetic input

III. FHR Terminology 32E

A. Three terminologies

    1. No uniform, narrowly defined, universally used terms to describe FHR patterns

    2. Stems, in part, from several limitations of FHR monitoring

       a. Lack of close relationship between nonreassuring FHR tracings and poor neonatal outcome in all but the most clinically extreme cases

       b. Difficulty inherent in interpreting dynamic and highly variable heart rate patterns

    3. In 1997 and 2008, U.S. National Institute of Child Health and Human Development (NICHD) held a Research Planning Workshop and proposed definitions for intrapartum FHR patterns

    4. All three sets of terminology are often used in the same hospital by nursing and medical staff

    5. In some settings, many or most clinicians not aware that there are three slightly different sets of terminology

B. Pre-1997 terminology 26B

    1. Baseline

       a. Beats per minute (bpm) value that the FHR oscillates around for 10 minutes or more

      b. Normal is 120–160

      c. Tachycardia: baseline of 160 or greater

      d. Bradycardia: <120

  2. Variability

      a. Long-term variability (LTV)

         i. Oscillation about the baseline that occurs with a frequency of 2–6 cycles per minute (Fig. 22.6)

        ii. Normal amplitude of change is 6–15 bpm (measured from peak to nadir of the oscillation)

      b. Short-term variability (STV)

        i. Beat-to-beat changes in pulse rate from one moment to the next

        ii. STV makes heart rate tracing look "jiggly" (see Fig. 22.6).

  3. Periodic changes (decelerations)

      a. Variable decelerations

        i. Variable in shape, duration, and timing with respect to contractions (Fig. 22.7 and Fig. 22.8)

        ii. Heart rate can often drop below 100 bpm and even 80 bpm

        iii. One classification scheme is given in Table 22.1

      b. Late decelerations

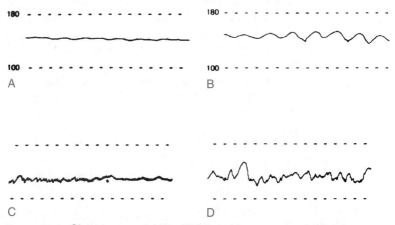

FIGURE 22.6 Short-term variability (STV) and long-term variability (LTV). *A,* Absent LTV, absent STV. *B,* Good LTV, absent STV. *C,* Good STV, absent LTV. *D,* Good LTV, good STV. (Redrawn from Zanini, B, et al: Am J Obstet Gynecol 136:44, 1980.)

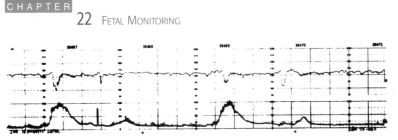

FIGURE 22.7 Tracing with mild variables (bottom portion represents contraction pattern). (From Freeman, RK and Garite, TJ: Fetal Heart Rate Monitoring. Williams & Wilkins, Baltimore, 1981, p 71.)

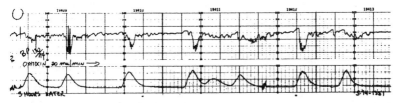

FIGURE 22.8 Tracing with moderate variables (bottom portion represents contraction pattern). (From Freeman, RK and Garite, TJ: Fetal Heart Rate Monitoring. Williams & Wilkins, Baltimore, 1981, p 71.)

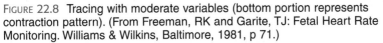

TABLE 22.1	Classification of Variable Decelerations		
BPM	**Duration (sec)**		
	<30	30–60	>60
>80	Mild	Mild	Moderate
70–80	Mild	Moderate	Moderate–severe
<70	Moderate	Moderate–severe	Severe

    i. Decreases in heart rate that are late-onset, mirror contractions in symmetry, and repetitive

    ii. May often be very mild in amplitude change

    iii. Typically occur in absence of accelerations

    iv. Controversy: not all obstetricians agree about definition of this term (in the pre- or non-NICHD usage); consensus appears to be that late decelerations assume significance only if they are repetitive, but there is debate about whether a single deceleration without repetition can be termed late

  4. Presumed causes of decelerations
   a. Early: head compression
   b. Variable: umbilical cord compression
   c. Late: uteroplacental insufficiency (reduced oxygen transfer to fetus)
 C. 2008 NICHD terminology[2] (Fig. 22.9 to Fig. 22.20)
  1. Baseline: mean FHR rounded to nearest 5 bpm for 10 minutes; must occur for no less than 2 minutes of 10-minute interval (does not have to be contiguous) and excludes episodes of:
   a. Periodic or episodic changes
   b. Periods of marked variability
   c. Segments of baseline that vary by more than 25 bpm

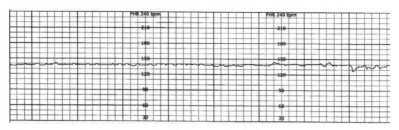

Figure 22.9 **Absent variability.** (From National Certification Corporation [NCC]: Applying NICHD Terminology and Other Factors to Electronic Fetal Monitoring Interpretation. NCC Monograph, Volume 2, No. 1, 2006.)

Figure 22.10 **Minimal variability.** (From National Certification Corporation [NCC]: Applying NICHD Terminology and Other Factors to Electronic Fetal Monitoring Interpretation. NCC Monograph, Volume 2, No. 1, 2006.)

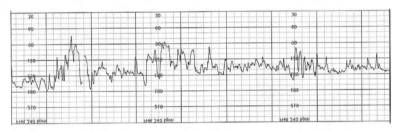

FIGURE 22.11 Moderate variability. (From National Certification Corporation [NCC]: Applying NICHD Terminology and Other Factors to Electronic Fetal Monitoring Interpretation. NCC Monograph, Volume 2, No. 1, 2006.)

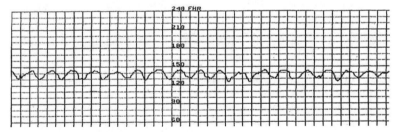

FIGURE 22.12 Marked variability. (From National Certification Corporation [NCC]: Applying NICHD Terminology and Other Factors to Electronic Fetal Monitoring Interpretation. NCC Monograph, Volume 2, No. 1, 2006.)

FIGURE 22.13 Sinusoidal pattern. (From National Certification Corporation [NCC]: Applying NICHD Terminology and Other Factors to Electronic Fetal Monitoring Interpretation. NCC Monograph, Volume 2, No. 1, 2006.)

2. Baseline variability (see Figs. 22.9–22.12)
   a. Fluctuations in FHR tracing that are irregular in amplitude and frequency over 10 minutes that exclude accelerations and decelerations (see below); described in bpm between peak and trough

1916-22

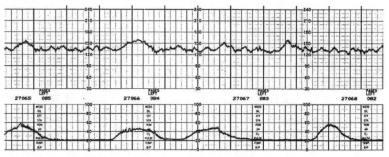

FIGURE 22.14 Normal rate. (From National Certification Corporation [NCC]: Applying NICHD Terminology and Other Factors to Electronic Fetal Monitoring Interpretation. NCC Monograph, Volume 2, No. 1, 2006.)

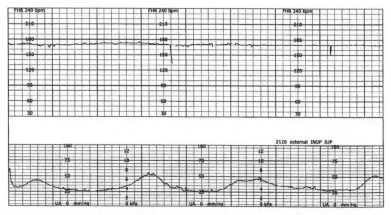

FIGURE 22.15 Tachycardia. (From National Certification Corporation [NCC]: Applying NICHD Terminology and Other Factors to Electronic Fetal Monitoring Interpretation. NCC Monograph, Volume 2, No. 1, 2006.)

        i. Absent: amplitude range undetectable
       ii. Minimal: detectable but 5 bpm or fewer
     iii. Moderate (normal): 6–25 bpm
     iv. Marked: >25 bpm
  3. Acceleration
     a. Visually evident abrupt increase in FHR from baseline
        i. Onset to peak <30 seconds
       ii. Duration: initial change from baseline to return to baseline

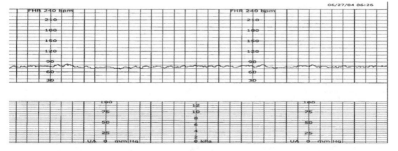

FIGURE 22.16 Bradycardia. (From National Certification Corporation [NCC]: Applying NICHD Terminology and Other Factors to Electronic Fetal Monitoring Interpretation. NCC Monograph, Volume 2, No. 1, 2006.)

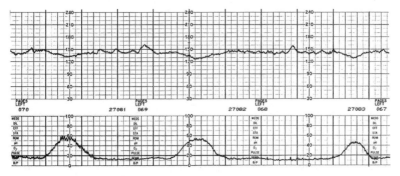

FIGURE 22.17 Early decelerations. (From National Certification Corporation [NCC]: Applying NICHD Terminology and Other Factors to Electronic Fetal Monitoring Interpretation. NCC Monograph, Volume 2, No. 1, 2006.)

    b. Duration
       i. At least 15 seconds
      ii. <2 minutes
    c. Gestational age
       i. 32 weeks or more: 15 bpm or greater amplitude increase
      ii. <32 weeks: 10 bpm or greater amplitude increase
  4. Prolonged acceleration: 2 to <10 minutes (if 10 minutes or more, it is a baseline change)
  5. Bradycardia: <110 bpm baseline (see Fig. 22.16)
  6. Tachycardia >160 bpm baseline (see Fig. 22.15)

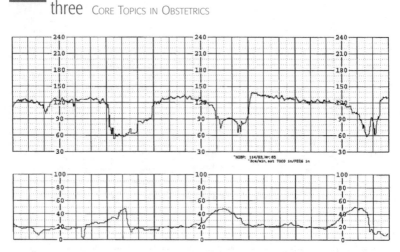

FIGURE 22.18 Variable decelerations. (From National Certification Corporation [NCC]: Applying NICHD Terminology and Other Factors to Electronic Fetal Monitoring Interpretation. NCC Monograph, Volume 2, No. 1, 2006.)

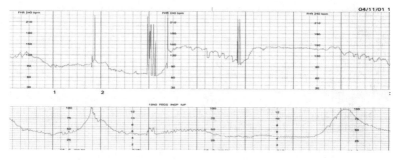

FIGURE 22.19 Prolonged deceleration. (From National Certification Corporation [NCC]: Applying NICHD Terminology and Other Factors to Electronic Fetal Monitoring Interpretation. NCC Monograph, Volume 2, No. 1, 2006.)

7. Decelerations (see Figs. 22.17–22.20): depth of deceleration determined in bpm from onset to nadir; recurrent if occur with 50% or more of contractions, intermittent if less often
   a. Early
      i. Gradual decrease (usually symmetrical) in FHR with return to baseline: onset to nadir >30 seconds

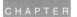

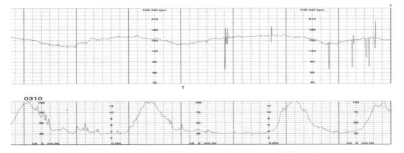

FIGURE 22.20 Late decelerations. (From National Certification Corporation [NCC]: Applying NICHD Terminology and Other Factors to Electronic Fetal Monitoring Interpretation. NCC Monograph, Volume 2, No. 1, 2006.)

   ii. Nadir of deceleration occurs at same time as peak of contraction: usually onset, nadir, and recovery coincident with start, peak, and resolution of contraction

  b. Late

   i. Gradual decrease (usually symmetrical) in FHR with return to baseline; onset to nadir >30 seconds

   ii. Nadir of deceleration occurs after peak of contraction: onset, nadir, and recovery usually occur after start, peak, and resolution of contraction

  c. Variable

   i. Abrupt decrease: <30 seconds from onset to nadir

   ii. Must be at least 15 seconds long and <2 minutes; must be at least 15 bpm deep

   iii. Commonly vary from contraction to contraction in onset, depth, and duration

  d. Prolonged

   i. ≥2 minutes and <10 minutes (if 10 minutes or more, is a baseline change)

   ii. Must be ≥15 bpm deep

 8. Sinusoidal: looks like sine wave with smooth, sine wave–like undulating pattern in FHR baseline at 3–5 cycles per minute that lasts 20 minutes or longer (see Fig. 22.13)

IV. Contraction Terminology (2008 NICHD)

 A. Normal: five contractions or fewer in 10 minutes, averaged over 30 minutes

B. Tachysystole: more than five contractions in 10 minutes averaged over 30 minutes

1. Should qualify as to presence of associated FHR decelerations
2. Clinical response may differ depending on whether contractions stimulated or spontaneous

V. Tracing Interpretation (2000 NICHD)

A. Components
   1. Baseline rate
   2. Baseline FHR variability
   3. Presence (or absence) of accelerations
   4. Presence (or absence) of decelerations
   5. Changes over time
   6. Uterine contractions

B. Three-tier FHR interpretation
   1. Category I: Normal
      a. Normal baseline
      b. Moderate variability
      c. Late or variable decelerations absent (early decelerations may or may not be present
      d. Accelerations present *or* absent
      e. Predictive of normal fetal acid-base status
   2. Category III: Abnormal
      a. Absent FHR variability *and*
         i. Recurrent late or variable decelerations
         ii. Bradycardia
      b. Sinusoidal pattern
      c. Predictive of abnormal fetal acid-base status; corrective actions include but not limited to maternal oxygen, change in maternal position, discontinuation of labor stimulation, treatment of maternal hypotension
   3. Category II: Indeterminate
      a. May represent appreciable fraction of tracings
      b. Not predictive of abnormal fetal acid-base status; warrants continued evaluation and observation

C. NICHD Report does not specify specific circumstances for performing a cesarean on basis of FHR tracing or specific time response to abnormal (category III) tracings; reassuring or normal (as defined by NICHD consensus statement):
   1. Normal baseline

2. Moderate variability

3. Presence of accelerations

4. Absence of decelerations

D. Predictive of current or impending fetal asphyxia severe enough to result in fetal injury or death

  1. Recurrent late or variable decelerations with absent FHR variability

  2. Substantial bradycardia with absent FHR variability

E. Many (most?) FHR tracings fall somewhere between normal and abnormal; for indeterminate no consensus exists for management; e.g.:[3]

  1. Late decelerations with moderate variability and accelerations

  2. Variable decelerations with slow return to baseline or late component

  3. Absent variability with no decelerations associated with contractions

  4. Fetal tachycardia without decelerations

F. Specific observations about heart rate tracing patterns

  1. Tachycardia may suggest fetal compromise, but not invariably so. Differential diagnosis includes prematurity, maternal fever, minimal fetal hypoxia, uterine tachysystole, drugs (atropine), arrhythmias, and hyperthyroidism.

  2. Decreases in variability occur frequently.

   a. Often due to sedation/labor narcotic analgesia

   b. Fetuses have "sleep" periods when variability reduced; periods quite variable in duration

  3. Acceleration is almost always associated with a fetus that is not hypoxic.

   a. Gentle scalp stimulation with finger often produces acceleration (overstimulation can produce vagal response and opposite result)

   b. Vibro-acoustic stimulation is alternative (special device placed over maternal abdomen)

G. Fetal scalp sampling 26C

  1. Intrapartum sample of fetal blood

   a. Plastic cone placed inside vagina with light source

   b. Small cut on scalp made with razor

   c. Fetal blood drawn up in capillary tube

d. Requires ruptured membranes and cervical dilation of at least 4 cm

2. pH analyzed in dedicated instrument

3. Interpretation
   a. >7.25: reassuring
   b. 7.20–7.24: repeat in 20 minutes
   c. <7.2: deliver

4. Falling out of favor; many maternity wards do not have the instrument because simple scalp stimulation can yield the same information; a 15-bpm rise for 15 seconds is strongly associated with a scalp pH above 7.25

VI. Treatment

A. Abnormal FHR patterns
   1. Delivery as quickly as possible
   2. Typically via cesarean section but if birth imminent, forceps or vacuum

B. Indeterminate patterns
   1. Oxygen
   2. IV hydration (treating hypotension)
   3. Placing mother on side (keep fetus from compressing vena cava)
   4. Changing maternal position
   5. Tocolytic therapy with beta agonist (terbutaline)
   6. Cessation of oxytocin infusion
   7. Saline infusion through IUPC to relieve umbilical cord compression

VII. Antepartum Monitoring (10D, 32D)

A. Indications
   1. Any pregnancy with fetal or maternal condition that is associated with increased risk of placental insufficiency or stillbirth
   2. No consensus on management for any specific condition chiefly due to lack of randomized, controlled trials comparing management schemes
   3. Examples
      a. Maternal: hypertension, diabetes, antiphospholipid syndrome
      b. Fetal: multiple gestation, post-term gestation, oligohydramnios, intrauterine growth restriction, subjective maternal report of decreased fetal movement

4. Initiation most commonly at 32–34 weeks but occasionally earlier, depending on circumstances

5. Frequency

    a. Generally no less than weekly

    b. Any change in maternal or fetal condition

B. Techniques

  1. Nonstress test

    a. Observation of FHR for 20 minutes

    b. "Reactive" two accelerations in 20 minutes

    c. "Nonreactive" absence of above; further evaluation indicated

  2. Contraction stress test

    a. Contractions induced via oxytocin infusion or nipple stimulation

    b. Test requires at least three contractions in 10 minutes

    c. Results

      i. Reactive or nonreactive as with NST

      ii. In addition

        (1) Negative: no decelerations

        (2) Suspicious: variable decelerations or late decelerations with <50% of contractions

        (3) Positive: late decelerations with 50% or more of contractions

    d. Avoid with prelabor, abruption, placenta previous

  3. Biophysical profile

    a. Five components; fetus observed by ultrasound for 30 minutes plus NST

    b. Each item present counts for two points

      i. Fetal tone: one or more episodes of flexion-extension-flexion

      ii. Fetal movement: three gross body movements in 30 minutes

      iii. Fetal breathing: one episode of rhythmic breathing

      iv. Amniotic fluid volume: 2-cm pocket in two perpendicular planes

    c. Reactive NST counts as two points

    d. Interpretation

      i. 8 or 10 points: normal

      ii. 6 points: should have further fetal evaluation or repeat in 24 hours

iii. 4 points or fewer: suggests need for delivery
4. Amniotic fluid index 26D
   a. Ultrasound assessment of amniotic fluid volume
   b. Sum of vertical heights of deepest pocket of each quadrant of uterus
   c. Oligohydramnios
      i. 5 cm or less
      ii. May be associated with intrauterine growth restriction or failing placenta
   d. Polyhydramnios
      i. 25 cm or more
      ii. Most commonly idiopathic
      iii. Also associated with gestational diabetes, fetal anomalies
5. Umbilical Doppler flow
   a. Doppler imaging of umbilical artery
   b. Abnormal
      i. Absent flow or reverse flow in artery during diastole suggests fetal compromise
      ii. Systolic to diastolic ratio >95th percentile for gestational age
   c. Not clinically useful except possibly in fetus with growth restriction
6. Maternal monitoring of fetal movement ("fetal kick count")
   a. Different paradigms: abnormal?
      i. <10 movements in 10 hours
      ii. Less movement in 1 hour than previously established norm for that patient
   b. Evidence mixed; not clearly effective in reducing stillbirths

VIII. Efficacy of Intrapartum Fetal Monitoring 26A
   A. Difficult to know: in the few studies that have looked at this, perinatal outcome was not improved with no monitoring as compared with intermittent auscultation
   B. Auscultation after a contraction
      1. Low risk
         a. First stage: every 30 minutes
         b. Second stage: every 15 minutes

2. High risk (definition variable)
   a. First stage: every 15 minutes
   b. Second stage: every 5 minutes
C. Compared with intermittent auscultation
   1. Overall cesarean section rate increased
   2. Cesarean section for fetal intolerance to labor increased
   3. Rate of operative vaginal delivery (both vacuum and forceps increased)
   4. Perinatal mortality rate not reduced
D. Normal fetal monitor tracing strongly associated with good neonatal outcome
E. Indeterminate fetal monitor tracing poor predictor of bad outcome: estimated that only 1 or 2 fetuses out of 1000 will develop cerebral palsy

IX. Intrapartum Asphyxia and Cerebral Palsy

A. American College of Obstetricians and Gynecologists[4] diagnostic criteria
   1. Umbilical artery metabolic or mixed academia—pH <7.00
   2. Persistent Apgar score of 3 or less for longer than 5 minutes
   3. Neonatal neurologic sequelae: seizures, coma, hypotonia
   4. Multiorgan system dysfunction: cardiovascular, gastrointestinal, hematologic, pulmonary, renal
B. Task Force on Cerebral Palsy and Neonatal Asphyxia of the Society of Obstetricians and Gynaecologists of Canada[5] added that, in addition to above, umbilical artery base deficit must equal or exceed 16 mmol/L

MENTOR TIPS

- It is important to note the key differences between the various nomenclature systems.
  Bradycardia is defined as either <120 or <110.
  2008 terminology does not distinguish between short-term and long-term variability.
  2008 terminology distinguishes decelerations by time of onset to time of nadir.
- Fetal monitoring has not been beneficial in substantially improving neonatal outcomes.

- Antepartum testing has very little evidence to support its usage or to support using one approach over another.
- Normal monitoring data are much better at predicting good outcome than are abnormal data at predicting bad outcome.

References

1. Stein Z, Susser M: Mental retardation. In Last JM, ed.: Public health and preventive medicine. New York, Appleton-Century-Crofts, 1980.
2. Macones GA, Hankins GDV, Spong CY, et al: The 2008 national institute of child health and human development workshop report on electronic fetal monitoring. Obstetrics and Gynecology 112:661–666, 2008.
3. Freeman RK: Problems with intrapartum fetal heart rate monitoring interpretation and patient management. Obstetrics and Gynecology 100:813–816, 2002.
4. ACOG Technical Bulletin 163: Fetal and neonatal injury. Washington, DC, American College of Obstetricians and Gynecologists, 1992.
5. Policy statement of the task force on cerebral palsy and neonatal asphyxia of the Society of Obstetricians and Gynecologists of Canada (part I). Journal of the Society of Obstetricians and Gynecologists of Canada 1267–1279, 1996.

Resources

ACOG Practice Bulletin 9. Antepartum fetal surveillance. Washington, DC, American College of Obstetricians and Gynecologists, October 1999.

ACOG Practice Bulletin 70. Intrapartum fetal heart rate monitoring. Washington, DC, American College of Obstetricians and Gynecologists, December 2005.

Freeman RK, Gartie TG, Nageotte MP: Fetal heart rate monitoring, 3rd ed. Philadelphia, Lippincott Williams & Wilkins, 2003.

Chapter Self-Test Questions

Circle the correct answer. After you have responded to the questions, check your answers in Appendix A.

1. Which is the most common adverse fetal outcome?

   a. Antepartum stillbirth

   b. Intrapartum stillbirth

   c. Mild mental retardation

   d. Cerebral palsy

2. Which is *not* a component of fetal heart rate monitoring?

   a. Baseline rate

   b. Baseline variability

   c. P–R interval

   d. Changes over time

3. Which is *not* a treatment for an indeterminate fetal heart rate tracing?

   a. Oxygen

   b. Position change

   c. Stopping oxytocin infusion

   d. Immediate delivery

4. Which is true about antepartum testing?

   a. Evidence-based protocols exist

   b. Indicated for maternal diabetes

   c. Can be used in midtrimester for fetal assessment

   d. Not generally used for fetal indications

See the testbank CD for more self-test questions.

DELIVERY

Michael D. Benson, MD

I. Vaginal Birth ⅡC

A. Novice performing delivery without immediate, experienced supervision (Fig. 23.1)

1. Do not break the bed or table.

2. Encourage the mother to push—she will want to anyway.

3. When the baby falls out on the bed between the mother's legs, use bulb syringe to clear mucus out of the mouth and nares, dry the baby, and double-clamp and cut the umbilical cord.

4. The placenta is usually expelled spontaneously within 20 minutes, after which the perineum can be inspected and lacerations repaired.

B. Active intervention

1. As the baby crowns, gently provide perineal counterpressure to facilitate gentle delivery and to prevent the head from "popping out" rapidly, causing lacerations.

2. As the perineum becomes increasingly distended, maintain steady counterpressure so the head eases out. Use a towel or a sponge with one hand to support the perineum in the midline. It is helpful to pinch the perineum together to prevent tears or extension of the episiotomy.

3. When the head emerges, allow it to rotate spontaneously to face either thigh.

4. Have mother briefly stop her conscious pushing efforts at this point. (Delivery may occur so quickly that time does not permit these steps.)

5. Use bulb syringe briefly to clear the mucus out of the nares and oropharynx.

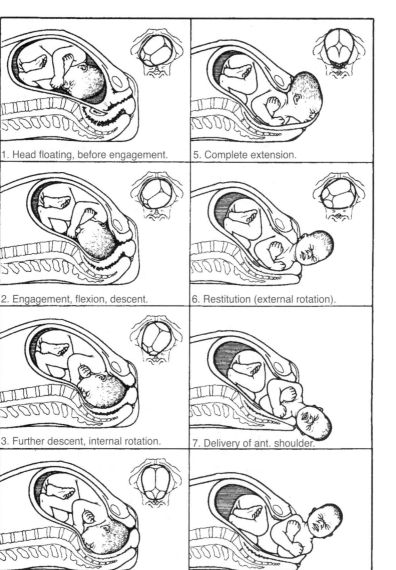

1. Head floating, before engagement.

5. Complete extension.

2. Engagement, flexion, descent.

6. Restitution (external rotation).

3. Further descent, internal rotation.

7. Delivery of ant. shoulder.

4. Complete rotation, beginning extension.

8. Delivery of posterior shoulder.

FIGURE 23.1 Orientation of the fetus through labor and birth. (Redrawn and adapted from Pritchard, JA and MacDonald, PC: Williams obstetrics, ed 16. Appleton-Century-Crofts, New York, 1980, p 397.)

6. Before delivery of the shoulders, slide a finger around the fetal neck beneath the symphysis to palpate for umbilical cord. If cord is there, lift it over fetal head or double-clamp and cut it.

7. Patient should resume pushing after mucus has been evacuated. Gently guide the baby downward so that the anterior shoulder delivers under the symphysis (Fig. 23.2)

8. Lift fetus upward so that the posterior shoulder does not lacerate the perineum. With the delivery of the shoulders, the baby will slide out quickly.

9. Grasp the newborn firmly but gently by the neck and both legs. Vigorous newborns can be placed on the mother's abdomen before or after cutting the umbilical cord.

10. Obtain any necessary cord blood samples while awaiting delivery of the placenta.

11. Spontaneous delivery of placenta usually occurs within 20 minutes. Inspect placenta on both sides for completeness and the number of vessels in the umbilical cord.

12. The cervix, vagina, and perineum should be inspected for lacerations.

    a. With a sponge stick in one hand, insert the other hand into the vagina, applying downward pressure on the posterior wall. An assistant may also gently retract the anterior vaginal wall with an appropriate retractor.

    b. The cervix can either be grasped with ring forceps or blotted dry to aid inspection. If the cervix cannot be seen, it is acceptable to palpate it circumferentially to be sure that there are no major lacerations, provided that there is not excessive bleeding. Palpation is often faster and less uncomfortable for the patient.

    c. After evaluation of the cervix, the vagina needs to be inspected visually, particularly in the area of the ischial spines, because tears are common there.

    d. The perineum should also be inspected, particularly in the area around the urethra. A rectal examination should be performed to be sure that there are no tears in the rectal-vaginal septum and to aid with inspection of the episiotomy or other perineal tears.

13. Perineal tears are classified as follows.

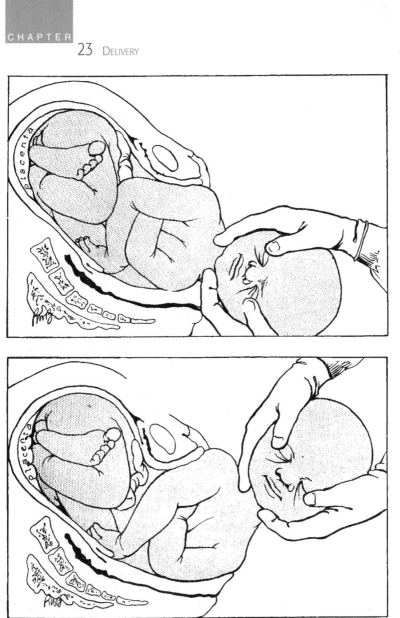

FIGURE 23.2 Delivery of anterior and then posterior shoulder (with gentle traction). (Redrawn and adapted from Pritchard, JA and MacDonald, PC: Williams obstetrics, ed 16. Appleton-Century-Crofts, New York, 1980, p 421.)

a. First-degree tear: break in skin or mucosa only

b. Second-degree tear: laceration that extends into submucosa.

c. Third-degree tear: involves anal sphincter; partial- or full-thickness

d. Fourth-degree tear: extends through sphincter into rectal mucosa

e. Superficial tears: do not need to be repaired unless there is bleeding that does not abate with pressure and time

14. Episiotomies have the following profile.`32G`

   a. Commonly or always done in the second half of the 20th century; studies have questioned practice

     i. Midline epsiotomies significantly increase both the risk of a third- or fourth-degree laceration and the subsequent risk of anal incontinence. However, they offer some protection against lacerations of the anterior perineum (near the urethra) and are less painful for recovery than mediolateral episiotomies.

     ii. Mediolateral episiotomies are associated with a lower rate of sphincter and rectal injuries.

   b. Should be done as close to head emergence as possible but prior to actual laceration developing

   c. Indications include occiput posterior presentation, shoulder dystocia, and operative vaginal delivery

15. Repair of an episiotomy or second-degree laceration is done as follows.

   a. Review of anatomy

     i. As the fetal head emerges, it compresses the posterior vaginal wall into the perineum so that they form a single plane.

     ii. Following birth, the perineum and vaginal wall resume their initial spatial orientation so that the vagina again forms a 60° angle with the perineum.

     iii. The different planes and tissue layers can be confusing.

     iv. The possibility of an episiotomy extension and the amount of the laceration should be carefully ascertained prior to the repair. Sometimes a rectal examination is helpful to assess integrity of the rectal mucosa and the anal sphincter. Even with an epidural, some sphincter tone is often present, permitting a better assessment of perineal integrity.

b. Suture material: absorbable

    i. Chromic (specially treated catgut): loses its tensile strength usually 50% by 1 week

    ii. Vicryl or Dexon: loses tensile strength over 4–6 weeks

c. Four layers need to be closed (Fig. 23.3, Fig. 23.4, and Fig. 23.5)

    i. Vagina

        (1) Start at the apex of the defect with 3-0 gauge suture.

        (2) Continue past the hymen to the point where the tissue changes from pink to normal flesh tone.

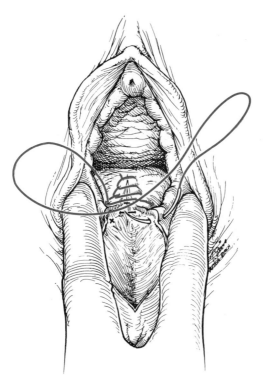

FIGURE 23.3 Reapproximation of vaginal mucosa (running suture). (Redrawn and adapted from Pritchard, JA and MacDonald, PC: Williams obstetrics, ed 16. Appleton-Century-Crofts, New York, 1980, p 432.)

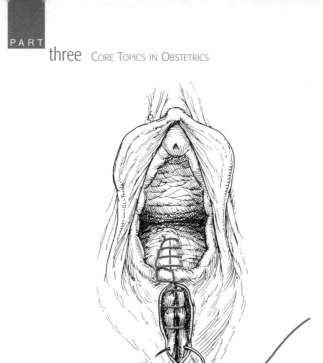

FIGURE 23.4 Interrupted sutures in deep perineum (bulbocavernosus muscle). (Redrawn and adapted from Pritchard, JA and MacDonald, PC: Williams obstetrics, ed 16. Appleton-Century-Crofts, New York, 1980, p 432.)

        (3) The suture is then not cut or tied but rather placed to the side so that it can be used.

    ii. Deep perineum

        (1) The shiny white sheath of the bulbocavernosus muscles is usually visible on either side of the midline episiotomy.

        (2) Three or four interrupted sutures of 2-0 material are placed in this layer.

        (3) Substantial bites of tissue are included on either side of the incision because this reapproximation provides significant strength.

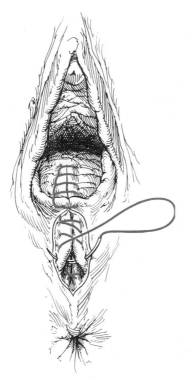

FIGURE 23.5 Reapproximation of superficial perineum. (This running suture can be a continuation of the suture from the vaginal mucosa repair. After this layer, the same suture strand can be used to finish the repair as a subcuticular suture.) (Redrawn and adapted from Pritchard, JA and MacDonald, PC: Williams obstetrics, ed 16. Appleton-Century-Crofts, New York, 1980, p 433.)

    iii. Subcutaneous tissue
        (1) The vaginal repair suture is brought out through the end of the repair underneath the skin.
        (2) The running suture is continued in the subcutaneous tissue in small vertical bites.
        (3) The running suture is tied at the end of the perineal incision if a subcuticular suture is not used.
    iv. Subcuticular suture: running mattress suture beneath the skin edge with 3-0 or 4-0 suture

C. Repair of third-degree lacerations

    1. Anal sphincter repair

        a. Identify torn ends of external anal sphincter; some physicians place Allis clamp on each end

        b. Types of repair

            i. End-to-end: most common

            ii. "Vest over pants": end of sphincter not sewn directly into opposing end but rather 1 cm or so proximal to torn end

            iii. Some studies show better result with "pants over vest" but not all

        c. Typically three figure-of-8 sutures of a 2-0 gauge absorbable suture

    2. Remainder of repair is same as with repair of episiotomy or second-degree laceration

D. Repair of fourth-degree lacerations

    1. For repair of rectal mucosa, 3-0 or 3-0–gauge suture used to close this layer in running, subcuticular fashion

    2. Occasionally perirectal fascia closed in a running fashion using 3-0–gauge suture

    3. Anal sphincter repaired as for third-degree lacerations

    4. Remainder of repair similar to that for second-degree lacerations

II. Forceps Delivery and Vacuum Extraction (11D, 32H-I)

A. Operative vaginal delivery to shorten the second stage of labor can be employed for maternal or fetal indications.

    1. Maternal:

        a. Prolonged second stage

        b. Maternal exhaustion: related to prolonged second stage, although occasionally used before the formal definition has been achieved

        c. Serious health conditions in which the parturient would benefit from a slightly abbreviated labor

            i. Uncommon

            ii. Significant heart or lung disease, neurologic illness, and pregnancy conditions such as severe pre-eclampsia

    2. Fetal: fetal intolerance to labor (including sudden fetal bradycardia, placental abruption, and prolapsed umbilical cord if occurring after patient fully dilated and close to delivery)

B. Usage
 1. Outlet forceps
   a. Sagittal suture has to be in anteroposterior plane (fetus within 45° of either direct occiput anterior or direct occiput posterior)
   b. Scalp must be visible without separating labia
 2. Low forceps
   a. Leading part of fetal skull at station +2 cm or more
   b. Can involve rotation of more than 45°
 3. Midforceps: application of forceps when fetal skull above +2 cm station
 4. High forceps: never done; refers to delivery of unengaged fetus (above 0 station)
C. Four features that distinguish forceps (Fig. 23.6)
 1. Blade: portion that grasps fetus
   a. Cephalic curve corresponds to shape of fetal head
   b. Pelvic curve conforms to general architecture of maternal pelvis
   c. Blades can be solid or hollowed out ("fenestrated") for firmer application/better traction
 2. Shank: connects blade to lock and handle; can either overlap or be separate

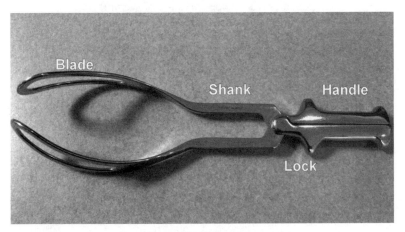

FIGURE 23.6 **Forceps.**

   3. Lock: portion that holds the two branches together
   4. Handle: part grasped by obstetrician
D. Technique
   1. Empty bladder.
   2. Using sutures and fontanelles, confirm exact position of
      the fetal vertex: left occipital anterior (LOA), right occipital
      anterior (ROA), left occipital posterior (LOP), right occipital
      posterior (ROP)
   3. Anesthesia: consider pudendal block if patient is not on
      regional anesthetic
   4. Application
      a. Blades designed for application to sides of fetal head rather
         than from front to back
      b. First blade placed over lower (posterior) side of head
      c. One hand positioned between vaginal wall and side of
         fetal head; other hand guides forceps blade around head
         and inside palm
      d. Procedure followed again for placement of second blade
      e. Blades have to be moved gently so they can lock
      f. Lock blades together
      g. Check/confirm placement; forceps blades should be lateral
         to the lambdoidal sutures in OA applications
      h. Apply traction during contraction such that blades follow
         axis of pelvis (inside curvature of sacrum)
      i. Traction is with moderate force, not pulling as hard as
         possible
      j. Often requires traction over several contractions
      k. As head emerges, remove blade one at a time
E. Vacuum extraction (Fig. 23.7)
   1. Same preparation steps as above
   2. During contraction, apply suction cup to top of fetal head (do
      not apply to side or face)
   3. Create vacuum by operating hand pump (varies by manufac-
      turer); gauges typically have clear indication as to desired
      vacuum pressure
   4. Apply traction during contraction; cup should be 2-3 cm in
      front of posterior fontanelle[i]

i   Miksovsky P, Watson WJ. Obstetric vacuum extraction: State of the art in the
new millennium. Obstetrical and Gynecological Survey, Volume 56, Number 11, 736–51.

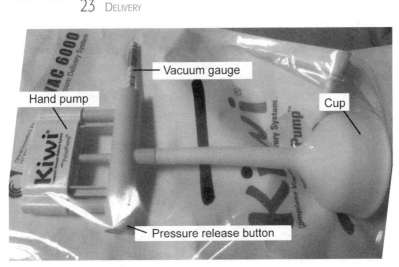

Figure 23.7 **Vacuum.**

5. Release pressure (but do not remove vacuum) at end of contraction (some obstetricians leave vacuum pressure on between contractions)
6. Vacuum will pop off to prevent too much traction; do not reapply if vacuum pops off after two to three times (not including faulty or incomplete application)
7. Release pressure, remove vacuum when head emerges

III. Cesarean Section 11D, 32L

A. Maternal and fetal indications
1. Maternal
   a. Cephalopelvic disproportion/failure to progress
      i. Failure to descend for 2 hours during second stage
      ii. Failure to make any change in station or dilation for 2 or more hours during active phase of labor (provided following criteria are met):
         (1) 4 cm dilated or more
         (2) Intrauterine pressure catheter documenting adequate contractions
         (3) Many physicians wait 3 or 4 hours to be sure patient not progressing

      iii. Failure to make any change in station or dilation during latent phase of labor: criteria for this indication vary widely among practitioners and institutions; generally, most obstetricians wait longer than for the active phase

b. If delivery necessary in the short term for maternal or fetal indications, cesarean delivery may be only choice if medical induction fails

c. Maternal hemorrhage: heavy obstetrical bleeding can be stopped only by delivery of fetus and placenta

d. Placenta previa

e. Repeat cesarean section (see Section IV, Vaginal Birth After Cesarean [VBAC])

f. Pelvic outlet obstruction
    i. Obstructing fibroids
    ii. Pelvic trauma or malformation

g. Maternal request ("elective cesarean"): somewhat controversial and generally discouraged; most obstetricians honor a request for a purely elective cesarean at term but only after extensive counseling; generally poses longer recovery for the mother than vaginal birth and higher risks of transfusion, infection, deep venous thrombosis, and damage to abdominal organs; offsetting these disadvantages are avoidance of perineal injury (with subsequent increased risk for incontinence); elective cesarean might be slightly safer for the fetus

  2. Fetal

    a. Malpresentation (breech, transverse lie)

    b. Extreme prematurity

    c. Fetal intolerance to labor (nonreassuring fetal heart tones)

    d. Predicted macrosomia (controversial)

    e. Multiple gestation

    f. Maternal active genital herpes infection

B. Preoperative preparation

  1. Nursing staff notified

  2. Anesthesia staff notified

  3. Written consent obtained; helpful to discuss risks and benefits in terms of mother and fetus

  4. Magnesium citrate given (liquid antacid): e.g., reflux common in pregnancy and patient may have eaten recently

5. Abdominal and pubic hair shaved
6. Foley catheter inserted
7. Complete blood count and type and screen sent off

C. Important preoperative considerations

1. Know the blood type and hemoglobin
2. Know the location and reason for all abdominal scars; gives an idea of the amount of scarring that will be encountered during incision
3. Patient weight and height help to anticipate abdominal wall thickness; harder to judge in pregnancy
4. Prophylactic antibiotics generally given unless elective, scheduled cesarean
   a. Double-check allergies before prescribing
   b. Drug of choice usually inexpensive first- or second-generation cephalosporin such as cephazolin (Ancef) 2 g IVPB
5. History of fibroids: ask the patient; a strategically placed fibroid can increase blood loss or make incision placement on the uterus more difficult
6. Check the last ultrasound report (if available) for placental location (may have to cut through an anterior placenta)
7. Determine if amniotic fluid has been clear or meconium-stained
8. Ensure whether patient wants tubal ligation; patients on public assistance may need special government papers signed 30 days in advance
9. If cesarean section is for cephalopelvic disproportion and head tightly molded in the pelvis, consider gently pushing up on the presenting part to dislodge it slightly; most easily done before patient prepared for surgery
10. If fetal well-being in question, notify pediatric personnel to be available in operating room

D. Performing cesarean

1. Entering abdomen: vertical incision
   a. Stay in midline, and stay in site of previous knife stroke.
   b. Make long, even strokes with knife.
   c. Fascia can be cut with knife throughout. Alternatively, a small incision with a knife can be made and extended upward and downward with Mayo scissors.

    d. The two rectus muscles can be separated bluntly for a primary section. Often, scar tissue will necessitate sharp dissection on subsequent sections.

2. Entering abdomen: transverse incisions

    a. Start at three fingerbreadths above symphysis to minimize chance of bladder injury

    b. Scarpa fascia often looks like fascia (rectus sheath)

    c. Once true fascia identified, put knife down for a moment and bluntly dissect fat and Scarpa fascia; this dissection neater and quicker on primary sections but not always possible on repeats; some surgeons do not like this blunt dissection

    d. Enter fascia by making two small incisions on either side of midline and gently connect them with additional knife strokes, using steady, even pressure.

    e. Extend fascial incision bilaterally with Mayo scissors

    f. There are two layers; they can be taken down separately or together by undermining first with scissors

    g. Lower layer may be closely adherent to muscle (which bleeds if cut); lower layer attaches to muscle more medially than upper layer—frequently the incision on this lower layer of fascia has to be curved upward to avoid this muscle at the lateral aspect of the incision

    h. Getting through the muscles and into peritoneal cavity

        i. Pfannenstiel incision (Fig. 23.8): after dissecting muscle off overlying fascia above and below incision, muscles can be separated bluntly or sharply in the vertical plane (harder to do on repeat section)

        ii. Modified Mallard incision (does not cut all the way across muscles): cut the medial two-thirds of rectus muscles transversely, carefully avoiding the epigastric vessels that run under the muscle; do not cut underlying, closely adherent peritoneum; frequently, the muscles are tightly adherent in the midline and difficult to separate them bluntly; make mini-Pfannenstiel incision (by dissecting muscle off fascia)

        iii. Entering peritoneal cavity

            (1) Make incision high as possible on peritoneal surface

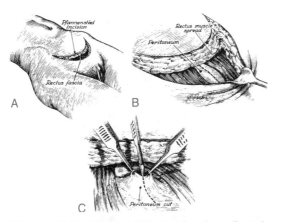

FIGURE 23.8 Pfannenstiel incision. *A,* Skin incision three fingerbreadths above the symphysis. *B,* Rectus muscles exposed, separated in the midline and sharply dissected from the overlying fascia, both above and below the incision. *C,* Incision into anterior peritoneum (entry into abdomen): site chosen away from bladder at inferior aspect of surgical field. (Redrawn and adapted from Wheeless, CR Jr: Atlas of pelvic surgery, ed 2. Lea & Febiger, Philadelphia, 1988, p 369.)

(2) Incision for vertical or Pfannenstiel is vertical; transverse for Mallard
   3. Dissect in layers when cutting through preperitoneal fat
   4. Entering the uterus (Fig. 23.9)
      a. Make incision in the vesicouterine peritoneum reasonably far away (cephalad) from bladder (not too low)
      b. Dissection of bladder off uterus
         i. Keep fingers well applied to uterine surface to gently push off bladder
         ii. Move fingers up and down, not side to side
         iii. If adhesions dense behind bladder, they may be sharply dissected with Metzenbaum scissors, keeping tips pointed toward uterus
      c. Uterine incision
         i. Should be approximately 6 cm long and made in steady, gentle strokes
         ii. For most term deliveries, incision should be made transversely in lower uterine segment (less vascular fibrous aspect of uterus)

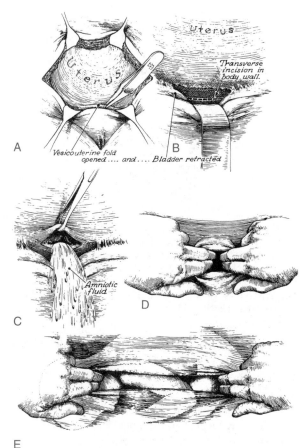

FIGURE 23.9 Entering the uterus: sharp and then blunt dissection (*A* to *E*). (Redrawn and adapted from Wheeless, CR Jr: Atlas of pelvic surgery, ed 2. Lea & Febiger, Philadelphia, 1988, p 219.)

   iii. Lap sponge can be held in the operator's nondominant hand to keep pressure along the incision to minimize bleeding into the incision

   iv. When only a few layers are left in the lower uterine segment, a single finger can be used to poke through

  v. Poke should be straight through the wall; if it does not go through easily, more cutting needs to be done with the knife.

  vi. Initial incision can be extended bluntly with fingers or with bandage scissors; curve incision up and lateral

5. Delivery

 a. Place hand inside of the uterus beneath the fetal head. Keep wrist straight, and do not use lower uterine segment as a fulcrum.

 b. Guide head gently up and outward toward the uterine incision.

 c. As the head emerges through the incision, fundal pressure is applied. Suction mouth and nares as the head is delivered.

 d. Manually remove placenta, or massage uterus to deliver placenta.

 e. Explore uterus after placental delivery.

6. Closing: up to seven layers to close

 a. Uterus: first layer (has to be placed)

 b. Uterus: second, imbricating layer; leaves uterus stronger for subsequent VBAC attempts; placement optional

 c. Visceral peritoneum: not commonly closed

 d. Parietal peritoneum: optional

 e. Fascia: closure necessary

 f. Subcutaneous tissue: closure reduces wound complications if greater than 2 cm

 g. Skin: closed with staples or dissolving sutures

7. Complications

 a. Blood loss requiring blood transfusion; average blood loss for vaginal delivery is estimated to be 300 mL and for a cesarean 800 mL

 b. Increased risk of endometritis; prophylactic cephalosporin typically administered once at time of cord clamping reduces but does not eliminate risk

 c. Increased risk of deep venous thrombosis; some obstetricians use compression boots, although no evidence this is beneficial

 d. Increase risk of damage to adjacent organs; bladder at risk

e. Maternal death; controversial; in a patient without coexisting significant morbidity, may not be excess risk of mortality over that of vaginal birth

IV. Vaginal Birth After Cesarean (VBAC) `22E, 32E`

A. Incision type

1. Safest is single prior lower cervical transverse uterine incision

2. Classical incision (uncommon): vertical incision over uterine fundus; VBAC contraindicated as this is most prone to rupture during labor (can rupture even before labor onset)

3. Lower cervical vertical (less common than lower cervical transverse): controversial

4. Risk of rupture increases with number of prior cesareans; most obstetricians consider vaginal birth only for those with a single prior lower cervical transverse incision

B. Maternal risks and benefits

1. Vaginal birth benefits

a. Shorter hospital stay

b. Less postpartum discomfort (usually, not always)

c. IF VBAC successful, less risk of infection, blood loss requiring transfusion, deep venous thrombosis

d. Risk of abnormal placentation, including location (placenta previa) and attachment to uterus (placenta accreta) increasing with rising number of cesareans

2. Risks

a. Uterine rupture rate (lower cervical transverse) roughly 1% (fetal injury, transfusion, emergency surgery, hysterectomy to control bleeding can be outcomes)

b. Failure to deliver vaginally with need for cesarean during labor; associated with higher risks than elective cesarean before onset of labor

c. Successful vaginal birth has risks not posed by elective cesarean; perineal injury with subsequent urinary or fecal incontinence

d. Some studies show higher overall rate of blood transfusion and infection for mothers attempting VBAC compared to elective, repeat cesarean before onset of labor

C. Fetal risks and benefits

1. Vaginal birth: no one has argued that fetus has lower morbidity or mortality from vaginal birth rather than elective cesarean; vaginal delivery may have benefits for mother and is warranted if fetal risks are low

2. Risks

a. Uterine rupture with attendant risk of death or permanent neurologic injury; between 1 in 500 and 1 in 1000; fetal morbidity can occur even in the best of circumstances with immediate recognition of uterine rupture and immediate delivery

b. Intolerance to labor, shoulder dystocia

D. Other considerations

1. Birth interval of fewer than 18 months associated with increased risk of rupture

2. Some evidence that two-layer closure of uterine incision with cesarean leads to stronger scar for subsequent labor

3. Prostaglandin induction associated with excessive risk of rupture and should not be used

4. Women with a history of cesarean for cephalopelvic disproportion may be at increased risk for a second failed attempt at vaginal delivery

5. Prior successful VBAC is no guarantee of uterine integrity with next labor, although it does suggest a relatively high probability of successful vaginal delivery on subsequent labors

---

 MENTOR TIPS

- Operative vaginal delivery should generally not be attempted unless one is confident that the fetus can be delivered vaginally. Although this confidence does not always guarantee success, a "trial of forceps" is very controversial. Failed forceps deliveries are associated with a higher risk of newborn neurologic injury. The use of a vacuum and forceps in sequence (or vice versa) should generally be avoided as well, although this can pose a management dilemma if the head is low and the mother is exhausted.

- Episiotomies were introduced as a result of speculation that they might reduce the risk of incontinence and large lacerations. After almost 100 years, there is some weak evidence that midline episiotomies might actually increase the risk of tears into the rectum. Still controversial, if an episiotomy seems like a good idea, many obstetricians are opting for medial-lateral incisions.

Resources

Cunningham FG, Leveno KJ, Bloom SL, et al: Williams obstetrics, 22nd ed. New York, McGraw-Hill, 2005.

Chapter Self-Test Questions

Circle the correct answer. After you have responded to the questions, check your answers in Appendix A.

1. Bladder should be emptied in advance of each of these deliveries *except:*

    a. Vacuum.

    b. Cesarean.

    c. Forceps.

    d. Vaginal delivery.

2. Which layers must be closed in a cesarean?

    a. Uterus and fascia

    b. Uterus and skin

    c. Peritoneum and fascia

    d. Fascia and skin

3. Which is *not* true about vacuum extraction?

    a. The effort should be stopped after three "pop-offs."

    b. The bladder should be emptied first.

    c. The vacuum should be released between contractions.

    d. The attempt should not exceed 10 contractions.

    e. None of the above.

4. Which correctly describes a third-degree laceration?

   a. Tears in either labia and the posterior vaginal mucosa

   b. Tear through vaginal mucosa, perineal skin, and bulbocavernosus muscles

   c. Tear through vaginal mucosa, deep perineum, and rectum

   d. Tear through vaginal mucosa, deep perineum, and into anal sphincter

See the testbank CD for more self-test questions.

24 CHAPTER

FETAL COMPLICATIONS

Michael D. Benson, MD

I. Multiple Gestation
A. Demographics, risk factors 20A
  1. Twinning
     a. Monozygotic (identical): one zygote divides into two embryos
        i. Rate is 3/1000 deliveries
        ii. Constant worldwide
        iii. Not heritable
        iv. Types
           (1) Diamnionic, dichorionic: division by 3 days
           (2) Diamniotic, monochorionic: division at day 3–8
           (3) Monamnionic, monochorionic: division after day 8
           (4) Conjoined: division after day 11–12
     b. Dizygotic (fraternal)
        i. Rate variable
           (1) Ethnicity
              (A) Asian 6/1000 deliveries
              (B) Caucasian 10/1000
              (C) African American 12/1000
              (D) In some tribes in Africa, can be as high as 60/1000
           (2) Increases with:
              (A) Advancing maternal age
              (B) Family history of patient or first-degree female relative with twins
              (C) Conception occurring within 30 days of stopping oral contraceptives

2. Higher-order gestations

    a. Spontaneous rates: each next order of multiples occurs at roughly 1/90th the rate of the prior order

        i. Triplets: roughly 1 in 6400

        ii. Quadruplets: roughly 1 in 500,000

        iii. Vast majority are polyzygotic rather than monozygotic

    b. Assisted reproduction

        i. Clomiphene citrate: 5%–8% risk of multiple gestations

        ii. Gonadotropins: 25% risk (10% higher-order multiples)

    c. Special cases

        i. Case reports of multiple gestations with different gestational ages: zygotes fertilized 4–8 weeks apart

        ii. Higher-order gestations can have any combination of events, e.g.:

            (1) Triplets: two zygotes, where one divided into two

            (2) Quadruplets: two zygotes, where both divided

B. Diagnosis `20C`

    1. Physical examination: can be suggestive, but not reliable

        a. Prior to advent of ultrasound, half of multiple gestations were diagnosed at time of delivery

        b. Increased fundal height and two audible fetal heart tones suggestive but not diagnostic (fetal heart tones of singleton pregnancy can often be heard in more than one location)

    2. Ultrasound: highly reliable, but not infallible

        a. Sensitivity greater than 95%

        b. Twins might be missed until delivery one in several thousand times (but not 1 in 100,000)

    3. In monochorionic twins, absence of membrane septum is important prognostic issue

    4. Zygosity determination (issue for same-gender twins only)

        a. Monozygotic twins often appear very different at birth

        b. In childhood, "are they as alike as two peas in a pod?" highly accurate for determining identical twins

        c. Blood typing and DNA typing diagnostic

C. Complications

    1. Prematurity

        a. Twins: average gestational age at birth is 35 weeks

        b. Triplets: average gestational age at birth is 32 weeks

2. Cerebral palsy: strongly associated with prematurity and low birth weight
   a. Singletons: 2–3/1000
   b. Twins: approximately 13/1000
   c. Triplets: approximately 45/1000
3. Miscarriage/intrauterine fetal demise/stillbirth
   a. Risk increased overall
   b. Second fetus delivered has substantially higher risk (diminished somewhat with electronic fetal monitoring)
   c. Rises substantially at term: twin gestations delivered by due date (rather than waiting up to 2 weeks after)
4. Congenital anomalies
   a. Increased two to three times overall
   b. Higher in monozygotic multiple pregnancies
   c. Amniocentesis can be done for each fetus (indigo Carmen commonly injected after fluid obtained to help ensure same fetus not sampled twice)
5. Other
   a. Demise of one fetus
      i. In first trimester, known as disappearing twin
      ii. Rarely can lead to coagulopathy
   b. Monochorionic twin gestation: survival uncommon due to high rate of cord accidents
6. Maternal complications 20B
   a. Anemia: fetuses are voracious consumers of iron and folate; supplementation advisable
   b. Hypertensive disorders of pregnancy
   c. Postpartum hemorrhage
   d. Maternal mortality increased two to three times
   e. Discomforts of pregnancy more common and worse (heartburn, edema, varicosities)
7. Discordant growth
   a. Definitions vary: most common is more than 20% difference in estimated weight
   b. Associated with higher stillbirth rate
   c. Etiology
      i. Congenital or chromosomal anomalies

      ii. Twin-twin transfusion syndrome

      iii. Idiopathic

   d. Treatment: premature delivery

8. Twin-twin transfusion syndrome

   a. More common among monozygotic twins

   b. Twins share same placental circulation

   c. One twin polycythemic; other anemic

   d. Dramatic discordancy in growth between twins

   e. High rate of intrauterine fetal demise

   f. Suggested by ultrasound

   g. Treatment: difficult; most common is premature delivery

D. Treatment 20D

  1. Antepartum monitoring: little evidence to suggest any specific protocol

    a. Weekly NSTs beginning at 32 weeks, biweekly at 36 weeks

    b. Ultrasounds every 3–4 weeks to assure concordant growth

    c. Weekly cervical examinations to check for cervical change (or fibronectin assessments)

  2. If premature delivery before 34 weeks looks likely, antepartum administration of steroids

  3. Mode of delivery

    a. More common among multiple gestations

    b. Vertex-vertex

      i. Plan vaginal delivery

      ii. Average time between deliveries is on the order of 20 minutes

    c. Non-vertex presentation second twin

      i. Controversial

      ii. Two patterns of practice:

        (1) Deliver all twins with non-vertex second twin via cesarean

        (2) Deliver vertex twin vaginally and, for second twin, internal version to convert to breech and then do breech extraction via grasping feet

      iii. Consensus in singleton pregnancies is breech presentation associated with higher rate of neurologic injury with vaginal birth; no clear consensus on multiple gestation

II. Abnormal Fetal Growth 31A-D

A. Intrauterine growth restriction (small for gestational age)

1. Definitions vary, but most common is estimated fetal weight below 10th percentile for gestational age

2. Etiology

  a. Maternal

   i. Substance abuse (tobacco use, alcohol abuse, drug abuse)

   ii. Diseases with significant effect on maternal health, specifically vascular health (e.g., hypertension, heart disease)

   iii. Severe malnutrition

   iv. Teratogens

  b. Fetal

   i. Multiple gestation

   ii. Congenital/chromosomal anomalies

   iii. Infection

3. Diagnosis

  a. Physical examination

   i. Fundal height/uterine size substantially less than predicted for gestational age

   ii. Poor sensitivity/specificity

  b. Ultrasound 32A

   i. Symmetrical: fetus symmetrically small; suggests early etiology, most commonly chromosome abnormality

   ii. Asymmetrical; head normally grown; abdomen small: suggests placental insufficiency

4. Treatment

  a. Bedrest often recommended but of no proven value

  b. Delivery

  c. To delay delivery as long as possible, antepartum fetal monitoring may be used to try to predict imminent danger more specifically

  d. Umbilical Doppler flow studies have been helpful in reducing perinatal death rates in this specific condition; abnormal findings:

   i. Systolic/diastolic flow greater than 3

   ii. Reversed arterial blood flow during diastole

e. No specific treatment to enhance fetal growth beyond assuring proper maternal nutrition

B. Macrosomia

   1. Definitions vary: common one is birth weight over 4000 g

      a. Top 10% of babies born in United States

      b. Birth weight increasing as maternal body mass index (BMI) increasing

      c. 4500 g: top 1.5% of birth weights

   2. Risk factors

      a. Largest single factor

         i. Elevated preconception BMI

         ii. Excessive maternal weight gain is close behind

      b. Gestational diabetes (probably not the case if diagnosed and well controlled)

      c. Multiparity

      d. Prior history

      e. Post-term gestation

   3. Diagnosis

      a. All methods of estimating fetal weight unreliable

      b. In some studies, maternal estimate more accurate

   4. Complications

      a. Increased rate of cesarean sections

      b. Shoulder dystocia

         i. Definition somewhat variable so incidence has to be treated somewhat skeptically

         ii. Risk is 1.4% overall

         iii. Risk over 4500 g may be 9% or higher

         iv. Gram for gram, risk of shoulder dystocia appears to be higher in gestational diabetics

         v. Majority of cases (and injuries) occur in infants <4000 g

III. Rh Isoimmunization

A. Etiology 19A

   1. Fetal-to-maternal blood transfusion resulting in maternal sensitization to red blood cell (RBC) antigens; resultant maternal antibodies can cross placenta and cause fetal RBC hemolysis

   2. A, B, O blood group

      a. Incompatibility most common

         i. Seen in type O mothers

      b. Can be seen on first pregnancy as many mothers have circulating anti-A or anti-B antibodies

      c. Most antibodies are IgM, which cannot cross placenta and therefore cannot harm fetal RBCs

      d. Most common newborn effects are neonatal anemia and jaundice

3. C, D, E (Rhesus) blood group

      a. Contains five antigens: C, c, D, E, e

      b. Confusing terminology

         i. Small "d" indicates absence of "D": not a specific antigen

         ii. Other antigenic variants include weak D: not significant cause of fetal disease

         iii. Rh-positive: refers to presence of D antigen

         iv. Rh-negative: absence of D antigen

      c. Most common and significant sensitizing antigen is the D antigen, which is absent in:

         i. Whites: 15%

         ii. African Americans: 5%–8%

         iii. Asian, Native Americans: 1%–2%

4. Other significant antigens

      a. Lewis and I antibodies commonly reported but do not cause hemolytic disease of newborn (primarily IgM)

      b. Kell antibodies can produce disease

         i. Often result from prior blood transfusion

         ii. Maternal antibody titers cannot be used to follow disease

5. Maternal antibodies cross placenta on next pregnancy and destroy fetal RBCs with resultant anemia, high output cardiac failure, and fetal death

6. Alloimmunization thought possible for 0.1 mL of fetal blood entering maternal circulation

7. Can occur at any point during pregnancy; of sensitized mothers:

      a. 7% in first trimester

      b. 16% in second trimester

      c. 29% in third trimester

      d. Most common at delivery: roughly half of cases

8. Risk factors 19C
    a. Miscarriage
    b. Amniocentesis
    c. Third-trimester maternal bleeding
    d. Manual removal of placenta
    e. Cesarean delivery
B. Screening and diagnosis 19D
    1. Screening
        a. Issue in Rh-negative mothers
        b. Antibody screen in early pregnancy and at 28 weeks (will pick-up D antibody)
    2. Diagnosis for those with detected D antibody
        a. Antibody titers
            i. Useful in those without a prior affected child
            ii. Absolute level of 1:8 or greater suggests fetal risk and further testing
            iii. Rising titer also suggests fetal risk
            iv. Generally tested at 4-week intervals
        b. Paternal blood type
            i. Can be determined to exclude possibility of at-risk fetal genotype
            ii. Determining certainty of paternity extremely problematic
                (1) Some studies show 10% of newborns born to married women are not genetically related to patient's husband
                (2) Patients often under considerable social pressure not to disclose true paternity
                (3) "Don't ask, don't tell"; if you do not ask, patient will never have to tell
        c. Fetal genotype can be determined directly via amniocentesis
        d. In utero determination of fetal anemia
            i. Historical
                (1) Determination of amniotic fluid bilirubin level by amniocentesis and spectral analysis at wavelength of 450 nm)
                (2) Lily graph: optical density at 450 nm as function of gestational age

(A) Zone I: unaffected
(B) Zone II: moderately affected
(C) Zone III: high risk for stillbirth
ii. Current: middle cerebral artery Doppler testing
(1) Specialized study
(2) Not useful for other conditions
(3) Significant anemia predicted by systolic flow 1.5 times multiple of median for given gestational age
iii. Other ultrasound findings of life-threatening fetal anemia
(1) Fetal hydrops: thickening of fetal skin signifying edema and heart failure
(2) Thickened placenta
e. Treatment: gestational age–dependent
i. Delivery
ii. Ultrasound-guided in utero transfusion via umbilical vein (cordocentesis: can also be used to check karyotype and hematocrit) `32C`
C. Prevention: passive immunization with anti-D antibody given to those with negative antibody screens `19B`
1. Term gestation
a. 300 mcg (standard U.S. dose) given at 28 weeks (RhoGAM)
b. Second dose within 72 hours of delivery
c. Does not work perfectly: risk reduced to 1 in 1000
d. Protects against transfusion of 15 mL of fetal blood
2. First-trimester abortion or miscarriage: 50 mcg; protects against transfusion of 2.5 mL of fetal blood (MICRogam)
3. Anti-D antibody originates from plasma of individuals with high titers
a. All plasma lots tested for HIV and hepatitis B and C
b. Processing removes all viral particles
4. Kleihauer-Betke test (hemoglobin acid elution test): some recommend for all Rh-negative mothers delivering Rh-positive babies to check for excessive fetal maternal hemorrhage (which might require more than one dose of RhoGAM)

IV. Stillbirth (Intrauterine Fetal Demise)
A. Definition: pregnancy loss after 20 weeks or 500 g
B. Demographics and risk factors

1. Causes 21A
   a. Second trimester
      i. Congenital anomalies
      ii. Chromosome errors (most common 13, 18, 21, X0)
      iii. Rh-alloimmunization
      iv. Infection
      v. Maternal endocrine disorders (diabetes, hypo- and hyperthyroidism)
   b. Third trimester: same as above and:
      i. Antiphospholipid antibodies
      ii. Trauma
      iii. Obstetrical conditions
         (1) Previa with hemorrhage
         (2) Abruption
         (3) Cord accidents
         (4) Labor events (outnumbered by antepartum events by 5:1 or 6:1)
         (5) Intrauterine growth restriction
         (6) Amniotic fluid embolism
         (7) Uterine rupture
         (8) Multiple gestation
2. Incidence: roughly 1 in 100 to 1 in 200 births in developed nations (much higher in developing countries)

C. Diagnosis 21B
1. Maternal report of movement neither sensitive nor specific
   a. Mothers commonly report absent movement for brief periods (even hours) when healthy, moving fetus is present
   b. Mothers report fetal movement hours or days after demise
2. Physical examination
   a. Presence of fetal heart tones can usually be distinguished from maternal pulse but not always, particularly if maternal pulse over 100
   b. Absence of heart tones strongly suggestive but on occasion they can be missed even when visible on ultrasound
3. Ultrasound most reliable diagnostic method; secondary findings include oligohydramnios, edema, and absent movement and respirations

D. Treatment 21C-E
1. Diagnostic workup to determine cause of demise

a. Autopsy
b. Pathologic examination of placenta
c. Karyotype
d. Kleihauer-Betke test of mother (to look for fetal-maternal hemorrhage)
e. Complete blood count with platelets
f. Diabetes screen
g. Antibody screen
h. Thyroid-stimulating hormone
i. Urine toxicology screen
j. Thrombophilia workup
    i. Lupus anticoagulant
    ii. Anticardiolipin antibodies
    iii. Antithrombin III
    iv. Protein C
    v. Protein S
    vi. Factor V Leiden
    vii. Methylenetetrahydrofolate reductase
k. Infection evaluation
    i. Placental cultures for suspected chorioamnionitis
    ii. Rubella titer (if not already done)
    iii. Rapid plasma reagin
    iv. Serologies (IgM, acute and convalescent IgG): cytomegalovirus, *Toxoplasma*, parvovirus
    v. Herpes simplex culture or polymerase chain reaction
2. Delivery
    a. Typically via induction of labor
    b. Intrauterine fetal demise can be cause of coagulopathy, but this is seen very rarely in current practice since several weeks have to elapse first
3. Maternal counseling
    a. Denial common initial reaction
    b. Grief expected, but obsessive thoughts months later may signal superimposed depression
    c. Mothers often blame themselves
    d. Helpful interventions (only if patient is so inclined)
        i. Giving parents opportunity to hold baby
        ii. Photographing baby for future
        iii. Perinatal loss groups

MENTOR TIPS

- Rate of monozygotic twinning is constant around the world; dizygotic rates vary considerably.
- Multiple gestation places fetuses at substantially increased risk for anomalies, prematurity, stillbirth, and cerebral palsy.
- Intrauterine growth retardation may result from maternal or fetal disease but often occurs in isolation.
- Little treatment is available for intrauterine growth retardation beyond deciding when to deliver.
- Macrosomia is most closely linked to elevated pre-conception BMI and excessive pregnancy weight gain.
- Rh-alloimmunization is rarely seen due to efficacy of passive immunization with anti-D antibodies.
- Rh-alloimmunization typically affects the next pregnancy.
- Doppler flow evaluation of middle cerebral artery has largely replaced serial amniocentesis determinations of bilirubin for assessment of fetal anemia.

Resources

ACOG Practice Bulletin 22. Fetal macrosomia. Washington, DC, American College of Obstetricians and Gynecologists, November 2000.

ACOG Practice Bulletin 12. Intrauterine growth restriction. Washington, DC, American College of Obstetricians and Gynecologists, January 2000.

ACOG Practice Bulletin 75. Management of alloimmunization during pregnancy. Washington, DC, American College of Obstetricians and Gynecologists, August 2006.

ACOG Practice Bulletin 4. Prevention of Rh D alloimmunization. Washington, DC, American College of Obstetricians and Gynecologists, May 1999.

Chapter Self-Test Questions

Circle the correct answer. After you have responded to the questions, check your answers in Appendix A.

1. Which is true about monozygotic twinning?

   a. More common than dizygotic twinning

   b. Rate varies among ethnic groups

   c. Varies with maternal age

   d. Rate does not depend on family history

2. Management of twin pregnancy:

   a. Antepartum monitoring derived from evidence-based data

   b. Consensus exists that breech second twin should be delivered vaginally

   c. Antepartum steroids appropriate if delivery anticipated before 34 weeks

   d. Cesarean recommended for vertex-vertex twins

3. Which treatments are *not* effective for intrauterine growth restriction?

   a. Bedrest

   b. Proper maternal nutrition

   c. Umbilical Doppler flow studies to monitor fetal well-being

   d. Delivery

4. Maternal isoimmunization:

   a. Affects fetuses in the next pregnancy.

   b. Risk increases as the pregnancy progresses.

   c. Passive immunization highly effective in preventing Rh-isoimmunization.

   d. All of the above.

See the testbank CD for more self-test questions.

25

THIRD-TRIMESTER BLEEDING

Michael D. Benson, MD

I. Abnormal Placentation

A. Overview: placenta can deviate from normal in various ways: location, attachment, and premature separation 23A

B. Abruption: premature separation of placenta from uterine wall; can vary considerably in severity and extent 27B

    1. Complicates about 1 in 200 pregnancies

        a. Risk factors (in order of relative risk, most to least) 27A

           i. Prior abruption: largest single risk factor; may increase risk by factor of 10 over those without such a history

           ii. Thrombophilias: probably second biggest risk factor (condition-specific; see Chapter 26)

           iii. Preterm premature rupture of membranes

           iv. Hypertension

           v. Cigarette use

           vi. Multiple gestation

           vii. Advancing maternal age

           viii. Cocaine use (risk not quantified)

        b. Maternal morbidity and mortality

           i. Typically related to life-threatening bleeding

           ii. Disseminated intravascular coagulation (see below): less than 10% of cases; not usually seen unless abruption is quite severe and fetus has died or is in immediate jeopardy

        c. Neonatal morbidity and mortality

           i. Significant cause of perinatal mortality (10%–15% of perinatal deaths)

           ii. Important cause of prematurity

           iii. Increased rate of neurologic injury among survivors for given gestational age

2. Diagnosis 23B-C

  a. Symptoms: can be highly variable; may include vaginal bleeding, uterine contractions, and abdominal pain

  b. Physical examination (also can be highly variable) (significant physical findings often not seen until process quite advanced)

    i. Uterine tenderness

    ii. Hemorrhagic shock

    iii. Nonreassuiring fetal heart rate tracing

    iv. Uterine contractions ranging from not noticed by patient to tetanic (continuous/constant)

    v. Vaginal bleeding ranging from none at all ("concealed abruption") to hemorrhage

  c. Laboratory test results, imaging: not usually helpful because none very sensitive

    i. Complete blood count

    ii. Coagulation studies

    iii. Ultrasound

      (1) Very poor at diagnosis because blood clots that may form between wall of uterus and placenta have appearance similar to that of placenta

      (2) Can help exclude placenta previa

3. Treatment: deliver or not to deliver 23D

  a. Bedrest generally recommended when continuing pregnancy, although efficacy doubtful

  b. Problems with planning treatment

    i. Clinical course may not be linear or predictable

    ii. Diagnosis often presumed as mild cases are very difficult to confirm

  c. Ideal treatment is always delivery of fetus and then placenta; cures problem for both mother and child

  d. If fetus significantly premature, conflict arises as to course of action to take for fetus (delivery remains safest for mother but she will generally place fetal well-being ahead of her own)

    i. Many abruptions can follow indolent course or start and stop

    ii. For significant prematurity, may be acceptable to observe mother closely in hospital to prolong gestation

C. Previa: abnormal location (placenta covers cervix and would deliver in advance of fetus) `27B`

1. Classification

a. Total: cervical internal os completely covered by placenta

b. Partial: os partially covered

c. Marginal: placental edge is at margin of os

d. Low-lying placenta: edge of placenta near cervical os but not covering it; most common definition is within 2 cm (clinically somewhat different than preceding three and can be associated with successful vaginal delivery; there can be significant subjectivity in ultrasound interpretations)

e. Vasa previa: isolated placental blood vessels course through amniotic membranes over cervical os

  i. Different condition than placenta previa

  ii. Large risk to fetus of hemorrhage and death but little risk to mother

  iii. Clinically difficult to distinguish fetal bleeding presenting vaginally from maternal bleeding

2. Incidence and risk factors `27A`

a. Roughly 1 in 300 pregnancies

b. Risk factors

  i. Increasing maternal age

  ii. Multiparity

  iii. Multiple gestation

  iv. Prior cesarean delivery: risk rises with each successive cesarean section (from 1 in 100 with second cesarean to 3 in 100 with sixth cesarean)[1]

c. Placenta previa associated with increased risk of abnormal placental attachment: accreta, increta, percreta

3. Morbidity and mortality `23D`

a. Maternal: chiefly related to potential for massive hemorrhage and occasional need to do cesarean hysterectomy to control bleeding (much more with accreta variants)

b. Perinatal

  i. Can be direct cause of fetal injury and death through maternal hemorrhage and resultant placental compromise

  ii. Greatest morbidity rate caused by need to deliver prematurely for maternal hemorrhage

4. Diagnosis relies on ultrasound

    a. More common at 20 weeks than at term; placenta generally carried upward as uterus grows and lower uterine segment elongates (this may be real or may simply appear to be the case as placenta margin becomes easier to identify; cause of this observation has never been clarified); placental attachment does not "move"

    b. If not covering the internal os at 20 weeks, placenta will not cover it later

    c. 60% of those covering os at 20 weeks will move away

    d. Physical examination can cause life-threatening hemorrhage in those with previa; vaginal examinations of those with bleeding in late second trimester or third trimester are not performed before ultrasound confirmation that the placenta is not covering internal os

  5. Treatment: cesarean delivery before labor or significant bleeding (if possible)

    a. Delivery required by heavy bleeding (preferably before hemorrhagic shock occurs)

    b. Heavy bleeding highly likely once labor begins; common protocol is to deliver by cesarean at 36 weeks if amniocentesis confirms fetal lung maturity and 1 week later if not

    c. Bedrest and avoidance of sex recommended if placenta covering os by 28 weeks

    d. Patients generally hospitalized for small bleeding episodes for varying times

      i. While in hospital, IV access maintained at all times

      ii. Crossmatched blood also kept available; typically 2–4 units packed red blood cells (RBCs)

    e. For previas covering prior surgical scars such as prior cesareans, possibility of accreta (see below) needs to be kept in mind

D. Accreta: abnormal attachment of placenta to uterine wall `27B`

  1. Definitions

    a. Accreta can refer generally to the condition but more specifically refers to placental attachment to myometrium superficially

    b. Increta: placental villi invade more deeply into myometrium

    c. Percreta: placental villi invade through myometrium

d. Surface area of placenta involved may vary

    i. Complete: entire placenta abnormally attached

    ii. Partial: several cotyledons

    iii. Focal: one cotyledon

2. Risk factors: typically conditions that lead to defective decidua formation at placental attachment site 27A

    a. Placenta previa (most important risk factor)

    b. High multiparity

    c. Prior uterine surgery

        i. Uterine curettage (remains very uncommon with this history alone)

        ii. Cesarean section[1]

            (1) Risk rises from 1 in 400 at first cesarean to 1 in 200 with third cesarean

            (2) At fourth cesarean risk is 1 in 50; sixth or more 1 in 15

3. Diagnosis

    a. Clinically at time of delivery; all or part of the placenta remains attached to uterus and cannot be removed

    b. Obstetrical hemorrhage common but variable depending on amount of placental involvement

    c. Typically requires pathology confirmation (uterine curettage, hysterectomy)

    d. Diagnosis before delivery

        i. Can have high degree of suspicion with placenta previa, particularly in presence of prior uterine scar (most commonly a cesarean)

        ii. Doppler flow ultrasound and magnetic resonance imaging help identify placental invasion of myometrium

4. Treatment 23D

    a. Most widely accepted treatment for accreta is hysterectomy

    b. Difficulty in diagnosis

        i. Requires a tissue sample; diagnosis can be suspected only in the absence of hysterectomy (uterine curettage not intended to remove muscle from uterus, so not known what the sensitivity or specificity of curettage is for detecting mild cases)

        ii. Condition probably more common (and not always recognized) than suggested by pathology

iii. Probably cases of accreta that do not require hysterectomy: patients who do not have heavy, uncontrollable bleeding (but these cases will not be identified as diagnosis cannot be made without hysterectomy)

c. Alternatives to hysterectomy

i. Embolization of pelvic arteries by interventional radiology

(1) Can be done emergently (depending on facility)

(2) Successful pregnancies have been reported

(3) In cases of high suspicion with scheduled cesareans (such as for previa covering previous scar) catheters can be placed preoperatively to facilitate treatment if hemorrhage should occur

ii. Leaving placenta in place

(1) Embolization has been reported with placenta in place

(2) Methotrexate has been used

(3) Controversial (little experience; risk of infection and sepsis)

II. Retained Placenta 27B

A. Diagnosis

1. Typically suspected when placenta remains undelivered after an arbitrary time has passed

a. Over 95% of patients deliver within 30 minutes

b. Delivery after this time associated with increased rate of transfusion and surgical procedures

c. Succenturiate lobe of placenta is separate portion typically connected to main body by thin segment of tissue or blood vessels and amniotic membranes

d. Internal exploration of uterus or ultrasound (or both)

2. May be first sign of accreta

B. Treatment

1. Manual removal

a. Place one hand through cervix into uterus and sweep cavity with fingers to snare placenta

b. More than one pass may be necessary

c. Helpful to have other hand on abdomen pressing down over fundus to identify anatomy

      d. Very uncomfortable for patient; helpful to have epidural in place or use IV sedation

      e. No data whether prophylactic antibiotics should be administered to prevent postpartum endometritis

   2. Curettage when portions of placenta remain after exploration

      a. Special sharp curette for obstetrics: banjo curette

      b. Large-bore 1.2 cm (and above) suction curette

C. Uterine inversion: on rare occasions, traction on umbilical cord in an effort to deliver placenta will deliver uterus (inside out) through the vagina; this can occur in absence of placenta accreta

   1. Heavy bleeding can result

   2. Replace uterus by pushing it back into original position

   3. Rarely, formal surgical procedure may be required:

      a. Laparotomy with traction on uterus from above with instruments

      b. Hysterectomy may be necessary

III. Uterine Atony `27B`

A. Most common cause of excessive bleeding due to failure of uterus to contract adequately and compress uterine vessels that supply placental site

B. Diagnosis suggested by soft, boggy uterus that fails to contract in association with heavier bleeding than anticipated

C. Risk factors `27A`

   1. Extremes of length of labor (both long and rapid)

   2. Chorioamnionitis

   3. Multiple gestation

   4. Oxytocin use

   5. Prior history

D. Treatment

   1. Medical

      a. Uterine massage

         i. External: massaging uterine fundus abdominally; occasionally requires sustained effort to keep uterus contracted

         ii. Bimanual massage: part of differential diagnosis of uterine atony is retained placenta so that during uterine exploration the uterus can be massaged with both hands

         iii. Bladder catheterization: full bladder may inhibit the uterus's ability to contract

b. Medication

 i. Oxytocin routinely administered after birth to reduce likelihood of atony

  (1) 10 units IM

  (2) 20 or 30 units in 1 L of IV fluid at 4-hour rate

 ii. Methergine: 0.2 mg IM or orally every 6 hours; avoid in hypertensives

 iii. 15-methyl prostaglandin F2 alpha: carboprost tromethamine (Hemabate)

  (1) Approved by United States Food and Drug Administration specifically for treatment of uterine atony

  (2) Dosing

   (A) 250 mcg IM

   (B) May administer up to 8 doses over 90 minutes

  (3) Side effects

   (A) Hypertension may be side effect (does not typically require treatment)

   (B) Gastrointestinal: nausea, vomiting diarrhea

   (C) Fever

 iv. Prostaglandin E2: 20-mg suppositories

 v. Prostaglandin E1: misoprostol (Cytotec); up to 1000 mcg rectally

2. Surgical

 a. Uterus in place

  i. Procedure directly on uterus; successful subsequent pregnancies have been reported

   (1) B-Lynch procedure: sutures of No. 2 chromic placed vertically along one lateral border, then traversing lower uterine segment and continuing vertically over other side of uterus[2,3] (Fig. 25.1)

   (2) Four 1-cm suture squares using dissolving sutures through anterior and posterior walls of uterus to plicate them together[4]

  ii. Uterine artery embolization generally done when vital signs stable and staff and facilities permit

  iii. Hypogastric (internal iliac) artery ligation has fallen out of favor due to time required, less than 50% effectiveness, and anatomy unfamiliar to most obstetricians

  iv. Uterine packing

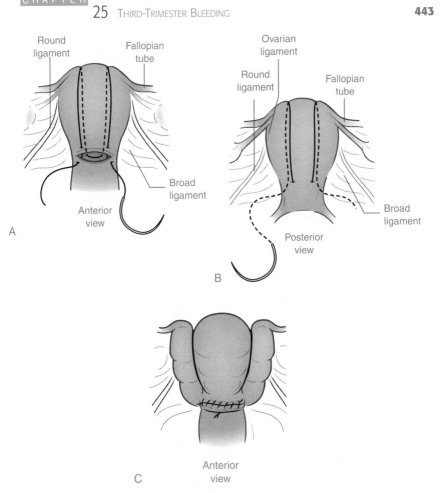

FIGURE 25.1 B-Lynch brace suture of uterus. *A* and *B,* Applying the suture. *C,* Result. (Redrawn from an image by Mr Philip Wilson, FMAA, AIMI, based on Dr B-Lynch's video record of an operation.)

(1) Largely replaced by other procedures
(2) Occasionally utilized with large gauze sponges or (better still) large Foley balloons
(3) SOS Bakri tamponade balloon
   (A) Permits up to 500 mL of volume
   (B) Hospital may not carry it
   (C) Manufacturer recommends avoiding in uterine atony, American College of Obstetricians and Gynecologists (ACOG) recommends it
(4) Concerns include infection and pressure necrosis in the case of the balloons if pressure prolonged

b. Hysterectomy
   i. Still occasionally necessary
   ii. List above does not mean that all alternatives should necessarily be tried before hysterectomy as bleeding may be considerable
   iii. For uterine atony, supracervical hysterectomy generally warranted (removing cervix adds time and risk without offsetting benefit)

IV. Birth Canal Lacerations 27B

A. Lower genital tract (see Chapter 23)
   1. Uncommon cause of hemorrhage; typically repaired with chromic or polyglycolic acid sutures (Vicryl, Dexon)
   2. More common with forceps (and possible vacuum extraction)
   3. Lacerations can occur anywhere along vagina or cervix
   a. Vaginal lacerations more common over ischial spines
   b. Cervical lacerations can be difficult to detect
      i. Can be grasped with ring forceps and inspected circumferentially; typically will need at least one assistant to hold retractors
      ii. Palpation of cervix can help find or exclude lacerations
   c. Rarely, arterial vessel can be torn below mucosa and substantial bleeding can occur; hidden from view between vagina and rectum; hematoma can spread upward into abdomen
      i. Can be suggested if patient has severe pelvic pain that is out of the ordinary
      ii. Can occasionally be palpated

B. Uterine rupture `27B-C`

1. Risk factors: prior uterine surgery, simultaneous induction of labor with prostaglandins and oxytocin (generally avoided as a result) `27A`

2. Uterine dehiscence: generally refers to separation of prior uterine surgical scar without causing symptoms (particularly excessive bleeding)

3. Uterine rupture during labor can cause immediate jeopardy to mother and fetus

    a. May be signaled by large variable decelerations, sudden increase in pain, sudden hypotensive or perceived change in fetal lie or position on abdominal examination (i.e., extremity poking through uterus into abdominal cavity)

    b. Treatment

        i. Deliver fetus immediately via laparotomy (cesarean)

        ii. Close uterine defect (typically very similar to cesarean delivery)

        iii. If occurs after delivery, patient will need exploratory laparotomy, which often resembles cesarean in terms of incision and closure

V. Obstetrical Disseminated Intravascular Coagulation (DIC) `27B`

A. Molecular mechanism: remains unknown; possibilities include:

1. Direct leak of pro-coagulants from pregnancy into maternal circulation

2. Leakage of fetal material into maternal circulation with activation of immune system and secondary activation of coagulation cascade

3. Direct damage to maternal endothelium resulting in release of pro-coagulants such as tissue factor

B. Associated with specific conditions `27A`

1. Abruption: complicates a minority of clinically severe abruptions (severe enough to require urgent delivery)

2. Intrauterine fetal demise (IUFD) (not commonly seen with modern practice): rare complication of IUFD in third trimester; does not result in labor for prolonged periods (weeks, months)

3. Amniotic fluid embolism (AFE): rare condition (perhaps 1 in 20,000 pregnancies)

  a. Diagnosis

   i. One or more signs/symptoms occurring very rapidly during pregnancy or within 48 hours of delivery

    (1) Cardiovascular collapse

    (2) Respiratory distress

    (3) DIC

    (4) Coma, seizures

   ii. Diagnosis made in absence of other specific explanations of signs/symptoms but does not preclude comorbid conditions (such as abruptions)

   iii. Autopsy: presence of fetal material in maternal pulmonary circulation (obtained from central line specimens in living patients more controversial)

  b. Treatment

   i. Supportive: directly at remedying specific medical condition

   ii. Delivery of fetus

    (1) AFE usually results in immediate and significant maternal compromise so fetus is typically in jeopardy

    (2) Fetal injury or death is commonplace if AFE occurs before delivery

C. Diagnosis

 1. Physical examination

  a. Blood starts oozing from any puncture sites (IV sites, phlebotomy sites, needle entrance wounds during suturing)

  b. Blood emerges from body orifices (nose, mouth, urethra, vagina)

  c. Blood fails to clot in red-top test tube within 10 minutes (or clot begins to dissolve within 60 minutes)

 2. Laboratory findings

  a. Elevated coagulation studies: prothrombin time (PT), partial thromboplastin time (PTT), and depressed platelets

  b. Decreased fibrinogen

   i. Normal levels in pregnancy 300–600 mg/dL

   ii. Levels below 150 mg/dL associated with clinical bleeding

    c. Elevated fibrin degradation products
       i. Generated when fibrin broken down by plasmin
       ii. Produced during thrombosis and inflammation
    d. Elevated D-dimer
       i. Generated when fibrin broken down by plasmin
       ii. More specific to thrombosis than fibrin degradation products because forms only after fibrin mesh cross-linked by factor XII
       iii. Interpretation requires clinical judgment
          (1) Also elevated with deep venous thrombosis and pulmonary embolus
          (2) Moderate elevations in pregnancy occasionally encountered in absence of disease

D. Treatment
   1. Typically requires delivery of all pregnancy tissue (fetus and placenta)
   2. Blood transfusion (often massive)
   3. Avoid heparin (theoretically would stop clotting but would cause abnormal bleeding with any disruption of vasculature, which is commonly encountered in obstetrical hemorrhage)
   4. Epsilon-aminocaproic acid
     a. Inhibits conversion of plasminogen to plasmin
     b. Reversal agent for heparin
     c. May prevent degradation of fibrin clot and possibly promote obstruction of small vessels and tissue ischemia
     d. Not recommended for obstetrical DIC

E. Complications
   1. Cardiopulmonary collapse/arrest due to blood loss
   2. Multiorgan failure may not be due directly to blood loss but rather to tissue ischemia resulting from microscopic thrombi obstructing small vessels
     a. Renal failure
     b. Hepatic failure
     c. Acute respiratory distress syndrome

F. Maternal cardiac arrest
   1. Do chest compression in left lateral tilt (place wedge under patient's back); helps avoid fetal vena cava compression and interference with cardiac preload
   2. Beyond 24 weeks or so, deliver fetus as quickly as possible

    a. Fetus may be viable, and delivery is fastest way to resume provision of oxygen

    b. Provides direct maternal benefit; fetus is significant consumer of oxygen

    3. Prognosis for mother and fetus poor and diminishes with time

VI. General Principles Regarding Blood Transfusion for Obstetrical Hemorrhage 23E-F

A. Decision to transfuse

    1. Definition of hemorrhage

        a. Blood loss of 500 mL after vaginal birth or 1000 mL after cesarean; no strong consensus

        b. Estimation of blood loss often difficult at delivery time

          i. Amount of amniotic fluid often difficult to assess

          ii. Blood often on bedding and floor

    2. Clinical considerations

        a. Is patient bleeding

        b. Is patient at risk for subsequent bleeding

        c. Signs or symptoms: most physicians defer transfusion if patient not symptomatic, even with low blood counts; signs or symptoms: dyspnea, headache, tachycardia, orthostatic changes (dizziness, drop in blood pressure, increase in pulse)

        d. Vital signs: pulse >100 in patient who has stopped bleeding and is afebrile may be sign of significant anemia

        e. Absolute hemoglobin: most physicians transfuse for hemoglobin under 5–6 g/dL prior to hospital discharge even if patient asymptomatic with normal vital signs

    3. Oral iron is alternative to transfusion in stable patient who has stopped bleeding

        a. Typically takes 10–14 days for clinical response

        b. Relationship between dose and nausea and constipation

        c. Can administer up to 300 mg ferrous sulfate three times daily although many patients cannot tolerate this dose

B. Initial steps

    1. Notify Nursing and Anesthesia that assistance may be required

    2. Establish two large-bore IV lines (18-gauge or greater; suitable for administering blood)

3. Provide aggressive crystalloid infusion (evidence colloid infusion, i.e. albumin, may be associated with increased mortality rate)

4. Obtain laboratory test results

   a. Complete blood count

   b. Clotting studies

   c. Type and crossmatch

      i. No fewer than two units packed RBCs and may be appropriate initially to request four or more

      ii. Most obstetric units obtain a tube of blood at admission specifically to have available in the laboratory; usually does not require a second blood draw for this purpose

      iii. Type and screen

         (1) Blood type determined

         (2) Screened for common antibodies

         (3) Takes 20–30 minutes

      iv. Crossmatch

         (1) Specific donor blood tested against recipient blood

         (2) Takes an additional 20–30 minutes

         (3) Risk of major transfusion reaction in those receiving type-and-screened blood (prior to getting blood crossmatched) <1 in 1000

C. Blood component replacement (all components should be blood type–compatible to reduce risk of transfusion reaction)

   1. Packed RBCs (240 mL) (contains RBCs, white blood cells [WBCs], and plasma; increases hemoglobin by 1 g/dL)

   2. Plasma clotting factors (both increase fibrinogen by 10 mg/dL)

      a. Fresh frozen plasma (250 mL) (contains fibrinogen, antithrombin III, factors V and VIII)

      b. Cryoprecipitate (40 mL) (contains fibrinogen, factors VIII and XIIII, von Willebrand factor)

   3. Platelets

      a. Platelets and RBCs, WBCs, and plasma

      b. 50 mL

      c. One unit can increase platelet count by 5000 to 10,000/mL

    d. Often supplied as platelet pack; 10 units; come from multiple patients

    e. Associated with development of antiplatelet antibodies, which can lead to increased platelet destruction on subsequent transfusions

  4. When to give clotting factors

    a. No formula (no evidence-based studies)

      i. Platelet transfusion may be considered for patients with platelets <20,000/mm^3 or those actively bleeding with <50,000/mm^3

      ii. Consider clotting component transfusion for:

        (1) Fibrinogen <100 mg/dL

        (2) PT or PTT >1.5 times normal

      iii. Clinical assessment may be faster than waiting for laboratory test results

        (1) Blood clot test (described previously)

        (2) Copious bleeding from minor trauma sites such as needle sticks

    b. Dilutional coagulopathy

      i. Administration of RBCs alone can, in theory, fail to replace clotting components and result in coagulopathy

      ii. Rarely seen (almost never for less than 10 units packed RBCs)

      iii. Treatment is same as that for DIC; replacement of clotting factors

D. Recombinant factor VIIa

  1. Acts on extrinsic coagulation pathway

  2. Dose: 50–100 mcg/kg every 2 hours until bleeding stops

  3. Effect seen within 10–40 minutes

  4. Limitations:

    a. Usage has little experience in obstetrics

    b. May increase subsequent risk of thromboembolism

    c. Very expensive (and may not be available)

E. Complications of blood transfusions

  1. Transmission of infectious disease

    a. HIV and hepatitis B and C

      i. Blood screened

      ii. Risk of HIV transmission roughly 1 per 500,000 per unit of donated blood

b. Other
  i. Malaria, babesiosis, Chagas disease; personal history or travel to endemic area precludes donation for period of time
  ii. Other infectious diseases sufficiently rare or benign that routine screening of blood not warranted (Ebola, Epstein-Barr virus, dengue fever)
c. Bacterial infection
  i. Mitigated by sterilization of blood
  ii. Risk increased if blood kept at room temperature for more than 4 hours
2. Disordered blood chemistry
  a. Hypocalcemia can occur in massive transfusion (more than one unit packed RBCs every 5 minutes)
    i. 3 g of citrate in every unit of packed RBCs
      (1) Citrate metabolized to bicarbonate
      (2) If not, calcium may drop; may lead to hypotension and arrhythmia
    ii. Treated with calcium chloride
  b. Acid-base disturbance
    i. Acid load: citric acid added as anticoagulant; RBCs produce lactic acid
    ii. Base load: citric acid metabolized to bicarbonate
    iii. pH disturbance usually not a major problem
  c. Potassium
    i. Stored RBCs have high potassium concentration
    ii. Hypokalemia from metabolic alkalosis (bicarbonate from citrate) more common than hyperkalemia
    iii. Can result in lethal arrhythmia
3. Transfusion reactions (can occur in up to 10% of recipients)
  a. Acute hemolytic reactions
    i. ABO-incompatible blood
    ii. Can occur within minutes; may be fatal
    iii. Reaction dose- and rate-dependent
    iv. Hemolysis: hypotension, oliguria, DIC, hemoglobinuria
  b. Delayed hemolytic reactions
    i. Reaction to primary exposure: weeks
    ii. Reaction to second exposure: days

  iii. Fall in hemoglobin, low-grade fever
  iv. Usually require no special treatment
 c. Febrile reaction: response to infused leukocytes
  i. 1% of transfusions
  ii. Acetaminophen
 d. Transfusion-related acute lung injury
  i. Pulmonary edema within 8 hours of transfusion; fever, dyspnea, cough
  ii. Stop transfusion, provide supportive care
  iii. Mechanism not known
  iv. Rare

MENTOR TIPS

- Uterine atony is most common cause of postpartum hemorrhage.
- Placenta previa should almost always be known in advance resulting from common use of second-trimester ultrasound.
- In cases of previa and prior cesarean, think accreta.
- Cesarean section increases risk for abnormal placentation subsequently, but absolute risk remains small.
- Tips on obstetrical DIC:
  It is rare.
  Initial presentation can be erratic; there may be bleeding from some sites and not others.
  Bleeding from suture site punctures is relatively common in absence of DIC.
  Blood should clot within 10 minutes and remain clotted in red-top for an hour.
  DIC is often associated with multiple organ failure, presumably due to microthrombi.
- One major reason for delivery in hospital and improved safety of childbirth is availability of blood; have clot available in blood bank at admission to Labor and Delivery.

References

1. Silver RM, Landon MB, Rouse DJ, et al: Maternal morbidity associated with multiple repeat cesarean deliveries. Obstetrics and Gynecology 107:1226–1232, 2006.

2. B-Lynch C, Coker A, Lawal AH, et al: The B-Lynch surgical technique for the control of massive postpartum haemorrhage: An alternative to hysterectomy? Five cases reported. British Journal of Obstetrics and Gynaecology 104:372–375, 1997.

3. B-Lynch C: Web site of the B-Lynch technique. http://www.cbl.uk.com/

4. Cho JH, Jun HS, Lee CN: Hemostatic suturing technique for uterine bleeding during cesarean delivery. Obstetrics and Gynecology 96:129–131, 2000.

Resources

ACOG Practice Bulletin 76. Postpartum hemorrhage. Washington, DC, American College of Obstetricians and Gynecologists, October 2006.

Chapter Self-Test Questions

Circle the correct answer. After you have responded to the questions, check your answers in Appendix A.

1. Which is the most common cause of postpartum hemorrhage?

    a. Uterine atony

    b. AFE

    c. Placenta accreta

    d. Retained placenta

2. Signs and symptoms of uterine abruption include:

    a. Abnormal fetal heart rate tracing.

    b. Vaginal bleeding.

    c. Uterine contractions.

    d. Abdominal pain.

    e. All of the above.

3. Which is a possible treatment for bleeding due to placenta accreta?

   a. Intrauterine tamponade with balloon or gauze

   b. Prostaglandin analogue

   c. Methotrexate treatment of placenta left in place

   d. Hypogastric artery ligation

4. Which procedure is falling out of favor for treatment of postpartum hemorrhage?

   a. Internal iliac artery ligation

   b. Balloon tamponade

   c. Uterine artery embolization

   d. Hysterectomy

See the testbank CD for more self-test questions.

MEDICAL COMPLICATIONS
OF PREGNANCY

Michael D. Benson, MD

I. Hypertension During Pregnancy

A. Definitions: all manifestations of gestational hypertension are presumptive until retrospectively confirmed by complete resolution of hypertension at 12 weeks postpartum) 8A, 18A, 29A

   1. Chronic hypertension: blood pressure (BP) of ≥140/90 (preferably on two occasions less than a week apart)[1]

      a. Before pregnancy or up to 20 weeks gestation

      b. New hypertension after 20 weeks gestation that persists for 12 weeks postpartum

      c. Classification

         i. Mild: BP 140/90 or greater

         ii. Severe: BP 180/110 or greater

   2. Gestational hypertension (also known as transient hypertension of pregnancy)[1]

      a. New hypertension in pregnancy

      b. No proteinuria

      c. Normotensive by 12 weeks

   3. Pre-eclampsia[1]

      a. Elevated BP

      b. Proteinuria of 300 mg per 24 hours

      c. Both required

   4. Severe pre-eclampsia:[2] pre-eclampsia with any one or more of the following:

      a. BP ≥160/110 (classically two occasions 6 hours apart while on bedrest)

    b. Proteinuria of 5 g or more in 24 hours (or 3+ or more two dipsticks at least 4 hours apart)

    c. Oliguria (<500 mL/24 hours)

    d. Cerebral (i.e., severe headaches) or visual disturbances

    e. Pulmonary edema or cyanosis

    f. Epigastric or right-upper quadrant pain (not attributable to other liver or gall-bladder disease)

    g. Abnormal liver function tests

    h. Thrombocytopenia (<100,000/mm^3 and not attributable to pre-existing or other causes)

    i. Fetal growth restriction

5. Eclampsia:[3] seizures in pre-eclamptic not attributable to other causes

6. Chronic hypertension with superimposed pre-eclampsia:[1] patients with chronic hypertension and one or more:

    a. New onset of proteinuria

    b. Hypertension with proteinuria before 20 weeks gestation

    c. Sudden increase in proteinuria that was present before pregnancy

    d. Sudden increase in BP that had otherwise been well controlled

    e. Thrombocytopenia (<100,000 platelets/mm^3)

    f. Elevated liver functions (alanine aminotransferase [ALT] or aspartate aminotransferase [AST])

7. HELLP syndrome (considered a unique variation of severe pre-eclampsia)

    a. **H**emolysis

    b. **E**levated **L**iver Enzymes

    c. **L**ow **P**latelets

8. Pre-eclampsia: atypical[4]

    a. Patients who are diagnostic outliers

        i. Abnormalities arise during pregnancy

        ii. Resolve postpartum

        iii. Not attributable to other disease processes

    b. Specific signs, symptoms, and laboratory abnormalities

        i. Hypotension and/or proteinuria presenting before 20 weeks or more than 48 hours postpartum

        ii. Other signs or symptoms of severe pre-eclampsia without hypertension or proteinuria or both

B. Mechanism of disease: remains unknown; efforts focusing on abnormal or defective cytotrophoblast invasion of endometrium, possibly related to immunologic issues

C. Epidemiology and risk factors 18B

   1. Background incidence for multigravidas (less after first-term pregnancy)

      a. Gestational hypertension 25%

      b. Pre-eclampsia 7.6%

   2. Rate of eclampsia (seizures)

      a. Pre-eclampsia (mild): 1%

      b. Severe pre-eclampsia: 3%

   3. Demographic or clinical factors that increase risk

      a. Chronic hypertension (adjusted odds ratio 2.66)

      b. Increasing body mass index (BMI): BMI >35 associated with adjusted odds ratio of 3.2

      c. Gestational trophoblastic neoplasia: 27% of those with hydatidaform mole develop pre-eclampsia (uncommon with early ultrasound recognition of molar pregnancy)

      d. Multiple gestation: risk 2–2.5 times higher

   4. Prevention

      a. Calcium supplementation: *Cochrane Review* says beneficial; National Institute of Child Health and Human Development (NICHD) trial suggests not

      b. Aspirin: who benefits and at what dose remain in dispute; may benefit subset of high-risk individuals

D. Diagnosis 18C

   1. Principally reliant on BP and urinary protein

   2. Symptoms (not reliable, generally occur only in severe pre-eclampsia or eclampsia)

      a. Headache (severe, unlike prior headaches)

      b. Visual changes

      c. Oliguria

      d. Right upper abdominal pain

   3. Laboratory evaluation: Table 26.1

E. Treatment 18D

   1. Three objectives

      a. Deliver the fetus; pregnancy-induced hypertension and all of its manifestations resolve, typically within hours or days

         i. Severe pre-eclampsia: efforts at delivery are initiated upon diagnosis of severe pre-eclampsia

TABLE 26.1	Laboratory Evaluation of Gestational Hypertension	
Lab Item	Value	Comment
Proteinuria	>300 mg per 24 hours (suggested by 1+ proteinuria on dipstick); >5 g in 24 hours consistent with severe pre-eclampsia	Required for diagnosis of pre-eclampsia
Platelet count	<100,00	Not sensitive or specific; needs to be placed in clinical context; other causes need to be ruled out such as idiopathic thrombocytopenia
ALT	Elevated	Not sensitive or specific; needs to be placed in clinical context; other types of liver or gallbladder disease need to be ruled out
AST	Elevated	Not sensitive or specific; needs to be placed in clinical context; other types of liver or gallbladder disease need to be ruled out
Creatinine	Elevated (>1.2)	Not sensitive or specific; needs to be placed in clinical context (particularly in those with renal disease or chronic hypertension)
Uric acid	Elevated (>5.9)	Not sensitive or specific
Hemoglobin	Elevated	Not sensitive or specific; needs to be placed in clinical context (relative to patient's previous prenatal hemoglobins)
Lactate dehydrogenase	Elevated	Not sensitive or specific
Bilirubin	Elevated	Not sensitive or specific; needs to be placed in clinical context; other types of liver or gallbladder disease need to be ruled out

(1) Maternal course unpredictable but can worsen precipitously

(2) In cases of significant prematurity, particularly less than 28 weeks, debate continues on appropriateness of continued observation to allow fetus time to mature

ii. Mild pre-eclampsia: deliver at term (>37 weeks) or with proof of fetal lung maturity

b. Prevent seizures

i. Consensus that severe pre-eclamptic patients should receive seizure prophylaxis with magnesium sulfate

ii. Most institutions treat mild pre-eclampsia also, although there is little direct evidence to support this (seizures can occur unpredictably but less common in this group)

iii. Magnesium administration

(1) Loading dose: 4–6 g IVPB over 20 minutes

(2) 2–3 g/hr by infusion pump; therapeutic serum levels: 4–7 mEq/L (4.8–8.4 mg/dL)

(3) Monitoring response

(A) Serum levels every 6 hours (not all institutions do this)

(B) Respiratory rate, deep tendon reflexes hourly; urine output (reduced output can raise magnesium levels)

(4) Toxicity:

(A) 10 mEq/L: deep tendon reflexes disappear

(B) 12–15 mEq/L: respiratory depression (can lead to respiratory arrest)

(5) Treatment of toxicity: calcium gluconate 1 g IV

(6) Mechanism of action (?): raises seizure threshold

c. Control BP

i. Pregnancy-induced hypertension and pre-eclampsia

(1) BP goals

(A) Systolic <160

(B) Diastolic <110 or 105

(2) Medications: Table 26.2

(3) Cautions: precipitous drop in BP can compromise blood flow to fetus

TABLE 26.2	Antihypertensives for Pre-eclampsia				
	Initial Dose	Repeat Dose	No Response	Mechanism	Cautions
Hydralazine	5 mg IV push	5-10 mg IV push every 20 minutes	After 20-30 mg, consider alternative drug	Vasodilation	
Labetalol	20 mg IV	40 mg IV 10 minutes later	80 mg IV 10 minutes later	Alpha- and beta-adrenergic blocker	Maximum dose 200 mg Avoid in asthmatics
Nifedipine	10 mg orally	10 mg in 20 minutes	Use alternative	Calcium channel blocker	
Nitroprusside	0.25 mcg/kg/min	May increase to 5 mcg/kg/min		Causes endothelial release of nitrous oxide, resulting in vasodilation	Do not use for more than 4 hours because fetal cyanide toxicity may occur

ii. Chronic hypertension without superimposed pre-eclampsia
  (1) Mild hypertension: no treatment recommended
  (2) Severe hypertension: treat for reduction of maternal morbidity
    (A) Drugs of choice: methyldopa or labetalol
    (B) Avoid
      (i) Atenolol (associated with growth restriction)
      (ii) Angiotensin-converting enzyme inhibitors (associated with fetal and neonatal death and renal failure)

F. Adverse outcomes⟨18E⟩
  1. Maternal: abruption, subcapsular liver hematoma, stroke, coagulopathy (thrombocytopenia), pulmonary edema, retinal detachments
  2. Fetal: prematurity (due to need for induction), intrauterine growth retardation, hypoxia

II. Gestational Diabetes ⟨9A-B, 17B⟩

A. Incidence, risk factors, and etiology
  1. New diagnosis in nondiabetic women
    a. 1%–2% several decades ago
    b. 6%–8% currently (impact of rising BMIs in population)
  2. Risk factors are traditionally cited, but with increased screening for gestational diabetes, they may not have meaning if the patient has had a normal result
    a. Prior stillbirth
    b. Prior fetus weighing more than 9 pounds
    c. Strong family history (first-degree relatives)
    d. Elevated BMI at start of pregnancy or excessive weight gain (a greater risk factor than any of the preceding and controllable to an extent)
  3. Hormones of pregnancy antagonize action of insulin; particularly human placental lactogen, which is produced by placenta in direct proportion to its weight
B. Screening
  1. Universal: all pregnant women receive screening test

2. Selective: some particularly low-risk women can be omitted from screening:
   a. Age <25 years
   b. Normal baseline BMI without excessive pregnancy weight gain
   c. No first-degree relatives with diabetes or personal history of impaired glucose metabolism
   d. No history of stillbirth, macrosomia in prior pregnancy
3. Screening test
   a. Glucose level 1 hour after 50-g glucose load (fasting or nonfasting)
   b. Screen cutoffs
      i. 140 mg/dL plasma
         (1) False negative: 20% of gestational diabetes will be missed
         (2) Positive: 15% (most will be false positives)
      ii. 130 mg/dL plasma
         (1) False negative: <10%
         (2) Positive—25% positive; (most will be false positives)
      iii. Some patients might benefit from more aggressive screening (those with BMI >35 or 40 and those with personal history of gestational diabetes requiring insulin in prior pregnancy) (no consensus)
         (1) In the first trimester
            (A) HbA_{1C}
            (B) Random glucose
            (C) Fasting glucose
         (2) 3-hour glucose tolerance test instead of 1-hour screen at 24–28 weeks

C. Diagnosis
   1. Gestational diabetes in women not known to have carbohydrate intolerance before pregnancy
      a. 3-hour glucose tolerance test
         i. Administered fasting
         ii. Fasting glucose drawn
         iii. 100-g glucose load administered orally
         iv. Glucose obtained at 1, 2, and 3 hours
         v. Two abnormal values define patient as gestational diabetic (Table 26.3)

TABLE 26.3

Diagnosis of Gestational Diabetes by Plasma Glucose Level Thresholds

	Carpenter/Coustan	National Diabetes Data Group
Fasting	95	105
1-hour postprandial	180	190
2-hour postprandial	155	165
3-hour postprandial	140	145

From Report of the Expert Committee on the Diagnosis and Classification of Diabetes Mellitus. Diabetes Care 2000; 23 (suppl1), S4—S19.

      vi. Threshold values are two standard deviations from study done by O'Sullivan and Mahan[5] above the mean but have not been validated in any other terms; no clinical trials using different thresholds have been performed

      vii. Many of the adverse consequences of gestational diabetes (fetal macrosomia in particular) can be seen with only one abnormal value

  b. Classification

      i. A1: glucose can be controlled with diet alone

      ii. A2: insulin required for control (some patients may not be gestational diabetics in the true sense as they might have long-standing carbohydrate intolerance identified only at time of pregnancy)

      iii. Control defined as:

         (1) Fasting <105 mg/dL

         (2) One hour postprandial <130 mg/dL

2. Preconception diabetes (patients on insulin or oral hypoglycemic agents before pregnancy)

  a. Classification

      i. Class B: onset at age 20 years or older and duration less than 10 years

         (1) Class B1: fasting glucose 130 or more

         (2) Class B2: adult onset (type II) diabetics (on insulin prior to pregnancy)

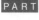

ii. Class D: diabetes of more than 20 years' duration or beginning before age 10 years

iii. Class F: concomitant nephropathy

iv. Class R: malignant retinopathy

v. Class H: heart impairment or disease

D. Risk of morbidity of untreated diabetes directly related to extent of glucose control; in those under good control, extent of excess risk small, if any

   1. Gestational diabetes

      a. Macrosomia

      b. Intrauterine fetal demise

      c. Polyhydramnios

      d. Newborn hypoglycemia and polycythemia

      e. Maternal diabetic ketoacidosis (with attendant risks for fetus)

   2. Preconception diabetes: pregnancy by itself does not advance or accelerate diabetes; risks of gestational diabetes apply as well as:

      a. Congenital anomalies

         i. Can be as high as 10%

            (1) Heart defects most common

            (2) Central nervous system (CNS) anomalies common (anencephaly, spina bifida, caudal regression syndrome), with caudal regression by far the most common

         ii. Related to how much HbA_{1C} elevation at start of pregnancy, although risk may be increased even with normal HbA_{1C}

         iii. Most common types of anomalies

            (1) Caudal regression

            (2) Situs inversus

            (3) Renal anomalies

            (4) Heart defects

      b. Diabetic retinopathy may progress in women under good control

      c. Prematurity

         i. Occasionally, diabetics need to be induced prematurely for fetal indications

         ii. Rate of spontaneous preterm labor increased

  d. Increased rate of miscarriage
  e. Increased risk of pre-eclampsia
  f. Delayed fetal lung maturity
   i. 1–1.5 week delay in phosphotidyl glycerol in diabetic pregnancies
   ii. Increased risk of respiratory distress syndrome at all gestational ages before term
 3. Excessive fetal weight/growth from any cause appears to be associated with substantially increased risk of childhood obesity and development of diabetes
E. Treatment
 1. Monitoring: typically four times daily via capillary finger testing using home glucose meters: fasting and three postprandial
  a. Plasma glucose 10%–15% less than whole blood; most current reflectance meters are calibrated for plasma
  b. Fasting <105 mg/dL (plasma)
  c. 1-hour postprandial <155 (plasma)
  d. 2-hour postprandial <130 (plasma)
 2. Diabetic diet: half the population can control glucose levels on diet alone; repeated counseling by dietitian can be helpful
  a. Three meals and three snacks; objective is to spread out calories over the day and avoid large caloric challenges
  b. 30% total calorie reduction for women with BMI 30 or greater
  c. Restrict carbohydrate calories to <40% of total calories
 3. Insulin: Table 26.4
  a. Commonly split dose
  b. Insulin pump becoming more common; requires at least four times daily capillary glucose monitoring
 4. Oral hypoglycemic agents
  a. Glyburide (Micronase)
   i. Very minimal placental transfer to fetus
   ii. Duration 4–8 hours
   iii. Take 30–60 minutes before meal
   iv. Comes as 2.5-mg tablets; maximum single dose 7.5 mg
   v. Hypoglycemia remains a risk
   vi. Not universally accepted among endocrinologists and obstetricians as treatment during pregnancy

TABLE 26.4		
Time Course of Insulin		
	Peak (Hours)	**Duration (Hours)**
Humalog	1	2
Regular insulin	2	4
NPH, lente insulin	4	8
Ultralente	8	20
Insulin glargine	5	<24

    b. Metformin
       i. Crosses placenta
       ii. Often used to treat infertility patients (particularly those with polycystic ovarian syndrome)
       iii. May reduce miscarriage rate in selected populations
       iv. Limited teratology and neonatal hypoglycemia information
       v. Use after first trimester remains experimental

5. Antenatal testing: no randomized controlled trials for any protocol
    a. Level II ultrasound at 18–20 weeks to check for fetal anomalies
    b. Risk related to amount of glycemic control and duration of diabetes
       i. Monitoring should begin at 28 weeks for those in poor control
       ii. Can start at 34 weeks for those in better control
    c. Types of monitoring
       i. Weekly or biweekly nonstress tests (NSTs) beginning at 32–36 weeks
       ii. Ultrasounds every 3–4 weeks to evaluate growth (to check for both intrauterine growth retardation and macrosomia)
       iii. Biophysical profile to supplement NST
       iv. Doppler flow study of umbilical vessels for suspected intrauterine growth retardation

6. Labor management

    a. Induction at 39 weeks for those on insulin

    b. Can defer delivery for those with A1 diabetes with excellent control but generally not past 42 weeks

    c. Cesarean section for those with estimated fetal weight of 4500 g or more: no method of estimating weight is very accurate (although recommended by American College of Obstetricians and Gynecologists [ACOG], has not proved to be very effective in reducing neonatal or maternal morbidity)

    d. Diet-controlled gestational diabetes

       i. Avoid glucose in IV solutions

       ii. Initial glucose and recheck 2 hours later; if <110 mg/dL (plasma); further glucose testing may not be necessary

    e. For those on insulin

       i. 5% dextrose IV at 100 mL/hr

       ii. Regular insulin infused at 0.5 units/hr

       iii. May increase up to 2.5 units/hr

       iv. Check glucose hourly

    f. Good glucose control (between 80 and 110 mg/dL plasma) reduces perinatal asphyxia and neonatal hypoglycemia

III. Infections During Pregnancy

  A. Sexually transmitted diseases (see also Chapter 9) `17D`

    1. HIV

    2. Herpes

    3. Syphilis

    4. Hepatitis B

  B. Perinatal group B streptococcal disease[6] `17D`

    1. Beta-hemolytic streptococci divided into different Lancefield groups, A–E; only A, B, and D cause disease

    2. Significant source of neonatal morbidity and mortality can result from group B sepsis

    3. Neonatal sepsis rate about 1 per 1000 in late 1990s before introduction of prophylactic antibiotic treatment

    4. Type of disease

      a. Early onset occurs in first 7 days; usually in first 2 days

        i. Mortality rate at term is 2% but can be up to 30% in premature infants

ii. Types of illness
    (1) Septic shock
    (2) Respiratory distress
    (3) Meningitis

b. Late onset occurs after first week
    i. Can come from maternal genital tract and nursery personnel
    ii. Most commonly meningitis; 50% suffer neurologic injury
    iii. Mortality 2%
    iv. Prevention strategies with maternal screening and intrapartum antibiotics not effective

5. Demographics of maternal colonization and newborn sepsis
    a. 10%–30% of women are colonized in rectum, vagina, or urinary tract; can be transient, chronic, or intermittent
    b. 75% of newborns born to colonized mothers are themselves colonized
    c. Sepsis only occurs in roughly 1% of colonized newborns; sepsis risk increases in those with:
        i. Prematurity
        ii. Maternal intrapartum fever (100.4°F or higher)
        iii. Ruptured membranes for 18 hours or more
        iv. Prior infant with group B streptococcus (GBS)
        v. GBS bacteriuria

6. Prevention
    a. Culture of vagina and rectum at 36 weeks for GBS (using specific culture media to maximize sensitivity)
    b. Women who do not need culture at 36 weeks (because they require antibiotic prophylaxis in any case)
        i. Culture not necessary in those with GBS bacteriuria at any point in pregnancy (any amount of colonization; normal threshold of 100,000 colonies does not apply)
        ii. Those with prior infant with GBS sepsis
    c. Intrapartum antibiotics (until delivery)
        i. Penicillin G 5 million units IV followed by 2.5 million units IV every 4 hours *or* ampicillin 2 g IV initial dose, then 1 g IV every 4 hours
        ii. Penicillin allergy

(1) Prior anaphylaxis or those with asthma that would make anaphylaxis more difficult to treat
   (A) Clindamycin 900 mg IV every 8 hours
   (B) Erythromycin 500 mg IV every 6 hours
(2) Those without high risk of anaphylaxis: cefazolin 2 g IV, then 1 g IV every 8 hours
(3) For GBS resistant to erythromycin and clindamycin: vancomycin 1 g IV every 12 hours

  d. Intrapartum prophylaxis for GBS not necessary for those with a negative culture in prior 5 weeks

C. Rubella 17D

1. Epidemiology
  a. Disease of childhood, caused by an RNA virus
  b. Most common in spring
  c. Vaccine became available in 1969; disease rate dropped by 99%
  d. Sporadic disease exists due to individual failures to receive vaccine
  e. Spread by respiratory droplets
  f. Incubation period 2–3 weeks
  g. Virus present in blood and nasal secretions for a few days before symptoms

2. Clinical disease
  a. Mild constitutional symptoms: malaise, headache, myalgias
  b. Rash: widely distributed, erythematous, maculopapular; not pruritic
  c. Symptoms short-lived; resolve within 3–5 days

3. Diagnosis
  a. IgM: peaks 7–10 days after onset of illness
  b. IgG: rises more slowly; remains elevated permanently, implies immunity

4. Congenital rubella infection
  a. Risk related to time of maternal infection
  b. 50% risk if maternal infection acquired in first 4 weeks after conception; 10% at 12 weeks, and 1% thereafter
  c. Anomalies
    i. Deafness (up to 75% of those infected)
    ii. Vision impairment (30%)

      iii. Neurologic defects (25%)

      iv. Heart defects (20%)

      v. Other: mental retardation, microcephaly

   d. Intrauterine diagnosis

      i. Placental and amniotic fluid cultures can detect virus but do not predict disease accurately

      ii. Ultrasound to check for anomalies most useful

 5. Prevention

   a. Vaccine is live virus; contraception should be used for 4 weeks afterward

   b. Not given to pregnant women but given immediately postpartum to those who are not immune (not a risk for nursing)

   c. Vaccination for those who do not have significant levels of IgG; screening for immunity and vaccination for those not immune can be done as part of preconception counseling

D. Cytomegalovirus: double-stranded DNA virus **17D**

 1. Childhood infection; typically asymptomatic

 2. Symptoms, if they occur, include malaise, fever, lymphadenopathy, hepatosplenomegaly

 3. Diagnosis

   a. Tissue culture of virus from urine, semen, saliva, breast milk

   b. Serology: IgM rises in acute phase; fourfold rise in IgG consistent with infection

 4. Prevention

   a. No vaccine

   b. Routine screening not reliable

   c. Because sexual transmission is one mode of spread, number of partners should be limited and condoms used

   d. Handwashing helpful

 5. No effective treatment

 6. In utero infection

   a. Risk

      i. Higher with primary infection rather than reactivation

      ii. 50% risk to fetus for mother who has primary infection

   b. Risk of injury highest in first trimester

   c. Morbidity: severe injury to 80% of survivors

      i. Hepatosplenomegaly

      ii. Microcephaly

      iii. Chorioretinitis

      iv. Hearing loss

      v. Intrauterine growth restriction

  d. Mortality as high as 30%

  e. Diagnosis of congenital infection

      i. Culture of amniotic fluid or placenta can demonstrate virus but not helpful for prognosis

      ii. Ultrasound can guide expectations for fetal outcome (but may be normal in first trimester); findings include microcephaly, intracranial calcifications, oligohydramnios, and hydrops

E. Varicella zoster virus (herpes family, DNA virus) `17D`

  1. Acute, primary disease: chickenpox

    a. Typically childhood illness

    b. Rash: macules and papules (highly pruritic) to vesicles and pustules

    c. Highly contagious

    d. Disease in adulthood more severe; can lead to potentially lethal viral pneumonia (onset 2–6 days after rash appears)

  2. Recurrent illness: herpes zoster (shingles); not linked to in utero infection of fetus or postpartum infections of newborns

  3. Maternal varicella

    a. Severity and mortality rate less with acyclovir treatment and current ability for respiratory support (pneumonia mortality rate can be as high as 28%)

    b. Complicates fewer than 1 in 1000 pregnancies

    c. Prevention

      i. Prior chickenpox or vaccination provides immunity

      ii. Immunity can be checked by serum varicella IgG

      iii. Those not immune at time of exposure can get varicella immune globulin

        (1) Needs to be administered within 96 hours of exposure

        (2) Probably does not protect fetus

      iv. Varicella vaccine (Varivax)

        (1) Attenuated live virus

        (2) Not recommended during pregnancy or for those planning to conceive

        v. Prognosis: serology and direct viral detection possible, but ultrasound more useful in predicting risk and nature of fetal injury

    d. Fetal varicella infection

        i. Typically at risk only in first 4 months of pregnancy

        ii. Risk ranges 1%–9% during this time

        iii. Sequelae include limb hypoplasia, cutaneous scarring, mental retardation, and CNS abnormalities

F. Parvovirus ("fifth disease"): single-stranded DNA virus `17D`

  1. Symptoms

    a. Typically occurs in children in late winter

    b. "Slapped cheek" appearance of rash, fever, malaise, mild joint pain

    c. Rash can wax and wane over months

    d. Transient aplastic crisis

        i. Limited to those with hemoglobinopathies

        ii. Anemia develops within 7 days of initial symptoms

        iii. Recovery usually complete

  2. Diagnosis

    a. Serial serum IgM and IgG antibodies (3 weeks apart)

    b. IgG remains elevated for life and usually denotes immunity (approximately 50% of adults are immune)

  3. Maternal infection

    a. Suggested by rising IgM

    b. Ultrasound most useful for determining fetal involvement; fetal hydrops (skin edema) most suggestive of serious infection; requires examination 10 weeks beyond symptoms to ensure fetal involvement not occurring

    c. Those with hydrops might benefit from in utero transfusion (via umbilical cord)

    d. Those without hydrops usually have no long-term sequelae

    e. Risk of fetal infection

        i. 10% before 20 weeks

        ii. <5% after 20 weeks

G. Toxoplasmosis `17D`

  1. Caused by *Toxoplasma gondii*

  2. Life cycle of microbe: trophozoite, cyst, and oocysts

  3. Oocyst can form only in cat intestines, excreted in feces; trophozoite can exist in mammals such as cows

4. Human infection through infected meat or food contamination by cat feces
5. Half of population has antibodies; more common in lower socioeconomic groups
6. Prevention
   a. Avoid stray cats and cat litter
   b. Avoid raw meat
   c. Clean and wash fruit and vegetables
7. Epidemiology of toxoplasmosis during pregnancy
   a. 5% of mothers seroconvert
   b. 3/1000 newborns show congenital infection
   c. 1/1000 has clinically significant infection
8. Diagnosis
   a. Detection of IgM
   b. Very high IgG
   c. Change of IgG from absent to present
   d. Serologic assays not standardized among laboratories
9. Fetal infection
   a. Highest risk in third trimester
   b. Morbidity can include seizures, mental retardation, ascites, hepatosplenomegaly
   c. Diagnosis
      i. Ultrasound abnormalities: microcephaly, hepatosplenomegaly, intracranial calcifications
      ii. Amniocentesis: polymerase chain reaction to identify viral DNA presence
10. Maternal treatment: reduces risk of fetal injury
    a. Spiromycin (available in United States through Centers for Disease Control and Prevention [CDC])
    b. Sulfadiazine
       i. Combination more effective
    c. Aggressive treatment at birth also helpful in reducing sequelae

IV. Anemia `8C, 9A-B, 17A`

A. Normal values during pregnancy: CDC definition
   1. First trimester: Hb $\geq$ 11
   2. Second trimester: Hb $\geq$ 10.5
   3. Third trimester: Hb $\geq$ 11

B. Common anemias

1. Iron deficiency

   a. Iron consumption by fetus highest in third trimester; iron-deficiency anemia more commonly seen here

   b. Laboratory findings

   i. Hypochromic, microcytic

   ii. Schistocytes seen

   iii. Mean corpuscular volume decreased

   iv. Serum iron and transferrin saturation decreased

   c. Treatment: increased dietary iron supplementation

   i. Iron absorption reduced if taken with food

   ii. Iron can cause nausea, constipation; stools turn black

   iii. Response seen in 2 weeks

2. Vitamin deficiencies

   a. Folic acid deficiency impairs DNA synthesis

   i. Diagnosis

   (1) Normochromic, macrocytic

   (2) Serum iron and transferring increased

   (3) Serum folate <3 mg/L

   ii. Treatment: folic acid supplementation (typically 500 mcg to 1.5 mg daily)

   b. B_{12} reduces conversion of ribonucleotides to deoxynucleotides

   i. Diagnosis

   (1) Normochromic, macrocytic

   (2) Serum iron and transferring increased

   (3) Serum B_{12} <50 pg/mL

   ii. Treatment: B_{12} supplementation (1 mg/wk IM)

C. Hemoglobinopathies: hemoglobin structurally flawed

1. Hemoglobin consists of four polypeptide chains, each with a heme moiety

   a. Two alpha chains

   b. Two beta chains or two gamma chains (hemoglobin A_2)

2. Heterozygous mutation states might confer some protection against malaria

3. More common among those of African, Mediterranean, and Southeast Asian descent; these groups should be offered carrier screening (hemoglobin electrophoresis); if both parents are carriers, should be offered genetic counseling for prenatal diagnosis

4. Heterozygous and homozygous mutations manifest by reduced hemoglobin and typically microcytic and hypochromic red blood cells

5. Several hundred specific gene mutations identified

6. Individuals can have more than one heterozygous mutation; can lead to spectrum of anemia severity

7. Heterozygous state can exist with thalassemias; generally produces clinically significant disease

8. Sickle cell anemia

    a. Heterozygous

    b. Mild anemia

    c. Not associated with poor reproductive outcomes or other increased medical risks

    d. More common among Africans

    e. Carrier rate among African Americans roughly 1 in 12

9. Sickle cell disease

    a. Homozygous

    b. Abnormal hemoglobin leads to shortened red blood cell life span

    c. Severe anemia with hemolysis

    d. Pain crises: red blood cells (sickle-shaped) occlude blood vessels

    e. Increased susceptibility to infection

    f. Treated with transfusions for severe anemia and pain crises

    g. Pregnant women generally transfused to keep hemoglobin above 6 g/dL

D. Thalassemia: normal hemoglobin produced at decreased rate

    1. Beta thalassemia: flawed production of beta hemoglobin chains; genes on chromosome 11

        a. Beta thalassemia major (Cooley anemia)

            i. Homozygous for gene mutation

            ii. Beta chains not produced

            iii. Alpha chains produced

                (1) Fetus can survive

                (2) After first few months of life, alpha chains precipitate; severe hemolysis results

                (3) Monthly blood transfusions required; average life expectancy 20–30 years

        b. Beta thalassemia minor: heterozygous

i. Extent of anemia and illness varies depending on amount of beta-chain production

ii. Microcytic, hypochromic anemia resembles iron deficiency but does not respond to iron

iii. Hemoglobin electrophoresis: elevated hemoglobin A_2

iv. Does not affect fertility or reproductive outcomes

2. Alpha thalassemia: presence or absence of two genes involved; flawed production of alpha hemoglobin chains; genes on chromosome 16

   a. Alpha thalassemia major: four genes deleted

   i. Homozygous for deletion of both genes

   ii. No chains produced

   iii. Incompatible with life; high cardiac output failure

   iv. Ultrasound: hydrops

   b. Hemoglobin H disease: three genes deleted

   i. Hemoglobin H and hemoglobin B produced

   ii. Marked hemolytic anemia results from hemoglobin H precipitating in red blood cells

   c. Alpha thalassemia minor 1 (alpha thalassemia "trait")

   i. Two genes deleted (designation confusing)

   ii. Mild hypochromic, microcytic anemia

   iii. Resembles iron deficiency anemia but does not improve with iron

   d. Alpha thalassemia minor 2 (alpha thalassemia "silent carrier")

   i. One gene deletion (designation confusing)

   ii. Clinically undetectable

   iii. Can be diagnosed by specific DNA gene mutation testing in those with family members who have the more clinically significant thalassemias

V. Heart Disease 17E

A. Physiology of normal pregnancy 8A, 9A-B

1. Blood volume

   a. Plasma increases by roughly 50%

   b. Red blood cells increase by 30%

   c. Hemoglobin per mL falls; this physiologic drop underlies the CDC redefinition of anemia for pregnancy

2. Resting pulse increases by average 10 beats/minute

3. Cardiac output increases by approximately 30%–50%

4. After 20 weeks or so, weight of fetus and uterus can compromise venous return to the heart in supine position (this is not a reason for women not to sleep on their backs, but it is an explanation why a few cannot tolerate it)

5. BP tends to decline in mid-trimester and then rise in third trimester

6. Systolic murmurs along left sternal border audible in almost all pregnant women

7. Uterine blood flow as percentage of cardiac output: nonpregnant, 1%–2%; pregnant, 17%–20%

B. Classification of cardiac status (New York Heart Association [NYHA] criteria)

1. Class I: uncompromised; no angina and no symptoms of cardiac insufficiency

2. Class II: slight limitation of physical activity; cardiorespiratory symptoms with ordinary activity

3. Class III: marked limitation of physical activity; cardiorespiratory discomfort with any activity

4. Class IV: severe compromised; cardiorespiratory discomfort can occur even at rest

C. Risk of mortality by condition (ACOG classification 1992)

1. Group 1: mortality rate 0%–1%
   a. Atrial septal defect
   b. Ventricular septal defect
   c. Tetralogy of Fallot corrected
   d. Mitral valve stenosis, NYHA class I and II

2. Group 2A: mortality rate 5%–15%
   a. Aortic stenosis
   b. Aortic coarctation without valve involvement
   c. Marfan syndrome with normal aorta

3. Group 2B: mortality rate 5%–15%
   a. Mitral stenosis with atrial fibrillation

4. Group 3: Mortality rate 25%–50%
   a. Pulmonary hypertension
   b. Aortic coarctation with valve involvement
   c. Marfan syndrome with aortic involvement

D. Specific cardiac conditions
   1. Valve disease

    a. Most women with significant valve dysfunctions have valve replacement before pregnancy

    b. Women with mechanical valves must be fully anticoagulated; heparin is drug of choice as warfarin is a teratogen

    c. Anticoagulation stopped just before delivery and resumed a few hours later

2. Cardiomyopathy

    a. General principles

        i. Heart failure and cardiomyopathy must be distinguished from conditions that existed prior to pregnancy

        ii. Increased cardiac output of pregnancy may unmask underlying heart disease

    b. Idiopathic hypertrophic cardiomyopathy

        i. Can be inherited as autosomal dominant but can also result from de novo mutation

        ii. Symptoms: angina, dyspnea, arrhythmia

        iii. Treatment focuses on maintaining venous return and avoiding hypovolemia

        iv. Vaginal delivery appropriate

        v. Not accelerated or brought on by pregnancy

    c. Peripartum cardiomyopathy

        i. Dilated cardiomyopathy

            (1) Occurs in last month of pregnancy or within 5 months of delivery

            (2) Occurs 1 per 3–4000 births

            (3) Left ventricular ejection fraction <45%

            (4) Prognosis highly variable and difficult to predict on basis of presentation

                (A) 20% die without heart transplant

                (B) 30% have partial recovery

                (C) 50% completely recover

            (5) For those who survive, risk of recurrence on subsequent pregnancies substantial (>20%)

    d. Prior ischemic heart disease; prognosis good if no ventricular dysfunction

3. Heritability of congenital heart defects

    a. Background rate of heart defects 0.5%–1%

    b. Rises to 3%–4% of offspring with first-degree relative with congenital defect

c. Among those with heart defects, concordant with other relative only about half the time

4. Infective endocarditis: antibiotic prophylaxis no longer recommended for vaginal or cesarean delivery[7]

VI. Asthma [17F]

A. No predictable course during pregnancy

1. Roughly one-third get better, worse, or stay the same in equal proportions

2. Response in prior pregnancy somewhat related to course in future pregnancies

B. Stages of asthma: blood chemistries

1. Mild: alkalosis

   a. Oxygen saturation normal
   b. Carbon dioxide increased

2. Moderate: alkalosis

   a. Oxygen saturation decreased
   b. Carbon dioxide saturation increased

3. Danger zone: pH normal

   a. Oxygen saturation decreased
   b. Carbon dioxide saturation normal

4. Severe: acidosis

   a. Oxygen saturation decreased
   b. Carbon dioxide saturation increased

5. FEV_1 best predictor of disease severity

   a. Mild: 65%–80% of predicted
   b. Moderate: 50%–64%
   c. Danger: 35%–49%
   d. Severe: <35%

6. Status asthmaticus: failure to respond to therapy within 30–60 minutes of treatment associated with increased maternal mortality rate

C. Treatment

1. Avoid F series prostaglandins and ergonovine if possible

2. Commonly used asthma medications are not teratogenic

3. Mild intermittent: inhaled beta agonists

4. Mild persistent:

   a. Inhaled beta agonists
   b. Inhaled Cromolyn
   c. Inhaled corticosteroids if no response

    5. Moderate persistent: preceding as well as oral theophylline and/or inhaled salmeterol

    6. Moderate severe: preceding as well as oral corticosteroids

    7. Intubation:

      a. $Paco_2$ >40 mm Hg

      b. Pao_2 <60 mm Hg

      c. Oxygen saturation <90%

      d. Maternal exhaustion

  D. Adverse outcomes:

    1. Fetus: generally not at increased risk unless disease severe

    2. Severe disease linked to increased maternal risk of pre-eclampsia; possible increased risk of pre-term labor and small for gestational age infants (no consensus in study data)

VII. Thrombophilia

  A. Physiologic changes in coagulation during pregnancy

    1. Increased venous stasis: direct compression of pelvic veins and vena cava by pregnancy

    2. General increase in almost all clotting factors

  B. Hypercoagulability results in two general clinical illnesses

    1. Venous thromboembolic (VTE) disease: manifests as deep venous thrombosis or pulmonary embolism

      a. Nearly half of patients experiencing VTE have specific thrombophilia diagnosed

      b. About half of those with a thrombophilia do not experience abnormal clotting without an additional risk factor such as pregnancy, surgery, oral contraceptive use, etc.

      c. Risk of VTE exists throughout pregnancy and into the postpartum period for 1–2 months

      d. Symptomatic VTE estimated to occur roughly 1 per 2000 pregnancies

      e. Maternal death rate from pulmonary embolism comprises roughly 15% of all U.S. maternal deaths

    2. Pregnancy complications

      a. Abruption

      b. Intrauterine growth retardation

      c. Placental infarction

      d. Recurrent miscarriage

  C. Inherited thrombophilias

    1. Specific types: Table 26.5

TABLE 26.5 **Inherited Thrombophilias**

Type	General Population Prevalence*	Diagnostic Tests	Relative Clotting Risk (Heterozygous State and Only One Type of Mutation)
Factor V Leiden mutation	2.7%	Factor V Leiden mutation test	Heterozygous state not clearly linked to abnormal clotting without antecedent history
Antithrombin III mutation	0.2%	Antithrombin III activity	Highly thrombogenic
Protein C deficiency	0.5%	Protein C activity	Highly thrombogenic
Protein S deficiency	0.08%	Protein S activity	Slightly thrombogenic
Hyperhomocysteinemia	1%–11%	Fasting homocysteine level**	Slightly to moderately thrombogenic; risk rises with level of homocysteine
Prothrombin gene mutation (G20210A)	2%–4%	Prothrombin G20210A mutation	Slightly thrombogenic

*Incidence of all inherited thrombophilias may vary widely depending on ethnic group
** If elevated, can test for methylenetetrahydrofolate reductase mutation; most common enzyme abnormality in underlying condition

2. All are autosomal dominant except hyperhomocysteinemia

3. Homozygous state much less common and much more thrombogenic

4. More than one mutation can exist in the same patient

D. Acquired thrombophilia: antiphospholipid antibody syndrome

   1. Definition rests on combination of clinical and laboratory findings; understanding of syndrome is evolving[8,9]

      a. Clinical manifestations

         i. Obstetrical

            (1) Three or more consecutive miscarriages before 10 weeks

            (2) One or more fetal deaths after 10 weeks without alternative explanation

            (3) Severe pre-eclampsia or placental insufficiency requiring delivery before 34 weeks

         ii. Thrombotic events: either arterial or venous without alternative explanation (e.g., trauma or heritable thrombophilia)

      b. Laboratory markers (two assays at least 6 weeks apart):

         i. Anticardiolipin antibody levels at least moderately elevated

         ii. Lupus anticoagulant present

   2. Diagnosis caveats

      a. Positive laboratory results in absence of the preceding strict clinical criteria have uncertain significance

      b. High prevalence of low titer levels of anticardiolipin antibodies; low levels are not disease markers

E. Management of VTE and thrombophilias during pregnancy

   1. General concepts of treatment

      a. Anticoagulants: low dose given without partial thromboplastin time (PTT) monitoring; adjusted dose titrated to prolongation of clotting assay

         i. Heparin

            (1) Every 12-hour subcutaneous dosing: hold dose during labor or before cesarean (particularly in anticipation of regional anesthesia)

            (2) Low dose

               (A) 5–10-K units throughout pregnancy

(B) 5-K, 7.5-K and 10-K units by trimester (PTT should be checked on 10 K to ensure it is not prolonged)

(3) Adjusted dose: 10-K units or more titrated to prolonged PTT

(4) Complications:

(A) Thrombocytopenia

(i) Common: non-immune and reversible

(ii) Uncommon: immune; may manifest in thrombosis

(B) Osteoporosis

ii. Low-molecular-weight heparin

(1) Every 12- or 24-hour subcutaneous dosing: hold dose during labor or before cesarean (particularly in anticipation of regional anesthesia)

(2) Low dose: enoxaparin 40 mg once or twice daily

(3) Adjusted dose: 30–80 mg every 12 hours titrated to increasing antifactor Xa levels

(4) Complications: thrombocytopenia and osteoporosis may be substantially reduced in comparison with heparin

iii. Warfarin: known teratogen, so not administered during pregnancy, but may be given postpartum to non-nursing mothers

b. Prophylaxis

i. Low dose

ii. Adjusted dose (full anticoagulation)

2. Who gets prophylaxis

a. Low dose

i. Those with a thrombophilia *and* an adverse pregnancy history that might be linked to abnormal clotting

ii. Those with prior history of deep venous thrombosis with or without a thrombophilia, related or unrelated to prior pregnancy

b. Adjusted dose

i. Those with diagnosis of antiphospholipid syndrome

ii. Most homozygous thrombophilias

iii. Heterozygous antithrombin III

c. Prophylaxis generally continues 6 weeks postpartum

3. Diagnosis of venous thromboembolism during pregnancy
   a. History and physical examination have poor sensitivity and specificity; even harder to diagnose during pregnancy because some amount of dyspnea and lower-extremity edema and pain common (universal?) during pregnancy
   b. Compression ultrasound of lower extremities: high sensitivity
   c. Computed tomography has largely replaced ventilation perfusion studies for diagnosis of pulmonary embolism
   d. Venography may be used for diagnosis of iliac or pelvic vein thrombosis but remains difficult diagnosis

VIII. Surgical Considerations During Pregnancy 170

A. Purely elective surgery generally postponed; not out of any specific documentation of teratogenicity of commonly used anesthetics and analgesics, but general principle to reduce fetal exposure to drugs wherever possible

B. Gravid uterus makes examination and clinical course of many diseases more difficult to assess

C. Pelvic inflammatory disease (PID) extremely rare during pregnancy but remains possible; PID in pregnancy is indication for inpatient treatment

MENTOR TIPS

- Classification of hypertensive disorder during pregnancy focuses on timing of onset of hypertension and presence or absence of proteinuria.
- Right upper quadrant abdominal pain can be the first symptom of severe pre-eclampsia. It can easily be mistaken for gallbladder disease if not investigated.
- Delivery "cures" gestational hypertension and related disorders.
- Risk of gestational diabetes is closely related to maternal starting BMI and total weight gain.
- Birth weight is even more closely related to maternal starting BMI and weight gain than the presence of gestational diabetes.
- Fetal injury due to maternal infection is uncommon, but the risks to the fetus are highly dependent on the specific infectious agent and the gestational age at time of infection.

- Pregnancy in those with heart disease should be a deliberate undertaking, as cardiac output can increase by up to 50%.
- Asthma is not a benign condition; respiratory compromise poses a threat to the fetus; the drugs used to treat asthma are safe during pregnancy.

References

1. National High Blood Pressure Education Program: Working group report on high blood pressure in pregnancy. American Journal of Obstetrics and Gynecology 183:51, 2000.
2. ACOG Practice Bulletin 22. Diagnosis and management of pre-eclampsia and eclampsia. Obstetrics and Gynecology 99:159–167, 2002.
3. Sibai BM: Diagnosis, prevention, and management of eclampsia. Obstetrics and Gynecology 105:402–410, 2005.
4. Stella CL, Sibai BM: Preeclampsia: Diagnosis and management of the atypical presentation. Journal of Maternal-Fetal Neonatal Medicine 19:381–386, 2006.
5. O'Sullivan JB, Mahan CM: Criteria for the oral glucose tolerance test in pregnancy. Diabetes 13:278–285, 1964.
6. Schrag S, Gorwitz R, Fultz-Butts K, et al: Prevention of perinatal group B streptococcal disease: Revised guidelines from CDC. Morbidity and Mortality Weekly Report 51 (RR-11):1–22, 2002.
7. Prevention of infective endocarditis: Guidelines from the American Heart Association. Circulation 116:1736–1754, 2007.
8. ACOG Practice Bulletin 68. Antiphospholipid syndrome. Washington, DC, American College of Obstetricians and Gynecologists, November 2005.
9. Wilson WA, Gharavi AE, Koike T, et al: International consensus statement on preliminary classification criteria for definite antiphospholipid syndrome: Report of an international workshop. Arthritis & Rheumatism 42:1309–1311, 1999.

Resources

ACOG Practice Bulletin 29. Chronic hypertension in pregnancy. Washington, DC, American College of Obstetricians and Gynecologists, July 2001.

ACOG Practice Bulletin 33. Diagnosis and management of preeclampsia and eclampsia. Washington, DC, American College of Obstetricians and Gynecologists, January 2002.

ACOG Practice Bulletin 30. Gestational diabetes. Washington, DC, American College of Obstetricians and Gynecologists, September 2001.

ACOG Practice Bulletin 64. Hemoglobinopathies in pregnancy. Washington, DC, American College of Obstetricians and Gynecologists, July 2005.

ACOG Practice Bulletin 20. Perinatal viral and parasitic infections. Washington, DC, American College of Obstetricians and Gynecologists, September 2000.

ACOG Practice Bulletin 19. Thromboembolism in pregnancy. Washington, DC, American College of Obstetricians and Gynecologists, August 2000.

Benson MD: Gestational hypertension. Point-of-care reference for the internet. British Medical Journal [in press].

Blanchard DG, Shabetai R: Cardiac diseases. In Creasy RK, Resnik R, Iams JD (eds): Maternal-fetal medicine: Principles and practice, 5th ed. Philadelphia, WB Saunders, 2004.

Gibbs RS, Sweet RL, Duff WP: Maternal and fetal infectious disorders. In Creasy RK, Resnik R, Iams JD (eds): Maternal-fetal medicine: Principles and practice, 5th ed. Philadelphia, WB Saunders, 2004.

Chapter Self-Test Questions

Circle the correct answer. After you have responded to the questions, check your answers in Appendix A.

1. A 38-year-old G2 P0010 patient's initial BP was 150/95. The BP remains consistent through most of her prenatal visits, although it drops slightly in the second trimester. On her prenatal visit at 28 weeks, she has 2+ proteinuria on dipsticks taken a day apart. Her diagnosis is:

    a. Mild pre-eclampsia.

    b. Chronic hypertension.

    c. Chronic hypertension with superimposed pre-eclampsia.

    d. Gestational hypertension.

2. Which is *not* true about gestational diabetes?

    a. Complications of untreated diabetes include an increased risk of intrauterine fetal demise, shoulder dystocia, and cesarean section.

    b. Good control of glucose may reduce fetal risk close to that of fetuses in nondiabetic mothers.

    c. Risk is more closely related to starting BMI than advancing maternal age.

    d. All statements are true.

3. Which infection does *not* typically present with a rash?

    a. Cytomegalovirus

    b. Varicella zoster

    c. Parvovirus

    d. Rubella

4. Which is true about heart disease during pregnancy?

    a. Systolic murmurs are commonplace in the absence of disease at term.

    b. Mitral stenosis with atrial fibrillation is associated with a 25%–50% mortality rate.

    c. Inherited heart abnormalities are typically the same defect across family members.

    d. Whereas cardiac output increases during pregnancy, percentage of flow to the uterus does not change.

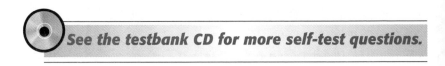

See the testbank CD for more self-test questions.

27

CHAPTER

COMPLICATIONS OF LABOR

Michael D. Benson, MD

I. Problems With Onset of Labor

A. Preterm birth

    1. Birth before 37 completed weeks (more than 21 days before estimated date of confinement [EDC])

    2. Incidence and risk factors

        a. 12.5% of all births

        b. Majority (70% or so) occur between 34 and 36 weeks

        c. Risk factors

            i. Prior preterm birth

                (1) Increases risk threefold for next pregnancy

                (2) Risk is 1 in 3 with two prior, consecutive preterm births

            ii. African-American ethnicity

                (1) Risk appears independent of educational attainment, socioeconomic status, access to medical care

                (2) Not seen in Africa

                (3) Cause not known

            iii. Multiple gestation

            iv. Maternal, fetal, or obstetrical disease necessitating induction

            v. Tobacco use

            vi. Polyhydramnios

    3. Etiology

        a. Cause for spontaneous labor at term or preterm not known

        b. Best speculation: both are related to inflammation (not necessarily infection)

    4. Three manifestations that may have inflammation as a common pathway

a. Preterm labor

b. Cervical insufficiency (incompetent cervix)

   i. Definition

     (1) Classically painless cervical dilation resulting in preterm delivery

     (2) With ultrasound assessment of cervical length, no longer seen as dichotomous condition

   ii. Diagnosis

     (1) Suggested by:

       (A) Two more midtrimester pregnancy losses

       (B) History of cervical trauma (chiefly cone biopsy)

       (C) Patient with advanced cervical dilation and effacement with membranes bulging though os before 37 completed weeks in absence of infection or contractions

     (2) Ultrasound: serial assessment of cervical length beginning at 16–20 weeks may be helpful in women with historical risk factors

   iii. Treatment: cervical cerclage

     (1) Elective ("prophylactic")

       (A) Suture of cervix at level of internal os placed at 12–13 weeks

       (B) No evidence of benefit (with exception of those with at least three midtrimester pregnancy losses)

     (2) Emergency cerclage: placed on urgent basis in patients with advanced, painless dilation

       (A) No randomized studies

       (B) Benefit unknown

c. Preterm, premature rupture of membranes

   i. Diagnosis: similar to diagnosis of spontaneous rupture of membranes at term `25A`

       (A) History: sudden gush and/or continuous leaking of fluid from vagina

       (B) Physical examination: sterile speculum

         (i) Amniotic fluid seen leaking from cervix or pooling in back of vagina

(ii) Fluid tests: nitrazine positive and fern positive

(iii) Alternatively, watery or white discharge that is clearly not amniotic fluid will be found to explain discharge

ii. Risk factors: `25B`

(1) Prior history increases risk

(2) 1%–2% of all pregnancies

(3) Factor in 20% of all perinatal deaths

iii. Management `25C-E`

(1) General principles

(A) 75%–90% of pregnancies delivered within 7 days

(B) Risk of chorioamnionitis increases as pregnancy progresses

(C) Chorioamnionitis in premature infants associated with long-term fetal injury

(D) Patients with evidence of chorioamnionitis (chiefly fever) generally delivered by induction of labor or cesarean as appropriate

(E) Cervical examinations associated with earlier time interval to delivery (in this specific circumstance of pre-term premature rupture of membranes [PROM])

(F) Fetal monitoring seeks evidence of cord compression or contractions that might be early sign of labor or chorioamnionitis

(G) If delivery does not appear imminent, patients generally transferred to antepartum floor and monitored periodically

(2) Before 24 weeks

(A) Survival rate and quality of life of survivors very poor

(B) Pulmonary hypoplasia and limb atrophy presumably from compression are unique complications at this gestational age

(C) Amount of remaining fluid may help with prognosis

(D) Some physicians and patients elect to induce and not resuscitate the newborn

(3) Before 32 weeks

  (A) Course of steroids (to accelerate fetal lung maturity and reduce risk in intraventricular hemorrhage)

  (B) Course of broad spectrum antibiotics

    (i) Duration of antibiotic treatment generally 3–7 days—limited evidence for ideal treatment length

    (ii) Ampicillin, ampicillin-sulbactam, and erythromycin used with benefit

(4) 32–34 weeks: antibiotics administered but steroids generally held

(5) 34 weeks and after

  (A) Chorioamnionitis risk believed to offset any additional benefit of expectant management

  (B) Fetus delivered via induction or cesarean according to obstetrical indications

5. Diagnosis 24

  a. Preterm labor

    i. Classically, regular increasing contractions with cervical dilation on serial examinations

    ii. In practice, often difficult to distinguish from frequent contractions that do not cause dilation

    iii. Patient descriptions include regular tightening, contractions, cramping, and "baby balling up"

  b. Cervical insufficiency: painless dilation of cervix leading to second trimester pregnancy loss

  c. Preterm PROM: rupture of membranes in absence of contractions

    i. Clear fluid gushing from cervix on speculum examination

    ii. Fern positive on microscopic examination

    iii. Nitrazine positive (basic pH)

6. Morbidity and mortality

  a. Survival rates as function of gestational age

    i. 24 weeks: 20%

    ii. 26 weeks: 50%

      iii. 34 weeks: survival rate similar to full term (within 1%)

  b. Neurologic injury

      i. <26 weeks: only 20% normal at 5 years

      ii. Strongest single clinical or demographic factor associated with cerebral palsy

7. Management 24D

  a. Clinical risk assessment

      i. Weekly cervical examinations neither beneficial nor harmful

      ii. Ultrasound assessment of cervical length not helpful in general population

      iii. Fetal fibronectin: swab of cervix without palpation of cervix

        (1) Negative test result: strongly predicts pregnancy will continue for another week

        (2) Positive test result: 30% deliver within a week

      iv. Bacterial vaginosis: although infection in general suspected to have a role in pre-term birth, neither screening nor antibiotic treatment for this diagnosis has been shown to have benefit

  b. Progesterone: for women with prior preterm birth

      i. 250 mg 17-alpha-hydroxyprogesterone caproate IM injection

      ii. Administer weekly

      iii. Start at 16–20 weeks

      iv. Continue through 36 weeks

      v. Results: placebo group, 55%; treatment group, 36%

  c. Tocolysis (inhibition of established labor)

      i. No agent has been shown to delay birth by more than 48 hours

      ii. Agents: beta-sympathomimetics (e.g., terbutaline), indomethacin, magnesium (latter is controversial)

      iii. Generally not given after 33 completed weeks due to minimal benefit

      iv. Generally reserved for women with demonstrated cervical change

  d. Corticosteroids

      i. Single course of steroids

        (1) Reduces risk of respiratory distress syndrome

> (2) May reduce rate of intraventricular hemorrhage by up to 50%
> (3) Generally must be given at least 48 hours in advance of birth to have benefit
>> ii. Benefit negligible after 34 weeks
>> iii. Generally given if tocolysis initiated
> **e.** Group B streptococcus (GBS) prophylaxis generally indicated for birth before 36 weeks for those in labor
> **f.** Treatments that do not work: bedrest, hydration, long-term tocolysis (beyond 1 or 2 days), ambulatory contraction monitoring, sexual abstinence

B. Post-term birth
  1. Pregnancies that continue 14 days past EDC `30A`
  2. Morbidity and mortality `30B`
    a. Fetal
      i. Perinatal mortality rate (antepartum stillbirth rate in particular) rises steadily after EDC and more quickly after 41 completed weeks
      ii. Increased rate of fetal macrosomia; however, inducing labor has not been shown to improve outcome
    b. Maternal
      i. Increased labor dystocia
      ii. Doubling of cesarean section rate
  3. Monitoring
    a. Because perinatal mortality rate rises, most obstetricians begin fetal monitoring at start of 41 weeks
      i. Biweekly nonstress test
      ii. Assessment of amniotic fluid index
    b. No randomized controlled trials to evaluate benefit
  4. Induction of labor `30C, 32F`
    a. Assessment of cervix
    b. Cervical status strongly associated with probability of successful labor induction
      i. Bishop score[1] is one way of assessing cervix (Table 27.1)
      ii. Bishop score of 5 or less suggests lower success rate of induction; cervical ripening agents (prostaglandins or extra-amniotic saline infusion [EASI]) may be good first step

TABLE 27.1

Bishop Score for Assessing Cervical Ripeness

Category	Points
Dilation	
<1 cm	0
1–2 cm	1
3–4 cm	2
5 cm or more	3
Effacement	
<40%	0
40–50%	1
60–70%	2
80% or more	3
Station	
Less than -2	0
-2 to -1	1
Engaged	2
+1 or more	3
Consistency	
Firm	0
Medium	1
Soft	2
Position of Cervix	
Posterior	0
Midposition	1
Anterior	2

From Bishop EH: Pelvic scoring for elective induction. Obstet Gynecol 1964;24:266–268.

    c. Agents/methods **22D**

      i. Oxytocin

        (1) Variety of protocols

        (2) Dose increased every 15–30 minutes until uterine contractions 2–3 minutes apart

(3) Oxytocin as IV infusion has half-life of minutes
(4) Starting dose
   (A) 0.5 milli-International Units (mIU) of oxytocin per minute
   (B) 1 or 2 mIU/min
(5) Increases
   (A) Double dose at 15-minute intervals until 16–20 mIU/min
   (B) Increase by 1- or 2-mIU increments
(6) Peak dose
   (A) Many protocols require physician notification to exceed 20 mIU/min
   (B) 30 mIU/min highest infusion rate in most protocols
(7) Decreasing or stopping infusions
   (A) For tachysystole
      (i) More than five uterine contractions per 10 minutes averaged over 30 minutes
      (ii) Response to oxytocin highly variable from patient to patient and with the same patient over time
         (a) Not uncommon to see two or three mild contractions back to back; increasing oxytocin infusion often causes these contractions to space out and become stronger
         (b) Not unusual to be able to stop the infusion at times because the patient will have adequate contractions spontaneously
   (B) Fetal intolerance to labor
      (i) With frequent or prolonged contractions, fetus may show signs of compromise; infusion commonly stopped
      (ii) Uncommon and if due to excessive contractions, usually easily addressed by temporarily stopping infusion
      (iii) Beta-sympathomimetics (e.g., terbutaline) may also reduce contraction frequency

(8) Oxytocin toxicity
  (A) Oxytocin has weak antidiuretic properties
    (i) Can rarely result in water intoxication
    (ii) Hyponatremia occurs, causing seizures and ultimately death
  (B) Not a clinical concern with commonly used doses of oxytocin
    (i) 20 or 30 units/1000 mL commonly infused over 4 hours postpartum to reduce bleeding (infusion rate of 125 mIU/min)
    (ii) Concern arises if infusion continues 8 hours or more
  (C) Key idea is that oxytocin infusion doses vary considerably by purpose and whether fetus remains within uterus
ii. Prostaglandins
  (1) PGE_1: Misoprostol (Cytotec)
  (2) PGE_2: Cervidil
iii. Artificial rupture of membranes
  (1) Labor ensues in 90% of patients within 24 hours
  (2) Not possible with unfavorable cervix
  (3) Most commonly used in conjunction with oxytocin
iv. EASI
  (1) Foley catheter placed through cervix; balloon-inflated
  (2) Saline infusion begun
  (3) Effective but not always possible with unfavorable cervix

C. PROM at term
  1. Rupture of membranes before onset of labor
  2. Occurs in up to 10% of term gestations
  3. Risk of chorioamnionitis related to time between rupture and delivery
    a. This consideration generally a reason for induction
    b. Risk is not so high that immediate induction required
  4. Give antibiotics for GBS colonization

II. Problems With Duration of Labor `22A`

A. See Chapter 21 for normal course of labor; no consensus on normal time course of labor in women with epidurals (probably longer)

B. American College of Obstetricians and Gynecologists (ACOG) definitions of prolonged second stage in patients with epidural anesthesia:

   1. First labor: >3 hours

   2. Second labor: >2 hours

C. Evaluation of women with prolonged labor `11E, 22A`

   1. Differential diagnosis

      a. Inadequate contractions

         i. No universally accepted definition partly because natural, successful labors vary widely

         ii. Best criterion is minimum contraction strength of 200 Montevideo units

           (1) Montevideo units: amplitude of contraction minus baseline uterine pressure summed for each contraction per 10 minutes

           (2) Can be determined only by intrauterine pressure catheter

      b. Cephalopelvic disproportion (CPD) `22B`

         i. Fetal skull cannot pass through maternal pelvis

         ii. May result from:

           (1) Fetal skeleton being too big

           (2) Maternal pelvis being too small

           (3) Fetal skeleton orientation not ideal for passage through maternal pelvis

         iii. Empirically determined diagnosis

           (1) Cannot be predicted in advance of labor

           (2) Clinical pelvimetry and x-ray measurements of maternal skeleton not proved to be of value

           (3) Pelvic dimensions change depending on maternal position

           (4) Fetal head dimensions change during labor ("moulding")

   2. Treatment of prolonged labor

      a. Medical management

         i. Rupture of membranes

         ii. Place intrauterine pressure catheter to determine contraction intensity in mm Hg

         iii. Oxytocin augmentation if indicated (commonly is)

      b. Cesarean section

      i. CPD diagnosed if:
         (1) Cervix at least 4 cm dilated
            (A) Excludes latent phase of labor
            (B) CPD uncommon before 4 cm
            (C) Arrest of labor with adequate contractions
                can occur before 4 cm dilation but much less
                consensus about how much time should elapse
         (2) Contractions adequate (> 200 Montevideo units
            consistently)
         (3) No change for at least 2 hours
            (A) No further cervical dilation
            (B) No further descent of fetal head
         (4) Minimum time of 2 hours; some evidence that 3 or
            4 hours might be more appropriate
   c. Operative vaginal delivery: forceps or vacuum
     i. Indicated for:
       (1) Second stage of labor longer than ACOG criteria
       (2) Maternal exhaustion (generally not considered
          before preceding time of indication has elapsed)
       (3) Fetal intolerance to labor
     ii. Criteria for low operative vaginal delivery are met
     iii. Vaginal birth seems highly likely

III. Malpresentation `11E, 22E`
  A. Incidence
    1. 96% of term fetuses vertex
    2. 3%–4% breech
      a. Frank: buttocks presenting, feet by head
      b. Footling (single or double): feet presenting
      c. Complete: fetus seated with feet at level of buttocks
    3. Small minority are transverse or oblique lie
  B. Risk factors include uterine anomalies, high parity, multiple
    gestation, oligo- or polyhydramnios, and congenital anomalies
  C. Diagnosis
    1. Physical examination: detects only half of breech
    presentations before onset of labor
    2. Ultrasound: most reliable
  D. Morbidity and mortality
    1. Transverse lie: cannot deliver vaginally
    2. Breech

       a. Increased risk of permanent neurologic injury for all types of breech presentation at all weights from vaginal birth

       b. Increased risk of congenital anomalies (up to 6%)

       c. Increased rate of perinatal mortality and umbilical cord prolapse

   E. Treatment

      1. Cesarean section

      2. External cephalic version: physical attempt to flip fetus

         a. Success rates

           i. Initially successful up to 60% of the time

           ii. Fetus can flip back to breech in interval between version and labor

           iii. Commonly done between 36 and 38 weeks

         b. Risks generally minimal; abruption has been reported

         c. Done in hospital

           i. IV established

           ii. Ultrasound before and after

           iii. Epidural and tocolytic drugs have been suggested but have not been shown to be of consistent benefit

         d. Contraindications include oligohydramnios, labor, and uterine anomalies; presence of uterine scar is controversial

IV. Shoulder Dystocia `11E, 22G`

   A. Definition, incidence, and risk factors

      1. Difficulty in passage of shoulder beyond pubic symphysis after delivery of head; precise definition variable so incidence has to be treated somewhat skeptically

      2. Risk 1.4% overall

      3. Risk over 4500 g may be 9% or higher

      4. Gram for gram, risk of shoulder dystocia appears to be higher in gestational diabetics

      5. Majority of cases (and injuries) occur in infants <4000 g

   B. Morbidity and mortality

      1. Fetal

         a. No injury

         b. Temporary injury

           i. Broken clavical or humerus

           ii. Loss of use of arm: brachial plexus stretch injury (Erb palsy)

        c. Permanent injury: Erb palsy (loss of use of arm)

        d. Perinatal asphyxia with central nervous system injury or death

    2. Maternal: hemorrhage, fourth-degree lacerations

C. Prevention

    1. ACOG recommendation[3]

        a. Offer cesarean to those with estimated fetal weights:

            i. >4500 g for gestational diabetics

            ii. >5000 g for general population

    2. Induction for suspected macrosomia (and to prevent further fetal growth) has not been shown to be helpful

D. Treatment

    1. Shoulder dystocia drill (although commonly taught, no evidence of benefits)[4]

        a. Call for help (nurses, pediatrician/nursery team, anesthesia)

        b. Gentle downward traction

        c. Drain bladder

        d. Episiotomy (large)

        e. Suprapubic pressure

            i. Downward pressure immediately above symphysis; disimpact shoulder from behind symphysis

            ii. Avoid fundal pressure at top of uterus

        f. McRoberts maneuver: sharply flex maternal legs upward onto maternal abdomen

        g. Woods corkscrew maneuver: rotate shoulder 180° in corkscrew fashion

        h. Deliver posterior shoulder

            i. Sweep posterior arm of fetus across chest

            ii. Deliver arm

            iii. Rotate posterior shoulder

            iv. Deliver anterior shoulder

        i. Fracture of clavicle or humerus

        j. Zavanelli maneuver: push head back into birth canal, deliver by cesarean (difficult to do)

V. Vaginal Birth After Cesarean (VBAC) `22F, 32M`

    A. No randomized controlled trials comparing maternal and neonatal outcomes for repeat cesarean versus VBAC

    B. Cesarean section rate increased 5%–25% between 1970 and 1988

1. Corresponds with spread of electronic fetal monitoring into clinical practice
2. Improvement in neonatal outcomes from higher cesarean rate not demonstrated
3. Maternal BMI also increased during this time (and continues to increase)

C. Two patients, three outcomes (Table 27.2)

TABLE 27.2		
	Risks of VBAC and Its Alternatives	
	Mother	**Fetus**
VBAC successful	Reduced: • Postoperative pain • Bleeding • Deep venous thrombosis (DVT) risk • Infection Increased risk of subsequent incontinence?	1 in 500–1000 risk of: • Perinatal death • Neurologic injury
VBAC failed	Greatest risks: • Postoperative pain • Bleeding • DVT risk • Infection Increased risk (small) in subsequent pregnancies of: • Placenta previa • Placenta accreta	1 in 500–1000 risk of: • Perinatal death • Neurologic injury Increased risk of infection Risk of laceration during surgery (risk low; consequences usually small)
Elective, scheduled repeat cesarean	Increased risk (compared with successful VBAC but less risk compared with cesarean during labor): • Pain • Bleeding • DVT • Infection Increased risk (small) in subsequent pregnancies of: • Placenta previa • Placenta accreta	Risk of laceration during surgery (risk low; consequences usually small)

D. Maternal risk highest for failed VBAC
  1. Patient incurs risk of attempting VBAC plus risks of cesarean
  2. Risks of cesarean after labor higher than risk of scheduled cesarean
  3. Prior cesarean for CPD associated with higher risk of failed VBAC
E. Risk of perinatal death or permanent injury for otherwise healthy baby at term
  1. Estimated to be between 1 in 500–1000 attempted VBACs[5,6]
  2. For perspective, Centers for Disease Control and Prevention recommend treating 30% of entire laboring population colonized with GBS to reduce risk of neonatal streptococcus disease from 1 in 1000 to 1 in 5000
  3. Generally related to rupture of uterus; emergency cesarean can rescue many, but not all, fetuses
F. Safest outcome for baby is scheduled, elective repeat cesarean
G. Candidates
  1. Only one prior cesarean
  2. Lower cervical transverse uterine incision
  3. Obstetrician immediately available in maternity unit with anesthesia and nursing staff sufficient for emergency cesarean
H. Factors that may increase risk of rupture
  1. Delivery interval less than 24 months
  2. Single-layer closure of cesarean incision
  3. Induction of labor
    a. Prostaglandin use substantially increases risk; contraindicated
    b. Oxytocin induction associated with moderate increased risk but oxytocin augmentation of established labor is not

VI. Special Fetal Considerations
A. Umbilical cord prolapse
  1. Occurring in perhaps 2–3 per 1000 deliveries, cord prolapse is an obstetrical emergency
    a. With the umbilical cord presenting, cord occlusion more likely and fetal compromise can be severe
    b. Risk factors: malpresentation, high presenting part, cervix dilated more than 2 cm
  2. Immediate delivery generally treatment of choice

3. Possibility of cord prolapse should be kept in mind when considering amniotomy with high presenting part

B. Meconium aspiration syndrome

  1. Fetal passage of meconium into the amnionic fluid occurs in up to 20% of all births

    a. Rate increases post-term

    b. Usually a benign event with no special significance

    c. Meconium passage is also seen in some fetuses experiencing compromise before or during labor

  2. This syndrome is a clinical condition in which meconium aspirated into bronchioles resulting in severe inflammation of airways and respiratory compromise

    a. Can be associated with long-term hypoxic injury and neonatal death

    b. Life-threatening version occurs perhaps 1 per 1000 births

    c. Meconium sterile but causes intense inflammatory response in airways

    d. Meconium aspiration may be result of pre-existing fetal compromise; not entirely clear if meconium aspiration cause of illness or partly a result of it

  3. Obstetrical intervention in presence of meconium

    a. Nursery team in delivery room to assist with suctioning and resuscitation if necessary

    b. Although infusion of saline into uterine cavity during labor has been suggested to "thin" the meconium, studies have not shown it to be beneficial

    c. See next chapter for additional steps

C. GBS colonization—CDC 2002 revised guidelines 17D

  1. Background

    a. Early onset GBS disease

      i. Approximately 30% of women at term are colonized

      ii. Maternal GI tract serves as reservoir for the organism.

      iii. Early onset disease can be severe with pneumonia and meningitis resulting

      iv. Fatality rate may reach 50% with significant number of survivors suffering permanent neurologic injury

      v. Early-onset disease occurs in roughly 1 per 1000 newborns of women who are not colonized versus 5 per 1000 born to women who are colonized

vi. Overall incidence of GBS sepsis was 2–3/1000 births (80% was early onset versus late onset)
  b. Risk factors: prematurity, maternal colonization, fever during labor of >99.5°F, ruptured membranes >12 hours
2. Prevention protocol
  a. All mothers screened at 35–37 weeks
  b. Screening done by culturing vagina and then rectum with cotton swab
  c. Antibiotic prophylaxis indicated for:
    i. Prior infant with GBS disease
    ii. GBS bacteriuria during current pregnancy
      (1) Bacteriuria defined as *any* GBS in urine (not traditional 100,000 colonies or more)
      (2) These women do not receive cultures; are assumed to be colonized
    iii. Positive screening cultures
    iv. Unknown cultures (or not done) *and*
      (1) Preterm delivery
      (2) Ruptured membranes for 18 hours or more
      (3) Fever of 100.4°F or higher
  d. Antibiotics to use (IV, stop after birth)
    i. Penicillin or ampicillin
      (1) Penicillin 5 million units IV, then 2.5 million units every 4 hours
      (2) Ampicillin 2 g initially, then 1 g every 4 hours
    ii. Penicillin allergic
      (1) If GBS known to be susceptible:
        (A) Clindamycin 900 mg IV every 8 hours *or*
        (B) Erythromycin 500 mg IV every 6 hours until delivery
      (2) If susceptibility not known
        (A) Vancomycin 1 g every 12 hours
  e. Prophylaxis not perfectly effective but does reduce incidence by up to 90%

MENTOR TIPS

- For preterm birth before 34 weeks, remember steroids and antibiotics (during labor).
- Tocolytics delay delivery by a few days (at most).
- Delivery after 33 weeks is generally not interfered with (beyond antibiotics during labor).
- Post-term gestation is associated with increased stillbirth rate.
- Breech babies are no longer delivered vaginally.
- Shoulder dystocia is difficult to predict.
- VBAC carries risk to fetus of 1 in 500–1000 of serious injury or death.

References

1. Bishop EH: Pelvic scoring for elective induction. Obstetrics and Gynecology 24:266–268, 1964.
2. Friedman EA: Labor: Clinical evaluation and management, 2nd ed. New York, Appleton-Century-Crofts, 1978.
3. ACOG Practice Bulletin 40. Shoulder dystocia. Washington, DC, American College of Obstetricians and Gynecologists, November 2002.
4. Hernandez C, Wendel GD: Shoulder dystocia. In Pitkin RM (ed): Clinical obstetrics and gynecology. Hagerstown, Pa., Lippincott, 1990, p 526.
5. Lydon-Rochelle M, Holt VL, Easterling TR, et al: Risk of uterine rupture during labor among women with a prior cesarean delivery. New England Journal of Medicine 345:3–8, 2001.
6. Landon MB, Hauth JC, Leveno KJ, et al: Maternal and perinatal outcomes associated with a trial of labor after prior cesarean delivery. New England Journal of Medicine 351:25, 2004.

Resources

ACOG Practice Bulletin 49. Dystocia and augmentation of labor. Washington, DC, American College of Obstetricians and Gynecologists, December 2003.

ACOG Practice Bulletin 13. External cephalic version. Washington, DC, American College of Obstetricians and Gynecologists, February 2000.

ACOG Practice Bulletin 10. Induction of labor. Washington, DC, American College of Obstetricians and Gynecologists, November 1999.

ACOG Practice Bulletin 55. Management of post-term pregnancy. Washington, DC, American College of Obstetricians and Gynecologists, September 2004.

ACOG Practice Bulletin 54. Vaginal birth after previous cesarean delivery. Washington, DC, American College of Obstetricians and Gynecologists, July 2004.

Chapter Self-Test Questions

Circle the correct answer. After you have responded to the questions, check your answers in Appendix A.

1. Which is helpful in assessing pre-term labor risk?

a. Weekly cervical examinations

b. Ultrasound assessment of cervical length

c. Fetal fibronectin

d. Screening for bacterial vaginosis

2. Which is *not* a complication of oxytocin infusion?

a. Fetal intolerance to labor

b. Seizures

c. Nausea

d. Tachysystole

3. Which is *not* true about malpresentation?

   a. Associated with higher perinatal mortality rate

   b. If external version works initially, reversion to breech is very uncommon

   c. Associated with higher rate of congenital anomalies

   d. Often missed by physical examination alone

4. Which is true of meconium aspiration syndrome?

   a. Amnioinfusion with normal saline to thin meconium is of established benefit.

   b. Having newborn nursery personnel present at delivery is recommended.

   c. Presence of meconium in amniotic fluid is indication for cesarean.

   d. It is clearly a cause (rather than a result) of perinatal asphyxia.

See the testbank CD for more self-test questions.

NEWBORN

Michael D. Benson, MD

I. Normal Newborn Care 8B

A. Fetal circulation

1. Fetal hemoglobin has greater affinity for oxygen than does adult hemoglobin; this allows for efficient absorption of oxygen at the maternal-fetal interface in the placenta.

2. Oxygen-bearing blood is transported by the venous circulation (placenta to fetus); deoxygenated blood is transported by arteries (fetus to placenta).

3. Key features of fetal circulation are the patent ductus arteriosus, which connects the right ventricle to the aorta, and the patent foramen ovale, which allows for oxygenated blood to flow from placenta to ductus venous and into the left atrium.

   a. Ductus arteriosus has low resistance

   b. Fetal pulmonary artery has high resistance

B. Transition to breathing air

1. Stimuli to breathe air

   a. Decrease in oxygen and increase in carbon dioxide at birth; stimulates respiratory efforts

   b. Physical stimulation

   c. Compression of chest during birth to force some fluid out of lungs

2. Physiologic changes of birth

   a. Fluid rapidly absorbed from alveoli and replaced by air

   b. Air inflow results in pulmonary artery dilation and pulmonary vascular resistance to drop

   c. Cord clamping eliminates low-resistance placenta and results in rise in systemic blood pressure

d. Closure of ductus arteriosus

    i. Rise in systemic blood pressure also occurs in aorta, reducing pressure gradient from right ventricle into aorta

    ii. Oxygenated lung produces bradykinin, which constricts ductus arteriosus

C. Apgar scores (Table 28.1) 12A

  1. First promulgated by anesthesiologist Virginia Apgar, this scoring system represented the first effort to assess the health of the newborn at a time when very little was being done to intervene for babies with poor respiratory efforts or slow pulses.

  2. The system was intended as a guide for newborn resuscitation, but it is important to recognize that the score is now obsolete; assessments of the compromised neonate (respiratory rate [RR], heart rate, and color) need to be performed every 30 seconds, not at 1 and 5 minutes.

  3. There is a weak (but some) association between depressed Apgar score at 5 minutes and subsequent morbidity and mortality; no association between 1-minute Apgar and subsequent morbidity.

D. Normal newborn vital signs and laboratory tests 12A

  1. Average weight 3.4 kg (7.5 lb) with average male baby 150 g heavier than average female

  2. Average length 20 inches

TABLE 28.1 Apgar Scores

Sign	0	1	2
Heart rate	Absent	Below 100	Over 100
Respiratory effort	Absent	Slow, irregular	Good, crying
Muscle tone	Flaccid	Some flexion of extremities	Active motion
Reflex irritability	No response	Grimace	Vigorous cry
Color	Blue, pale	Body pink, extremities blue	Completely pink

3. Normal temperature range: 36.5°–37°C axillary
4. Pulse: 120–160 (lower when sleeping, higher when crying)
5. Respiratory rate: 30–60
6. Blood pressure: not routinely measured
7. Laboratory values
   a. Glucose: >40 mg/dL (some debate about definition of hypoglycemia)
   b. Hemoglobin: 14–20 g/dL
   c. White count: 13–38 $\times$ 10^6/mcL
8. Umbilical cord gas values: Table 28.2

II. Routine Newborn Screening and Prophylaxis 12B

A. Screening
   1. Universally required screening (all states): phenylketonuria, hypothyroidism
   2. Commonly screened metabolic disorders: galactosemia, homocystinuria, maple syrup urine disease, congenital adrenal hyperplasia, hemoglobinopathies

TABLE 28.2	Normal Cord Blood Values and Interpretation of Gases	
Normal Cord Blood Values		
	Artery	Vein
pH	7.27	7.34
Pco$_2$ (mm Hg)	50.3	40.7
Hco$_3$- (mEq/L)	22.0	21.4
Base excess (mEq/L)	-2.7	-2.4
Interpretation of Gases		
Respiratory Acidosis	Metabolic Acidosis	
Low pH	Low pH	
High Pco$_2$	Normal to high Pco$_2$	
Normal base excess	High base excess	

From Riley RJ, Johnson JWC: Collecting and analyzing cord blood gases. Clin Obstet Gynecol 26:13, 1993.

3. HIV: although state laws vary, many states require newborn screening if maternal HIV status unknown

4. Babies at extremes of weight for gestational age are often screened for hypoglycemia and/or polycythemia

B. Disease prophylaxis

1. Blindness prevention

   a. Gonococcal ophthalmia neonatorum: acceptable prophylaxis in first hour of life includes silver nitrate or erythromycin and tetracycline ointments

   b. Chlamydial conjunctivitis: not effectively prevented with preceding agents; conjunctivitis in first month of life may be *Chlamydia* and might require specific treatment

2. Hepatitis B (now mercury-free) vaccine: first of three doses initiated in first few hours after birth (babies born to mothers who are carriers also receive immune globulin)

3. Vitamin K: typically given IM in first hour of life (helps to prevent coagulopathy from vitamin K deficiency)

C. Jaundice: risk for kernicterus (and brain damage) determined by bilirubin level and day of life; screening often done by bilirubin cutaneous meter, which can be followed by serum bilirubin level if indicated

D. Infection

1. Mother with diagnosis of chorioamnionitis: complete blood count (CBC) blood cultures obtained; antibiotics depending on clinical circumstance

2. Maternal group B streptococcus colonization: no special follow-up if mother received two doses of prophylactic antibiotic with one occurring within 4 hours of birth; if not, CBC and blood cultures sometimes obtained

III. Circumcision 32N

A. Benefits and risks

1. No clear medical indications for circumcision; procedure increasingly uncommon except in United States

2. Possible medical benefits

   a. Reduces risk of HIV transmission from female to male 40%–60% in high-risk populations

   b. Reduces risk of penis cancer (rare in any event)

   c. May reduce risk of other sexually transmitted diseases and penile inflammatory conditions

3. Risks
    a. Death; loss of penis 1–2 per million cases
    b. Infection, bleeding, meatal scarring
4. Some residency programs transferring responsibility for circumcision to pediatrics residency although there may be some concern about liability insurance and volume after residency

B. American Academy of Pediatrics recommends use of local anesthetic for circumcisions
  1. Local block
    a. 1% lidocaine without epinephrine
       i. 0.2–0.4 mL injected at base of penis at 2 o'clock and 10 o'clock (lateral to the easy-to-identify dorsal vein), near the two dorsal nerves of the penis; not to exceed 0.8 mL total
      ii. Stabilize skin at base of penis first with gentle traction
     iii. Advance needle 2–5 mm through the skin in posteromedial direction
     iv. Aspirate first to ensure needle not intravascular
      v. Injection will result in two small, practically continuous blebs at the base of the penis
     vi. Anesthesia should be achieved within 2–3 minutes
    b. EMLA cream: anesthetic cream (mixture of lidocaine 2.5% and prilocaine 2.5%) on the penis 1–2 hours prior to procedure
  2. Pacifier soaked in glucose solution might provide additional relief

C. Technique: several available; use of Gomco (bell) clamp described here (Fig. 28.1)
  1. Wash the penis with antiseptic, and drape the area. Administer the lidocaine at this point if you plan to use it.
  2. Grasp the foreskin at 11 o'clock and 1 o'clock with two hemostats. The urethral meatus is difficult to find, because the foreskin is somewhat folded over it. By grasping the foreskin in approximately the right location with hemostats and then applying gentle upward traction, you can confirm that you have appropriate placement of the hemostats.
  3. Slide a closed hemostat oriented transversely just underneath the foreskin at 12 o'clock. Be careful to keep the tips pointed

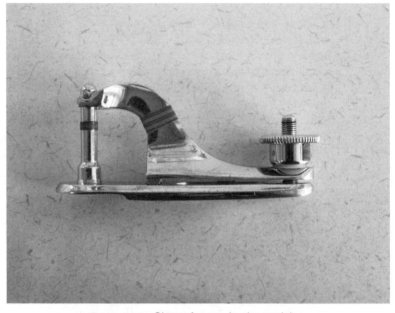

FIGURE 28.1 Clamp for use in circumcision.

outward, away from the penis itself. Advance gently until resistance is encountered. Spread the tips, and withdraw slowly. This method serves to free up any loose adhesions between the foreskin and the glans penis. As the hemostat is being withdrawn, the glans can be visualized to confirm the anatomy. This step can be repeated several times until the foreskin slides more easily along the glans.

4. Clamp the foreskin with the hemostat at 12 o'clock. The tips of the hemostat should be even with the bottom of the glans. Allow the clamp to remain on the skin for 30 seconds or so.

5. Cut along the foreskin at 12 o'clock with a scissors in the groove created by the clamp. The bleeding should be minimal, because the clamping step crushes the larger blood vessels.

6. With the help of the hemostats still affixed at 11 o'clock and 1 o'clock, slide the foreskin back below the glans. This step further breaks up adhesions.

7. Insert the appropriately sized bell under the foreskin and over the glans. It is helpful to use a third hemostat at 12 o'clock to pinch the foreskin together at the base of the bell to prevent the bell from sliding out.

8. Remove the hemostats at 11 o'clock and 1 o'clock.

9. Take the flat base of the clamp, and slide the bell portion through the hole at the end of the base. Gently affix the two prongs at the top of the bell protector to the receptacle on the clamp.

10. Look below the base of the clamp at the penis. The outline of the glans should be faintly discernible. Be sure that the skin is not too taut or loose. Small adjustments in the amount of foreskin can be made at this point by gently pushing the tissue up or down through the loose clamp arrangement with 2×2 gauze.

11. Tighten the large nut at the end of the clamp. This method pulls the bell up against the clamp. This step is irreversible, because it crushes the blood vessels. It is important to be sure that the nut is turned as tightly as possible, because hemostasis depends on this step.

12. Use a knife blade without a handle to cut off the foreskin distal to the clamp (above). It is important to get all the foreskin off and leave smooth edges. Otherwise the circumcision will leave a ragged edge of skin around the glans.

13. Loosen the clamp and gently slide the bell off the penis. Bleeding should be minimal. Should bleeding persist from specific arterioles, silver nitrate on a wooden applicator can be applied gently to the site for hemostasis.

14. Dress the wound with Vaseline and then dry gauze.

IV. Newborn Resuscitation (Fig. 28.2)

A. There is increasing emphasis in hospitals across the United States to have every person who commonly attends deliveries receive training in neonatal resuscitation as described by a collaboration between the American Heart Association and the American Academy of Pediatrics. 12c

B. Basic steps of resuscitation

1. Step 1: Immediately (seconds) after birth
   a. Full-term?
   b. Clear amnionic fluid?
   c. Breathing or crying?
   d. Good muscle tone?

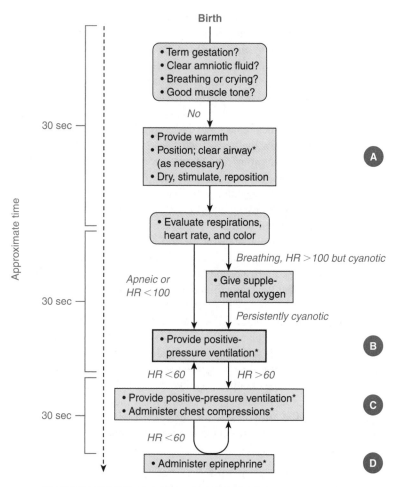

*Endotracheal intubation may be considered at several steps.

Figure 28.2 Neonatal resuscitation. (Redrawn and adapted from American Heart Association and American Academy of Pediatrics: Neonatal resuscitation textbook, 5th ed. AAP, 2006.)

2. Step 2: If answer to any of preceding is "no":

   a. Provide warmth.

   b. Attend to airway.

      i. Position in sniffing position, avoiding flexion or hyperextension (Fig. 28.3).

      ii. Suction airway if necessary with bulb or wall suction.

         (1) Mouth first

         (2) Nares second

   c. Dry and warm; do not leave baby in wet blankets.

   d. Stimulate (rub back or flicking soles of feet); do not shake.

   e. Reposition to help ensure airway is open.

3. Step 3:

   a. Evaluate three things at 30 seconds after birth (not 1 minute); this is not an Apgar score

      i. **Respirations:**

         (1) Good chest movement

         (2) Rate and depth of breathing should increase with gentle stimulation

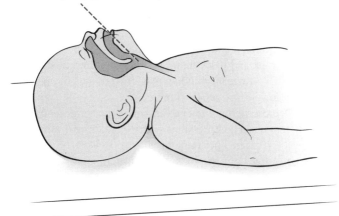

Correct—Line of sight clear (tongue will be lifted by laryngoscope blade)

FIGURE 28.3 Sniffing position for clear airway. (Redrawn and adapted from American Heart Association and American Academy of Pediatrics: Neonatal resuscitation textbook, 5th ed. AAP, 2006.)

      ii. **Heart rate:** should be greater than 100 beats per minute

      iii. **Color:** trunk should be pink (blue hands and feet are normal and not suggestive of hypoxemia)

  b. Intervene

      i. If apneic or pulse <100: provide positive pressure ventilation at 40–60 breaths per minute

      ii. If breathing and pulse >100 but has central cyanosis: give free-flowing oxygen

4. Step 4

  a. Evaluate RR, pulse, and color at 30 seconds

  b. If heart rate remains below 60, begin chest compressions at rate of 90 per minutes, alternating with 30 breaths per minute

5. Step 5

  a. Evaluate RR, pulse, and color at 30 seconds

  b. If heart rate remains below 60, give epinephrine

C. If meconium present at delivery (or in amniotic fluid prior to delivery)

  1. Baby immediately vigorous (RR, pulse, color): bulb or wall suction the mouth and then the nares

  2. Baby NOT immediately vigorous: intubate baby and suction trachea directly; withdraw tube and suction again until little or no meconium recovered

D. Chest compressions (Fig. 28.4)

  1. Placement of fingers

    a. Thumb technique: grasp baby with both hands around trunk and place thumbs over lower third of sternum

    b. Two-finger technique: place two fingers of one hand over lower third of sternum

  2. Depress sternum to one-third anteroposterior diameter of chest

  3. Rate of 90 compressions with 30 breaths per minute

    a. 120 events per minute

    b. Three compressions with pause for ventilation

E. Three pieces of equipment to provide positive pressure ventilation to newborns

  1. Self-inflating bag (Fig. 28.5)

    a. Remains inflated at all times

    b. Fill spontaneously after being squeezed

    c. Requires oxygen reservoir attached at end to deliver high oxygen concentration

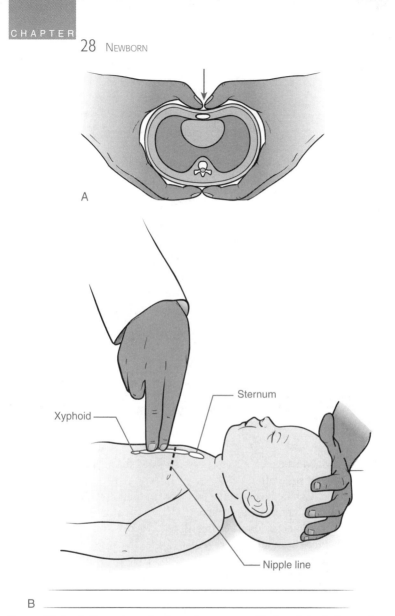

A

Sternum

Xyphoid

Nipple line

B

FIGURE 28-4 *A,* Correct application of pressure with thumb technique of chest compressions. *B,* Correct finger position for chest compressions.

(continued on page 520)

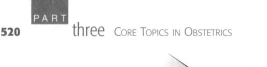

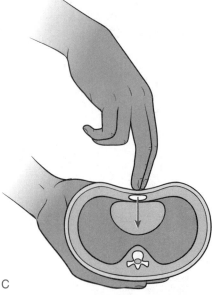

C

FIGURE 28.4 (continued) *C,* Correct application of pressure with two-finger technique. (Redrawn and adapted from American Heart Association and American Academy of Pediatrics: Neonatal resuscitation textbook, 5th ed. AAP, 2006.)

     d. Most have oxygen source attached for neonatal resuscitation
     e. Can deliver positive pressure ventilation without compressed gas source
     f. Cannot administer free-flow oxygen
  2. Flow-inflating bag (Fig. 28.6)
     a. Only fills with compressed gas source
     b. Flow control valve to regulate pressure
     c. Looks like deflated balloon
     d. Can deliver free-flow oxygen
  3. T tube (Fig. 28.7)
     a. Requires compressed gas
     b. Must set maximum pressure, peak inspiratory pressure, and positive end-expiratory pressure (PEEP)

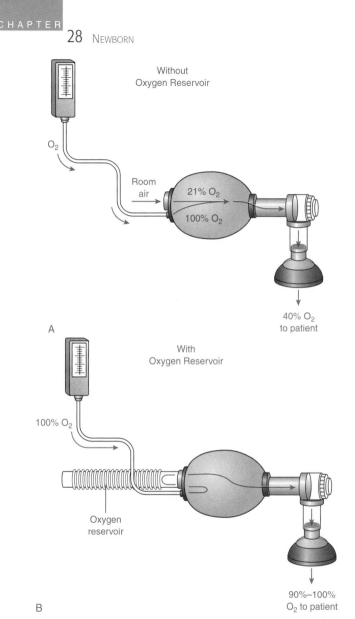

FIGURE 28.5 *A,* Self-inflating bag without oxygen reservoir delivers only 40% oxygen to the patient. *B,* Self-inflating bag with oxygen reservoir delivers 90%–100% oxygen to the patient. (Redrawn and adapted from American Heart Association and American Academy of Pediatrics: Neonatal resuscitation textbook, 5th ed. AAP, 2006.)

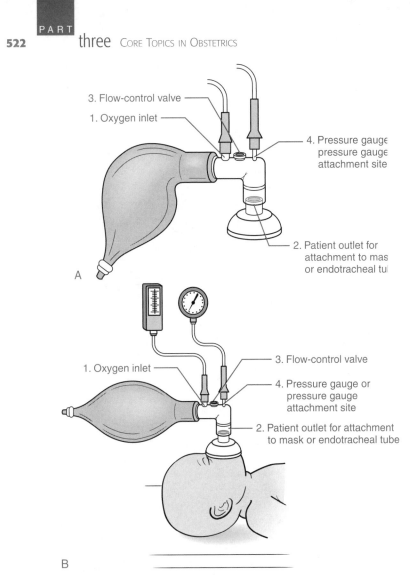

FIGURE 28.6 *A,* Parts of a flow-inflating bag. *B,* Flow-inflating bag attached to oxygen source and pressure manometer. (Redrawn and adapted from American Heart Association and American Academy of Pediatrics: Neonatal resuscitation textbook, 5th ed. AAP, 2006.)

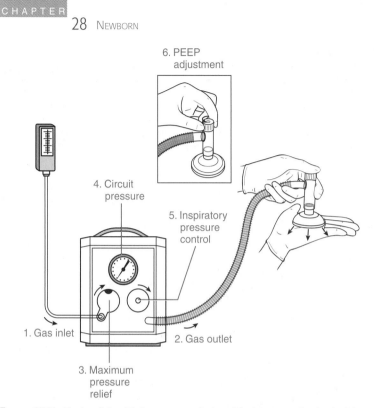

FIGURE 28.7 **Parts of the T-piece resuscitator. (Redrawn and adapted from American Heart Association and American Academy of Pediatrics: Neonatal resuscitation textbook, 5th ed. AAP, 2006.)**

    c. Positive pressure; alternately occlude and open hole in PEEP cap

    d. Can deliver free-flow oxygen

  F. Key points about endotracheal intubation (Table 28.3 lists correct size of tube by size of neonate)

    1. Indications

      a. Suctioning of meconium

      b. To facilitate ventilation during chest compression or with several minutes of bag-and-mask ventilation

      c. To administer epinephrine in absence of intravenous (IV) access

TABLE 28.3	Endotracheal Intubation Tube Sizes for Neonates		
Weight (Typical Gestational Age in Weeks)	Tube Size (mm) (Inside Diameter)	Suction Catheter Size (French)	Approximate Depth of Insertion (cm) (From Upper Lip)
<1000 g (<28 wk)	2.5	5 or 6	6–7
1–2 kg (28–34 wk)	3.0	6 or 8	7–8
2–3 kg (34–38 wk)	3.5	8	8–9
>3 kg (term)	3.5–4.0	8 or 10	9–10

2. Technique (Fig. 28.8)
   a. Place newborn in sniffing position and deliver free-flow oxygen during procedure
   b. Use laryngoscope to expose glottis by placing blade to right of mouth and displacing tongue to left
   c. Lift blade upward to expose vocal cords (upside-down V)
   d. Suction if necessary
   e. Insert tube into right side with curve in horizontal plane
   f. Slide tube through vocal cords until vocal cord guide is at level of cords
   g. Hold endotracheal tube in place while removing laryngoscope
3. Checking placement
   a. CO_2 detector shows exhaled CO_2
   b. Breath sounds over both lung fields but not over stomach
   c. Water vapor with exhalation
   d. Chest moves with each breath
   e. Vital signs improve
G. Orogastric tube; use with prolonged ventilation to prevent distention of stomach
   1. Length is sum of distance from bridge of nose to tip of earlobe and then to a point halfway between xyphoid process and umbilicus
   2. Use 8F feeding tube
   3. Insert tube through mouth; use 20-mL syringe to drain stomach
   4. Remove syringe and allow tube to vent

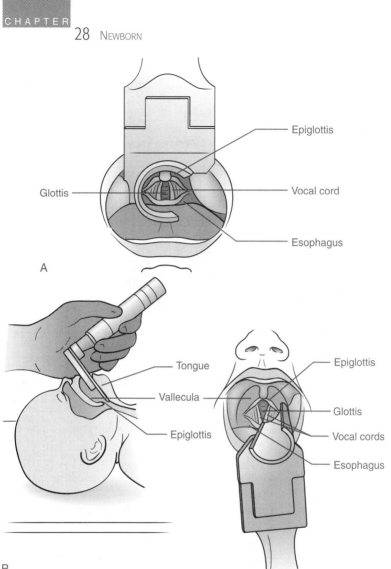

FIGURE 28.8 *A,* Laryngoscopic view of glottis and surrounding structures. *B,* Identification of landmarks before placing endotracheal tube through glottis. (Redrawn and adapted from American Heart Association and American Academy of Pediatrics: Neonatal resuscitation textbook, 5th ed. AAP, 2006. *A* originally based on Klaus M, Fanaroff A: Care of the high-risk neonate. Philadelphia, W.B. Saunders, 1996.)

H. IV access
   1. Cut umbilical cord 1–2 cm above skin perpendicular to cord
   2. Place 3.5-5F catheter that has been prefilled with normal saline (to eliminate air in the line) into umbilical vein (larger than the two arteries)
   3. Advance 2–4 cm until blood can be aspirated with attached syringe
   4. Can give 10 mL/kg of normal saline or O-negative blood over 5–10 minutes

I. Epinephrine
   1. Concentration 1:10,000 (0.1 mg/mL)
   2. IV preferred (0.1–0.3 mL/kg)
   3. Endotracheal tube: 0.3–1 mL/kg
   4. Give rapidly
   5. Use after 30 seconds of ventilation followed by 30 seconds of chest compression if heart rate still <60

J. Narcan (naloxone)
   1. Respiratory depression needs to be treated with assisted ventilation and oxygen as appropriate; first and foremost
   2. If respiratory depression suspected from narcotics
      a. Narcan 0.1 mg/kg IV or IM (works faster IV); 1 mg/mL solution
      b. Indicated only if:
         i. Maternal narcotics were administered within 4 hours of delivery *and*
         ii. Respiratory depression remains after positive pressure ventilation has restored normal color and heart rate

K. Ethics of newborn resuscitation
   1. Same ethical principles as for adults (see Chapter 3)
   2. Parents can act as surrogate decision makers for their children
   3. Where death or high risk of morbidity is likely, resuscitation should be withheld with an occasional exception for parental wishes
   4. Where the prognosis is uncertain, parent wishes regarding resuscitation should generally be honored
   5. Resuscitation may be ended after 10 minutes of absent heartbeat despite full effort

MENTOR TIPS

- Apgar scores remain important for the medical record, but they are obsolete as a guide for resuscitation. The assessment begins immediately, and assisted breathing begins in 30 seconds if needed, not at 1 minute.
- For newborn resuscitation, the same ABCs apply as for adults: airway, breathing, circulation, and so on.
- Many newborn problems can be anticipated; have extra personnel in the delivery room to assist with newborn (meconium, chorioamnionitis, prematurity).
- Tips on circumcision:

   Low risk, low benefit, although evidence is growing that it can provide significant protection against HIV infection and transmission.

   Use local anesthesia.

   You only have one chance to do it right. Do not attempt to take off just a little bit more, because this can be more difficult than it would appear.

   It is sometimes difficult to tell how much is enough and not too much. As a rule, you want the skin of the penis to end at the glans. It rarely will. More commonly it ends a millimeter or so above or below the glans.

   The penis can look bruised and edematous afterward. This will heal normally.

Resources

American Heart Association and American Academy of Pediatrics: Neonatal resuscitation textbook, 5th ed. AAP, 2006.

Chapter Self-Test Questions

Circle the correct answer. After you have responded to the questions, check your answers in Appendix A.

1. Which of the following is *not* true about fetal circulation and respiration?

   a. Oxygen saturation is higher in the fetal veins than in the arteries.

   b. The ductus arteriosus permits blood to bypass the pulmonary circulation.

   c. Air breathing is assisted by a fall in pressure of the ductus arteriosus.

   d. Rise in systemic blood pressure decreases flow through the ductus arteriosus.

2. Which is *not* true about circumcision?

   a. Local anesthetic should be used.

   b. The procedure may protect against HIV transmission.

   c. It is easily revised if too much foreskin is left on.

   d. Risks include bleeding and infection.

3. Which is *not* assessed during resuscitation?

   a. Pupil dilation

   b. Respirations

   c. Heart rate

   d. Color

4. Which is *not* true about epinephrine?

   a. Correct IV dose 0.3–1 mL/kg

   b. Concentration is 1:10,000

   c. Can be given IM

   d. Appropriate to use after 30 seconds of assisted ventilation if heart rate still <60

See the testbank CD for more self-test questions.

ANSWERS TO SELF-TEST QUESTIONS

Below are the answers to the self-test questions that appear at the end of most chapters.

Part I: The Basics

Chapter 1: Clinically Relevant Anatomy

1. c. T11–L2, S1–S3
Response: The nerve roots that mediate labor pain are not contiguous.
2. b.
Response: Levator ani. All the other three muscles are actually part of the perineal body.
3. The pelvic brim is circumference of plane dividing pelvis into true and false; consists of arcuate line (line that divides ala of ilium from body), pectineal line, and upper margin of pubis
4. The pelvic outlet is plane from bottom of pubis to tip of coccyx
5. The differences (8) between the female and male pelvises are:
Less massive
Ilia less sloped
Anterior iliac spines more widely separated (more lateral prominence of hips)
Pelvic inlet larger and more nearly circular
Sacrum shorter and wider
Sciatic notches wider and shallower
Pelvic outlet wider
Coccyx more movable

Chapter 2: History and Physical Examination

1. d. Lymphatic
Response: The lymphatic system is classified under hematologic/
lymphatic/immunologic and does not stand alone. This is not a
scientific distinction but rather a legalistic formula to provide codified
billing.
2. e. All of the above.
3. d. The American Medical Association created this classification system
at the request of United States Health Care Financing Administration.
4. c. Prior medical treatment belongs in the History of Present Illness but
is not a symptom descriptor.

Chapter 3: Legal and Ethical Issues

1. c. Decline to write the note, explaining that you can do so only for
patients who are both examined and actually have a medical illness.
Response: Although it will be unpopular with the patient and her mother
(and they might leave the practice), professional integrity is "dearly
bought and cheaply sold." In the long term, an easy compromise of
integrity might cause the patient to wonder how reliable both your
advice and medical records are.
2. b. Abandon the attempt and repeat it only after accommodations for
the patient's comfort have been made.
Response: Although the patient has autonomy, the physician has as well.
Just because the patient desires a specific course of action does not mean
the physician has to comply if it is against his or her better
judgment. This is an example of the conflict between two ethical
principles: autonomy and beneficence.
3. a. Disclose the error to the patient and explain what remedial steps are
being taken.
Response: This case underscores the importance of the ethical principal
of veracity. Some would argue that medical errors need not be disclosed
or volunteered if no injury results. This position is arguably valid and not
entirely inconsistent with the imperative of veracity. However, in this
specific case, an injury did result: the patient experienced pain because
the anesthetic was not infusing. Furthermore, it is not clear that infusing
an antibiotic intended for IV administration into the epidural space is
entirely benign.

4. a. Contact the police department of the municipality in which she
resides and have the police secure immediate psychiatric evaluation
in the closest emergency room—voluntarily or involuntarily

Response: Beneficence prevails over confidentiality. The patient is
verbalizing very specific threats of harm against another, and a phone
conversation cannot provide enough information to determine the
seriousness of this risk. Emergency psychiatric evaluation will protect the
patient against committing a violent act that will potentially have a huge
negative impact on her life as well as protect a member of society at large
from possible injury.

5. b. Respect her wishes while continuing to try to have her change her
mind. See the following discussion.

Response: This is an example of a case with no very good or obvious
choice. Fortunately, this scenario is incredibly rare. If the patient is
competent, in general the correct answer is **b.,** although attempting at the
same time to get an emergency court order to permit surgery would not be
a bad thing. (The decision would be medically moot for the fetus because
it would come too late, but it might be legally helpful.) The point here is
that if patient autonomy means anything, the patient has to be permitted
to refuse life-, limb-, or even fetus-saving interventions no matter how
irrational or ill-advised doing so might seem to the physician. The
complication in this case is that there are two patients with competing
interests.

Chapter 4: Succeeding in Your Clerkship

1. c. Have staff call him back and advise him that you would be happy to
talk with him as long as his wife calls and gives her consent for you
to talk with him.

Response: You must not give the results or even acknowledge that a test
was done. For example, you cannot even be sure the pregnancy is his.
Simply calling him back directly and refusing to answer any questions
places you in an adversarial position and could confirm that his wife had
an appointment. The best thing to do is to communicate through a third
party—your staff.

2. e. a. and b.

Response: Neuroanatomy has its uses and some tangential relation to
obstetrics and gynecology, but embryology and breast and pelvic anatomy
are much more important.

3. d. All of the above

4. c. Tell her you do not know but that you will look it up and let her know in a few minutes.

Response: It is best not to convey information about which you are not sure. The best doctors know what they do not know.

Part II: Core Topics in Gynecology

Chapter 5: Menstrual Cycle

1. a. Pregnancy cannot occur before first period.

Response: This is often the case but not always true.

2. a. Defined as the absence of secondary sexual characteristics by age 14 years

Response: This is how primary amenorrhea is defined.

3. d. Complete precocious puberty usually has a cause.

Response: Complete precocious puberty is usually idiopathic.

4. a. Pregnancy

Response: Pregnancy is by far the most common cause of amenorrhea among those listed.

Chapter 6: Menopause

1. b. Heart disease

Response: Heart disease is responsible for 50% of all deaths in the United States of both genders.

2. d. Endometrial biopsy

Response: The endometrial biopsy is the only test listed that actually obtains a tissue sample for histologic evaluation.

3. b. Decreased libido

Response: Testosterone is the only exogenous substance clearly proven to increase female libido. Concerns remain about its long-term safety.

4. d. Decreases colon cancer risk, increases breast cancer risks

Response: Estrogen substantially decreases colon cancer risk and long-term use moderately increases breast cancer risk. It also substantially increases uterine cancer risk in the absence of progestins.

Chapter 7: Contraception

1. c. Remove the IUD regardless of her pregnancy plans.
Response: Leaving the IUD in is associated with bad pregnancy outcomes but not always. It is better to remove it and then follow the patient's wishes.

2. d. a. and b.
Response: Yasmin can cause elevations in potassium in high-risk patients and impair carbohydrate metabolism (slightly). Oral contraceptives do not worsen rheumatoid arthritis and may help it.

3. d. Weight gain.
Response: Weight gain is a progestational and androgenic effect.

4. b. Depo-Provera
Response: Depo-Provera rivals the effectiveness of tubal ligation.

Chapter 8: Abortion and Sterilization

1. a. : 99.5% at 1 year, 98% at 10 years

2. e. Second-trimester medical abortion with intrauterine installation of medication.
Response: This method takes longer and has a safety profile similar to that of surgical procedures.

3. c. Round ligament
Response: It can easily be confused with the fallopian tube as they have a similar appearance and are in proximity. Positive identification is made by virtue of seeing the tubes' fimbriated ends.

4. a. Essure
Response: Essure can be done without sedation and with a minimum of local anesthetic injected into the cervix.

Chapter 9: Sexually Transmitted Infections

1. d. Molluscum contagiosum

2. a. Herpes

3. d. Begin treatment with levofloxacin 500 mg orally once daily for 14 days and metronidazole 500 mg bid for 14 days while awaiting laboratory results.

4. c. Azithromycin

Chapter 10: Infertility, Endometriosis, and Chronic Pelvic Pain

1. d. All of the above
Response: All of the above should be included in the initial evaluation.
2. c. Expectant management
Response: Each of steps in evaluation should be undertaken except for "expectant management." There is no reason to believe the patient will improve with the passage of time alone.
3. c. Involves the transfer of embryos into the uterus via the cervix
Response: GIFT stands for gamete intrafallopian transfer and does not place the embryos within the uterus. The unfertilized gametes are transferred into the fallopian tube, where they undergo fertilization.
4. d. All of the above
Response: Each factor listed can result in chronic pelvic pain.

Chapter 11: First-Trimester Bleeding

1. d. Ovarian cancer
Response: Ovarian cancer is the least likely cause of irregular vaginal bleeding, partly because it is uncommon before menopause but also because vaginal bleeding is not a common symptom. However, gestational trophoblastic neoplasia is sufficiently rare that it comes in as a close second, although it almost always causes abnormal bleeding.
2. d. Chorionic villi cover entire embryo
Response: This does not take place until day 12.
3. b. Hyperemesis gravidarum is thought to have a psychological component reflecting the woman's ambivalence about pregnancy
Response: Although poorly understood, hyperemesis gravidarum probably does not have a major psychological component in most women afflicted with it.
4. a. Well-controlled hypertension
Response: All of the issues listed are risk factors for miscarriage except well-controlled hypertension.

Chapter 12: Breast Disease

1. d. Arrange to have lump biopsy (fine-needle aspiration, core biopsy, open biopsy)
Response: A persistent, palpable lump needs to be biopsied even if the mammogram is reassuring.

2. b. Intraductal papilloma
Response: Patients with a bloody nipple discharge invariably think they have cancer when, in most cases, it is a benign intraductal papilloma.
3. b. Median age is in early 50s
Response: The median age is the early 60s; the disease is most commonly postmenopausal.
4. b. Weight
Response: Weight is the only demographic on this list not utilized by the Gail model.

Chapter 13: Incontinence and Pelvic Organ Prolapse

1. b. *S. saprophyticus*
Response: *Klebsiella* and *E. coli* are not gram-positive, and streptococcus is not a common cause of community-acquired pyelonephritis.
2. a. Urinalysis and culture
Response: It is important to establish at the outset that the patient does not have bacteriuria.
3. d. Immune response to mesh itself
Response: Meshes are typically made of prolene, a nondissolving suture material that has been used for decades and evokes very little hypersensitivity.
4. d. Mild cystocele
Response: However counterintuitive, cystoceles are not a common cause of urinary retention.

Chapter 14: Vulvar and Vaginal Symptoms

1. a. Faint, fishy odor
Response: Normal vaginal secretions have very little odor.
2. a. Scaling suggests psoriasis
Response: Skinfold rash suggests tinea, for which butenafine is the preferred treatment. Contact dermatitis is a diagnosis of exclusion.
3. e. All of the above
Response: Each one of these illnesses can present with a vulvar ulcer.
4. b. Incision, drainage, and placement of Word catheter
Response: This is the least invasive procedure for a first-time abscess. The patient does not need antibiotics.

Chapter 15: Cervical Disease and Human Papillomavirus

1. c. It shifts outward with pregnancy.
Response: Columnar epithelium matures into squamous epithelium, and the original squamous columnar junction is the distal edge of the transformation zone. A beefy red cervix can look peculiar to the novice but is usually nothing more than a transformation zone extending outward on the cervical portion.
2. d. Cervical dysplasia usually leaves no visible lesion on examination.
Response: The key idea is that premalignant lesions of the cervix do not generally have signs or symptoms.
3. d. All of the above
Response: Each is true for a diagnostic excisional procedure.
4. b. HPV testing recommended for use by college student health services
Response: It is important not to test college women for HPV (except as a reflex test for ASCUS) because a large number (half?) would test positive at some point. In this age group, the virus is usually cleared quickly.

Chapter 16: Gynecologic Neoplasms

1. b. Cervix
Response: Cancers of the vulva, uterus, and ovary are surgically staged. Uterine cancer can be clinically staged, but surgical staging is considered superior. Cervical cancer remains clinically staged.
2. a. Thecoma
Response: A stromal tumor arises from the stroma, the supporting architecture of the ovary. A Brenner tumor and an endometrioid tumor are neoplasms of the epithelium whereas an endodermal sinus tumor arises from germ cells.
3. a. Repeat the ultrasound in 4 weeks
Response: The most likely explanation for the cyst is normal physiology. A CA-125 has a high rate of false-positives and false-negatives. The *BRCA* mutations are needed for a family history of ovarian cancer (first-degree relatives), and laparoscopy is too invasive at this point in the workup.
4. d. Ovarian
Response: Rank order of total annual deaths (not lethality) is ovarian, endometrial, cervical, and vulvar.

Chapter 17: Specific Gynecologic Procedures, Techniques, and Instruments

1. a. Uterine artery, cardinal ligament, uterosacral ligament
Response: This is the order in which these structures are encountered on the uterus, moving from top to bottom.
2. d. 1
Response: The designation "-0" is equivalent to a negative number. A 3-0 suture is smaller than a 2-0 suture. Without the "-0" designation, larger numbers indicate a larger suture.
3. c. Polydioxanone
Response: Tevdek is braided Dacron, and prolene is polypropylene. Along with nylon, these are not absorbable.
4. d. Harmonic scalpel
Response: The lower temperature needed for coagulation is a potential advantage of the harmonic scalpel. This quality tends to reduce heat transfer to adjacent structures.

Chapter 18: Emotional and Sexual Health in Women

1. c. Most clinically useful diagnostic tool is patient history
Response: The history is by far the most useful tool. Whereas some physicians find daily mood or symptom charting useful for several months before starting therapy, most patients have a pretty good idea of the timing and nature of their symptoms. Many also do not have the patience to chart daily for months.
2. a. Cyclic oral contraceptives
Response: Noncylic oral contraceptives can be helpful, however.
3. c. Mechanism of sexual preference is well understood
Response: The underlying biologic mechanism of sexual identity and preference is poorly understood.
4. c. X-ray of limbs to check for fractures
Response: Specific diagnostic testing for traumatic injury is guided by the history and physical and is not standard for all patients.

Part III: Core Topics in Obstetrics

Chapter 19: Prenatal Care

1. a. Asthma
Response: Asthma does not affect pregnancy, nor is it affected by pregnancy.
2. c. 16
Response: At 12 weeks the uterus is just at the top of the symphysis, whereas at 16 weeks it is midway between the symphysis and the umbilicus.
3. d. Monitoring fetal movement has not been shown to reduce stillbirth rate
Response: Maternal monitoring of fetal movements has been shown to reduce the stillbirth rate.
4. c. Combination birth control pills can be started before the patient leaves the hospital.
Response: Generally, estrogen-containing contraceptives are not started until 4 weeks after delivery due to concern about hypercoagulability.

Chapter 20: Obstetrical Genetics

1. c. Patent ductus arteriosus
Response: This is an anatomically normal fetal structure that does not close properly after birth.
2. a. Cleft palate
Response: Cleft palate appears to be a multifactorial disorder.
3. a. Dilantin
Response: Dilantin is a known teratogen; the other drugs are not suspected of causing birth defects.
4. a. Fragile X syndrome
Response: The incidence of fragile X is not increased in Jewish populations.

Chapter 21: Labor

1. c. Observe for several hours and recheck cervix as needed. Permit ambulation, clear liquids, and intermittent monitoring.
Response: It is not clear if the patient is (or will be shortly) in labor. Therefore, further observation is warranted, with a cervical recheck in a few hours.

2. d. All of the above

Response: Hypotension due to vasodilation is a common physiologic response to an epidural. Medication, IV fluid, and side tilt are all appropriate.

3. d. All of the above

Response: Labor is a retrospective, somewhat arbitrary diagnosis and is often simply associated with arrival at the hospital.

4. d. The data included corrections for the use of oxytocin labor augmentation and epidural administration.

Response: The Friedman data come from the 1950s and early 1960s and do not reflect the widespread use of epidural analgesia and use of oxytocin infusions via computerized pumps.

Chapter 22: Fetal Monitoring

1. c. Mild mental retardation

Response: Mild mental retardation occurs 20–30 per 1000 births, whereas antepartum stillbirth and cerebral palsy occur at the rate 5 per 1000, intrapartum at 1 per 1000.

2. c. P–R interval

Response: The P–R interval is not displayed or assessed during fetal monitoring.

3. d. Immediate delivery

Response: In general, immediate delivery is not a treatment for an indeterminate fetal heart rate tracing, at least not before other steps are taken.

4. b. Indicated for maternal diabetes

Response: Although very few evidence-based protocols exist, fetal monitoring is believed to be helpful in the third trimester for maternal diabetes and fetal indications.

Chapter 23: Delivery

1. d. Vaginal delivery

Response: Emptying the bladder reduces the risk of trauma in each of these procedures except spontaneous vaginal delivery.

2. a. Uterus and fascia

Response: The uterus must be closed to control bleeding, and the fascia requires closure for abdominal integrity. Many obstetricians do not close the peritoneum (either surface), and the skin can be left to close by secondary intention if infection is an issue.

3. e. None of the above.

4. d. Tear through vaginal mucosa, deep perineum, and into anal sphincter
Response: Tear into the rectum is a fourth-degree laceration.

Chapter 24: Fetal Complications

1. d. Rate does not depend on family history
Response: Monozygotic twinning is infrequent and constant among ethnic groups and all ages.

2. c. Antepartum steroids appropriate if delivery anticipated before 34 weeks
Response: The only true statement concerns the administration of steroids for delivery anticipated before 34 weeks.

3. a. Bedrest
Response: Although occasionally recommended, bedrest has not been shown to help intrauterine growth retardation.

4. d. All of the above

Chapter 25: Third-Trimester Bleeding

1. a. Uterine atony
Response: Uterine atony is by far the most common cause of postpartum hemorrhage. Retained placenta comes in second, and accreta is probably third, although still quite uncommon.

2. e. All of the above

3. c. Methotrexate treatment of placenta left in place
Response: All except methotrexate can be used. Methotrexate might be a consideration if a small amount of placenta is left behind in the absence of active bleeding, but it would not be a treatment for acute bleeding. Hysterectomy (not listed) is often required to control bleeding with accreta.

4. a. Internal iliac artery ligation
Response: Internal iliac artery ligation is falling out of favor due to concerns over efficacy and familiarity of obstetricians with ligating the vessel (which is generally not done by obstetricians for any other reason).

Chapter 26: Medical Complications of Pregnancy

1. c. Chronic hypertension with superimposed pre-eclampsia
Response: The elevated blood pressures at the start of pregnancy suggest
that the patient has chronic hypertension. The finding of proteinuria in the
third trimester makes the diagnosis of superimposed pre-eclampsia.
2. d. All statements are true.
3. a. Cytomegalovirus
Response: Varicella zoster, parvovirus, and rubella commonly present
with a rash.
4. a. Systolic murmurs are commonplace in the absence of disease at term
Response: The mortality rate of mitral stenosis with atrial fibrillation is
5%–15%. Inherited heart abnormalities are not typically the same across
family members. The percentage of blood flow to the uterus dramatically
increases with pregnancy.

Chapter 27: Complications of Labor

1. c. Fetal fibronectin
Response: A normal fetal fibronectin result is highly reliable in predicting
the absence of labor in the next 7 days. Cervical examinations, bacterial
vaginosis screening, and ultrasound measurement of cervical length have
not been shown to be helpful in predicting preterm labor.
2. c. Nausea
Response: Fetal intolerance to labor from tachysystole, seizures from
hyponatremia, and tachysystole are all potential complications of
oxytocin.
3. b. If external version works initially, reversion to breech is very
uncommon
Response: Reversion to breech follows 50% of successful versions.
4. b. Having newborn nursery personnel present at delivery is
recommended
Response: Amnioinfusion is not a proven benefit. Meconium by itself
is not an indication for cesarean section, and meconium's causal
relationship with perinatal asphyxia remains uncertain.

Chapter 28: Newborn

1. c. Air breathing is assisted by a fall in pressure of the ductus arteriosus.
Response: The fetal veins bring oxygenated blood to the heart. Air breathing is assisted by a rise (not a fall) in pressure in the ductus arteriosus.

2. c. It is easily revised if too much foreskin is left on.
Response: Circumcisions are not easily revised if too much foreskin is left on.

3. a. Pupil dilation
Response: Pupil dilation is the only item listed not routinely assessed during resuscitation.

4. c. Can be given IM
Response: Epinephrine can be given IV or by the endotracheal tube; it is not given by the IM route.

B

ABBREVIATIONS

Abbreviation	Complete Term
ACE	angiotensin-converting enzyme
ACOG	American College of Obstetricians and Gynecologists
ACS	American Cancer Society
ACTH	adrenocorticotropic hormone
AFE	amniotic fluid embolism
AFP	alpha-fetoprotein
ALT	alanine transaminase
APGO	Association of Professors of Gynecology and Obstetrics
AROM	artificial rupture of membranes
ART	assisted reproductive technology
ASC	atypical squamous cells
ASCCP	American Society for Colposcopy and Cervical Pathology
ASC-H	atypical squamous cells, cannot exclude HSIL
ASC-US	atypical squamous cells of uncertain significance
BBT	basal body temperature
BCA	bichloroacetic acid
BMI	body mass index
BP	blood pressure
BPD	biparietal diameter
BPM	beats per minute
BRCA-1, BRCA-2	breast cancer genes
BUN	blood urea nitrogen
BV	bacterial vaginosis
CBC	complete blood count
CC	chief complaint
CDC	[U.S.] Centers for Disease Control and Prevention
CEE	conjugated equine estrogens

CF	cystic fibrosis
CIN	cervical intraepithelial neoplasia
CLE	continuous lumbar epidural
CMV	cytomegalovirus
CNS	central nervous system
CPD	cephalopelvic disproportion
CPP	chronic pelvic pain
CSF	cerebrospinal fluid
CT	computed tomography
CVS	chorionic villus sampling
CXR	chest x-ray
DCIS	ductal carcinoma in situ
DES	diethylstilbestrol
DHEA	dehydroepiandrosterone
DHEAS	dehydroepiandrosterone sulfate
DIC	disseminated intravascular coagulation
DMSO	dimethylsulfoxide
DNA	deoxyribonucleic acid
DSM-IV-TR	*Diagnostic and Statistical Manual of Mental Disorders,* 4th Edition, Text Revision
DTR	deep tendon reflex
DUB	dysfunctional uterine bleeding
DVT	deep vein thrombosis
EASI	extra-amniotic saline infusion
ECC	endocervical curettage
EDC	estimated date of confinement
EE	ethinyl estradiol
ELISA	enzyme-linked immunosorbent assay
EMB	endometrial biopsy
EMG	electromyography
EMTALA	[U.S.] Emergency Medical Treatment and Active Labor Act
EPDS	Edinburgh Postnatal Depression Scale
ET	estrogen therapy; embryo transfer
FAS	fetal alcohol syndrome
FDA	[U.S.] Food and Drug Administration
FEV_1	forced expiratory volume in 1 second
FHR	fetal heart rate
FHT	fetal heart tone
FIGO	International Federation of Gynecology and Obstetrics
FISH	fluorescent in situ hybridization
FSH	follicle-stimulating hormone

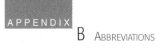

FTA-ABS	fluorescent treponemal antibody absorbed
GAG	glycosaminoglycan
GBS	group B streptococcus
GI	gastrointestinal
GIFT	gamete intrafallopian transfer
GnRH	gonadotropin-releasing hormone
GTN	gestational trophoblastic neoplasm
GU	genitourinary
HBIG	hepatitis B immune globulin
HCG, hCG	human chorionic gonadotropin
HDL	high-density lipoprotein
HELLP	Hemolysis, Elevated Liver enzymes, Low Platelets (syndrome)
HIPAA	[U.S.] Health Insurance Portability and Accountability Act
HIV	human immunodeficiency virus
HMG, hMG	human menopausal gonadotropin
HNPCC	hereditary nonpolyposis colorectal cancer
HPI	history of present illness
HPV	human papillomavirus
HRT	hormone replacement therapy
HSG	hysterosalpingogram
HSIL	high-grade squamous intraepithelial lesion
HSV	herpes simplex virus
HT	hormone therapy
HUMI	Harris-Kronner Uterine Manipulator Injector
IBS	irritable bowel syndrome
IC	interstitial cystitis
ICSI	intracytoplasmic sperm injection
ICU	intensive care unit
IFE	internal fetal electrode
IGF	insulin-like growth factor
IM	intramuscular
ITP	idiopathic thrombocytopenic purpura
IUD	intrauterine device
IUFD	intrauterine fetal demise
IUGR	intrauterine growth restriction
IUI	intrauterine insemination
IUPC	intrauterine pressure catheter
IV	intravenous
IVF	in vitro fertilization
IVPB	intravenous piggyback
KTP	potassium-titanyl-phosphate

LAM	lactational amenorrhea method
LCIS	lobular carcinoma in situ
LDH	lactate dehydrogenase
LDL	low-density lipoprotein
LEEP	loop electrosurgical excision procedure
LH	luteinizing hormone
LLETZ	large-loop excision of the transformation zone
LMP	last menstrual period
LOA	left occiput anterior
LOP	left occiput posterior
LSIL	low-grade squamous intraepithelial lesion
LTV	long-term variability
LUNA	laparoscopic uterine nerve ablation
MAO	monoamine oxidase
MCV	mean corpuscular volume
MP	micronized progesterone
MPA	medroxyprogesterone acetate
MRI	magnetic resonance imaging
MTHFR	methylenetetrahydrofolate reductase
NAAT	nucleic acid amplification test
NICHD	[U.S.] National Institute of Child Health and Human Development
NIH	[U.S.] National Institutes of Health
NSAID	nonsteroidal anti-inflammatory drug
NST	nonstress test
NTD	neural tube defect
OAB	overactive bladder
OCP	oral contraceptive pill
OHSS	ovarian hyperstimulation syndrome
OR	operating room
OTC	over-the-counter
PAPP-a	pregnancy-associated plasma protein A
PCOS	polycystic ovarian syndrome
PCR	polymerase chain reaction
PDE	phosphodiesterase
PDS	polydioxanone suture
PE	pulmonary embolism
PEEP	positive end-expiratory pressure
PEPI	Postmenopausal Estrogen/Progestin Interventions trial
PGE	prostaglandin E
PGY	postgraduate year (PGY-1, PGY-2, etc.)
PI	protease inhibitor

PID	pelvic inflammatory disease
PIH	pregnancy-induced hypertension
PMDD	premenstrual dysphoric disorder
PMH	past medical history
PMS	premenstrual syndrome
POP-Q	pelvic organ prolapse quantification system
PRBC	packed red blood cell
PROM	premature rupture of membrane
PT	prothrombin time
PTT	partial thromboplastin time
PUBS	percutaneous umbilical cord blood sampling
RBC	red blood cell
RNA	ribonucleic acid
ROA	right occiput anterior
ROP	right occiput posterior
ROS	review of systems
RPR	rapid plasma reagin
RR	relative risk; respiratory rate
RTI	reverse transcriptase inhibitor
SD	standard deviation
SERM	selective estrogen receptor modulator
SLE	systemic lupus erythematosus
SNRI	serotonin-norepinephrine reuptake inhibitor
SROM	spontaneous rupture of membrane
SSRI	selective serotonin reuptake inhibitor
STD	sexually transmitted disease
STI	sexually transmitted infection
STV	short-term variability
SUI	stress urinary incontinence
TCA	trichloroacetic acid
TENS	transcutaneous electrical nerve stimulation
TNM	tumor, node, metastasis
TPN	total parenteral nutrition
TP-PA	*T. pallidum* particle agglutination
TRALI	transfusion-related acute lung injury
TSH	thyroid-stimulating hormone
TVT	tension-free vaginal tape
UTI	urinary tract infection
VBAC	vaginal birth after cesarean
VDRL	Venereal Disease Research Laboratory
VEGF	vasoactive endothelial growth factor
VIN	vulvar intraepithelial neoplasia
VTE	venous thromboembolism

vWF	von Willebrand factor
WBC	white blood cell
WHI	Women's Health Initiative
YAG	yttrium-aluminum-garnet (laser)
ZIFT	zygote intrafallopian transfer

Key Contacts and Notes

Physician Contacts

NAME	CONTACT
Dr	Home phone:
	Mobile phone:
	Pager:
	Other:
Dr	Home phone:
	Mobile phone:
	Pager:
	Other:
Dr	Home phone:
	Mobile phone:
	Pager:
	Other:

Community Resources and Phone Numbers

NAME/PROGRAM	PHONE NUMBERS
Sexual and Physical Abuse	
Substance Abuse	
Communicable Diseases (HIV, Hepatitis, Others)	
Homeless Shelters	
Child/Adolescent Hotlines	
Suicide Hotlines	
Hospitals (General, Veterans, Psychiatric)	
Medicare	
Medicaid	
Other	

Facility Phone Numbers

NAME/PROGRAM	PHONE NUMBERS
Main	Phone:
	Fax:
Laboratory	Phone:
	Fax:
Radiology	Phone:
	Fax:
Physical therapy	Phone:
	Fax:
ECG/EEG	Phone:
	Fax:
Outpatient Scheduling	Phone:
	Fax:
Emergency	Phone:
	Fax:
Operating Suite	Phone:
	Fax:
Admissions	Phone:
	Fax:
Billing	Phone:
	Fax:
Medical Records	Phone:
	Fax:
Medical Staff Office	Phone:
	Fax:
Other important numbers	Phone:
	Fax:

Formulary Notes Specific to Your Facility

Other Important Information

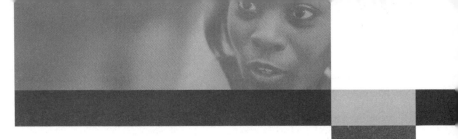

INDEX

Note: Page numbers followed by "b," "f," and "t" indicate boxes, figures, and tables, respectively.

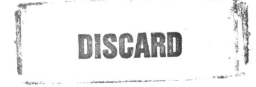